J. Meites

Estrogen Target Tissues and Neoplasia

Estrogen Target Tissues and Neoplasia

Edited by Thomas L. Dao

The University of Chicago Press
Chicago & London

The University of Chicago Press, Chicago 60637
The University of Chicago Press, Ltd., London
© 1972 by The University of Chicago
All rights reserved. Published 1972

Printed in the United States of America

International Standard Book Number: 0-226-13632-9
Library of Congress Catalog Card Number 76-182870

Contents

Preface *vii*

Acknowledgments *xi*

Mode of Action of Estrogens on Target Tissues I
---

1. Molecular Biology of Estrogen Regulation of Target Tissue Growth and Differentiation *Bert W. O'Malley and A. R. Means* *3*
2. Estrogen Receptors and Hormone Dependency *Elwood V. Jensen, George E. Block, Sylvia Smith, Kay Kyser, and Eugene R. DeSombre* *23*
3. Human Breast Cancer as a Steroid Hormone Target *Stanley G. Korenman* *59*
4. Hormonal Regulation of Histone Phosphorylation *Roger W. Turkington* *69*
5. Effect of Hormones on Histone Acetylation *Paul R. Libby* *85*
6. Discussion *Guy Williams-Ashman, Chairman* *101*
7. Summary *Guy Williams-Ashman, Chairman* *119*

Metabolism of Steroids by Mammary Cancer II
---

8. Paraendocrine Behavior of Human Breast Cancer *John B. Adams and Michael Wong* *125*

9 Transformation of Steroids by Mammary Cancer Tissue *Keith Griffiths, D. Jones, E. H. D. Cameron, E. N. Gleave, and A. P. M. Forrest* 151
10 Metabolic Transformation of Steroids by Human Breast Cancer *Thomas L. Dao, R. Varela, and Charles Morreal* 163
11 Steroid Sulfate Formation in Human Breast Tumors and Hormone Dependency *Thomas L. Dao and Paul R. Libby* 181
12 Studies on Adrenal Estrogen Sulfotransferase *John B. Adams, Roger K. Ellyard, and Joyce Low* 201
13 The Influence of Sulfation on Estrogen Metabolism and Activities *Samuel C. Brooks, B. A. Pack, and L. Horn* 221
14 Discussion *Mortimer Lipsett, Chairman* 237
15 Summary *Mortimer Lipsett, Chairman* 251

The Relation of Estrogens and Prolactin to Tumorigenesis of the Mammary Gland III

16 Hormonal Influence upon Normal, Preneoplastic, and Neoplastic Mammary Gland *Leonard J. Beuving and Howard A. Bern* 257
17 The Relation of Estrogen and Prolactin to Mammary Tumorigenesis in the Rat *Joseph Meites* 275
18 Estrogens and Prolactin in Mammary Cancer *Olof H. Pearson, A. Molina, T. P. Butler, L. Llerena, and H. Nasr* 287
19 Estrogen and Induction of Mammary Cancer *Dilip Sinha and Thomas Dao* 307
20 Effect of Brain Lesions on Mammary Tumorigenesis *Clifford W. Welsch* 317
21 Induction of Mammary Cancer in Rats of Long and Evans Strain *Charles B. Huggins, Hisao Oka, and George Fareed* 333
22 Discussion *Kenneth DeOme, Chairman* 345
23 Summary *Kenneth DeOme, Chairman* 355

List of Participants 357
Index 359

Preface

This volume is an account of the proceedings of the Workshop on Estrogen Target Tissues and Neoplasia which was held at the Roswell Park Memorial Institute in Buffalo, New York, on June 4th and 5th, 1970. The objective of this gathering of experts in the fields of hormone action and mammary neoplasms was to consider in perspective some recent advances in the basic biochemistry and physiology of estrogens and other hormones that may relate to the problem of human breast cancer.

Among the various steroid hormones capable of inducing both normal tissue growth and neoplasia, none have such diversified effects as the estrogens. If administering an estrogen under appropriate circumstances can cause the development of a malignant tumor that otherwise would not have arisen, the estrogen can be classified as a carcinogen.

The induction of malignant changes in target tissues is a perplexing phenomenon, since estrogens can evoke remarkable effects on several types of normal target tissues. It is not at all clear whether any of these actions may cause the subsequent development of neoplasia.

The introduction of the concept of "hormone dependence" of certain neoplasms by Charles Huggins represented a breakaway from the previously accepted notion of the autonomy of tumors; it evolved from recognition of the relationship between hormonal target tissues and their neoplastic counterparts. In the strict sense, the term hormone dependence is only operational, because we still know very little about the mode of action of sex hormones at a molecular level. We observe regression of breast cancer after excision of the ovaries or adrenals, but we understand almost nothing about the mechanism of regression. Nearly three decades after Huggins formulated the notion of hormone dependence, we remain very much in the dark about the precise interactions between hormones and their normal target tissues which bear on any neoplastic transformations.

In recent years, significant advances have been made in at least three areas of investigation which may be especially important for the ultimate understanding of hormones and tumor development.

Studies on intracellular macromolecules with a high and stereo-specific affinity for estrogens have revealed the existence of specific protein "receptors" in estrogen responsive tissues such as uterus, vagina, anterior pituitary, and, of particular interest, in mammary tumors of rats and humans. Although the binding of estrogens to these proteins does not "explain" the action of these hormones, the mere absence or presence of these macromolecules in tumor tissue is of obvious importance. A major question is whether this relates unequivocally to the hormone responsiveness of the neoplasms.

The persistence of estrogenic substances in urine of breast cancer patients after both ovaries and adrenals have been removed has led several investigators to search for the site(s) of production of these estrogens. Over the last few years, convincing evidence has been gathered that certain tumors contain a variety of enzyme systems that catalyze metabolic transformations of steroid hormones. Of special interest are studies on the capacity of tumors to synthesize sulfate esters of sex hormones, and apparently to convert certain steroid precursors into physiologically active hormones. Confirmation and extension of these findings will doubtless increase our understanding of the nature of hormone-dependent tumor tissue.

Not least important is the substantial progress achieved over the last decade in understanding the relation of estrogens and prolactin to tumorigenesis in the mammary gland. Recent advances in this area have rested heavily on methodological developments, notably the introduction of reliable radioimmunoassay procedures for prolactin in the blood plasma of rodents. Although the role of estrogens and prolactin in tumor formation has not yet been clearly defined, the new knowledge of the interdependence of prolactin and estrogen in growth of mammary cancer may well improve the treatment of human breast cancers.

The first section of this book deals with the action of estrogens on target tissue. The molecular biology of estrogen action is discussed in terms of influences of the hormones on enzymic processes involved in

Preface

RNA transcription or translation, estrogen-binding proteins, and enzymatic acetylation and phosphorylation of histones. The clinical implications of the presence or absence of specific estrogen-receptor proteins in human breast cancer tissue are also considered.

The second section is mainly concerned with the metabolism of steroid hormones by human mammary cancer tissues. Two important aspects of this problem are discussed: the transformations and possible biosynthesis of steroids and the formation of steroid sulfate esters in breast cancer. The clinical significance of the apparent "paraendocrine" behavior of mammary cancer tissue and its capacity to form steroid sulfate esters are reviewed in detail.

The third section considers a controversial but important subject in mammary tumorigenesis; namely, whether estrogens or prolactin are primarily involved in the pathogenesis of breast cancer.

Acknowledgments

I wish to thank Dr. Williams-Ashman, Dr. Lipsett, and Dr. DeOme for accepting my invitation to lead the different sessions, and also for their invaluable contributions in suggesting many of the speakers at the conference.

Like many other human undertakings, the conference could not have been successful or the volume published without personal sacrifice and sustained effort by many people. First, I want to pay special tribute to the participants, who worked hard to prepare their manuscripts and to submit them on schedule. The help of my colleagues, Dr. Dilip Sinha, Dr. Paul Libby, Dr. Charles Morreal, and Dr. Fred Rosen in transcribing the discussions is gratefully acknowledged. I wish to thank my secretaries, Mrs. Ann Licata and Miss Shirley Matyas, for their help in getting the manuscripts ready for publication.

I am particularly grateful for the generous contributions by the Mary Flagler Cary Charitable Trust Fund toward the publication of this volume.

But most important of all, I wish to acknowledge a long-time friend and the former director of our institute, Dr. James T. Grace, whose sustained interest and effort contributed greatly to the success of the conference. How regrettable it is that Dr. Grace was not able to come to welcome the participants, an occasion he had greatly looked forward to. He was incapacitated by an automobile accident that killed his wife Betty. A tragic event befell a wonderful family, and particularly sad is the great loss to our institute.

Mode of Action of Estrogens on Target Tissues   I

Bert W. O'Malley and A. R. Means

Molecular Biology of Estrogen Regulation of Target Tissue Growth and Differentiation — I

INTRODUCTION

Breast cancer is known to be hormone-responsive, since appropriate endocrine modification can lead to either stimulation or regression of breast tumors. In most species, estrogen stimulates fat deposition and development of the ductal system in the mammary gland. At present, however, there is a major need for more precise information concerning the molecular mechanisms of estrogenic reproduction, growth, differentiation, and neoplasia in cells of higher organisms. Since malignancy may well be due to the inability to maintain the differential status quo in a given tissue (1), it is imperative that we be able to define in chemically precise terms the mechanism of normal tissue differentiation. Once the biochemistry of the intracellular changes which occur during normal estrogen-mediated growth has been elucidated, we may more rationally explore the altered control mechanisms in neoplastic states of disordered growth.

THE OVIDUCT AS A MODEL SYSTEM FOR THE STUDY OF ESTROGEN ACTION

Much of the literature on the mechanism of estrogen uses the rat uterus as a model system. Indeed, estrogens have been demonstrated to stimulate glandular proliferation of female reproductive tissues and also to exert major effects on all classes of RNA in the target organs of a castrate female rat (7-9). There is good evidence that

The authors are affiliated with the departments of Obstetrics and Gynecology, Medicine, Biochemistry, and Physiology at the Vanderbilt University School of Medicine.

estrogen acts in the target tissue by initially combining with a specific cytoplasmic intracellular receptor molecule followed by transfer to its nuclear site of action (see chapter 2). This response might best be considered a primary growth response which eventually leads to cell hypertrophy. Estrogen certainly acts to restore and maintain functional differentiation of the uterus and to stimulate the uterine cell to maximal performance of its genetic capabilities. Although estrogen could also regulate the initial expression of gene function during embryogenesis of the uterus, it is difficult, utilizing the castrate uterine system, to show the induction of new proteins or the appearance of new metabolic functions not previously demonstrable in the uterus of the intact animal.

On the other hand, the chick oviduct allows us to demonstrate the events described above and thus emerges as one of the most desirable systems for the study of estrogen-mediated tissue growth and differentiation. The oviductal mucosa of the newborn chick consists of a thin layer of pseudostratified columnar epithelium which rests upon a dense layer of polygonal cells (5, 6). Furthermore, the state of differentiation is maintained until approximately 100 days of age, at which time morphologic changes begin to occur in response to endogenous estrogen (7). But at any time during this period of relative quiescence, administering estrogen initiates the process of cytodifferentiation and the oviduct mass increases over a thousandfold in response to continual estrogen injections (6). Thus in this system we are able to provide a lifetime of estrogen in only a few months and yet mimic quite precisely the normal process of cytodifferentiation and biochemical specialization which occurs in the adult laying hen. In fact, this response of the chick oviduct to estrogenic stimulation is one of the few instances where marked cytodifferentiation is not restricted to the period of embryogenesis.

Administering estrogens to the immature chick results in differentiation of three distinct cell types from the homogenous population of primitive mucosal cells (7, 8). Two of these new cell types—the tubular gland cells and the goblet cells—synthesize cell-specific proteins which are easily measured by biochemical and immunochemical assays (9–11). Thus ovalbumin and lysozyme synthesis by the tubal gland cell and avidin synthesis by goblet cells can be utilized as biochemical markers for cytodifferentiation. Employing these techniques, we have followed sequentially the cytodifferentiation of the primitive epithelial cells of the immature oviduct in response to estrogen. It has

Molecular Biology of Estrogen Regulation

been demonstrated that, indeed, the appearance of epithelial tubular gland cells correlates with the onset of two new biochemical capacities—the ability to synthesize ovalbumin and the ability to synthesize lysozyme (5, 11, 12). In this manner we have developed a system where morphologic differentiation and biochemical specialization occur coordinately in response to estrogen treatment.

Since it is reasonable to hypothesize that estrogen controls target-tissue growth by regulating the synthesis of key enzymes and structural proteins, we have searched for the earliest specific enzymic

TABLE 1: EFFECT OF THE INJECTION OF 17 β-ESTRADIOL ON OVIDUCTAL ORNITHINE DECARBOXYLASE IN THE IMMATURE CHICK

Time after 17β-Estradiol (10 μg, intravenously)	Ornithine Decarboxylase Activity (pmoles $^{14}CO_2$/30 min/ 100 μg protein)
0	3
20	2
60	9
120	66
240	92

NOTE: Oviducts were removed at the time indicated and assayed for enzyme activity as described previously (14, 17).

response to this steroid. Our studies have demonstrated that estrogen induces an early stimulation of synthesis of oviductal ornithine decarboxylase. The rapidity of this effect on oviductal decarboxylase forces us to consider the possibility that it may play a role in initiating the estrogen-mediated growth response in target cells (17).

Estrogenic Induction of a Specific Enzyme (Ornithine Decarboxylase) before Initiation of Cell Growth

Injecting 17β-estradiol into 6-day-old chicks (table 1) resulted in a rapid induction of ornithine decarboxylase activity in oviduct target tissue (17). Similarly, incubating oviduct slices with DES in tissue culture medium (table 2) again induced decarboxylase, DES resulted in a similar elevation of the enzyme and the induction was completely blocked by cycloheximide (17).

Polyamines have been implicated in a multitude of diverse biological reactions. These compounds have been reported to stimulate DNA and RNA synthesis, protect RNA from degradation, maintain optimal polysomal protein synthesis, and replace Mg^{+2} requirements for protein synthesis. It is possible that a chemical effector of growth could stimulate ornithine decarboxylase and cause subsequent accumulation of polyamines which would then favorably and nonspecifically alter the internal cellular milieu for rapid synthesis of nucleic acid and proteins, the prerequisite for cell growth.

TABLE 2: EFFECTS OF DIETHYLSTILBESTROL ON ORNITHINE DECARBOXYLASE ACTIVITY OF CHICK OVIDUCTS IN VIVO

Incubation Additions	Ornithine Decarboxylase Activity (pmoles $^{14}CO_2$/30 min/ 100 µg protein)
Control	20
DES	314
DES+cycloheximide	2
Control+serum	17
DES+serum	285

NOTE: Oviducts from immature chicks were incubated in tissue culture medium (199 with Hanks's salts) for 3.5 hr at 37° C in 95% O_2, 5% CO_2. DES (5 µg/ml) and cycloheximide (25 µg/ml) were added to appropriate flasks. Serum from immature chicks was added to appropriate flasks at a final concentration of 10%. Tissue was assessed for ornithine decarboxylase activity as described previously (14, 17).

Chemical induction of growth in certain other cell types has been associated with a marked early stimulation of ornithine decarboxylase activity and synthesis of putrescine and polyamines. Partial hepatectomy or administration of growth hormone results in elevated ornithine decarboxylase activity in rat liver (13). Epidermal growth factor also induces an increase of ornithine decarboxylase activity in mouse skin or chick embryo epidermis cultures (14). Finally, estrogen has been reported to effect a significant increase in spermidine concentration in the ovariectomized rat uterus (15), and testosterone has been shown to cause an increase in ornithine decarboxylase activity in castrate rat prostatic tissue (16).

Estrogenic Control of Oviduct Translation

In addition to the induction of specific oviduct proteins estrogen has also been demonstrated to stimulate the overall synthesis of protein in this organ (10, 18). Since the appearance of new cell types must, indeed, be coordinated with major changes in the population of proteins, and since all proteins are synthesized upon cell polyribosomes, we have investigated changes which occur in these particles

TABLE 3: CHANGES IN OVIDUCT CONTENT OF RIBOSOMES DURING ESTROGEN-MEDIATED GROWTH AND DIFFERENTIATION

	Polyribosomal Protein	
Days of Estrogen	(μg/mg oviduct)	(μg/oviduct)
0	0.63	12.02
1	1.10	39.11
4	1.70	320.31
7	2.01	998.85
10	1.67	786.49

NOTE: Immature Rhode Island red chicks were given daily subcutaneous injections of diethylstilbestrol in sesame oil (5 mg/0.1 ml). Oviducts were removed and homogenized and ribosomes were isolated as previously described (19, 20). Protein was determined by the method of Lowry et al. (22). Purity of the ribosomal preparations as determined by RNA/protein ratio (0.8–1.0) and ratio of A $260/280_{nm}$ (1.55–1.65).

during estrogen-mediated differentiation of the immature chick oviduct. Accordingly, we have recently reported the isolation and characterization of oviduct polyribosomes with respect to structure, function, and peptide products synthesized in vitro (19).

Estrogen brings about an increase in the synthesis of oviduct ribosomes within 1 day after it is administered to the immature chick (table 3). Moreover, this increase can be seen whether data are expressed as μg per mg oviduct or as total μg polyribosomal protein per oviduct. For at least 7 days of hormone treatment the oviduct content of polyribosomes continues to increase, but by 10 days it has begun to decline. Thus, as morphologic differentiation begins to occur new ribosomes are available to support the synthesis of new proteins which presumably are necessary for this process. At first glance the apparent decline in ribosome content at 10 days of estrogen may seem curious. However, it should be noted that cytodifferentiation—that is, the appearance of new cell types—is complete by about 9 days of hormone treatment. In this context the decline at 10 days becomes understandable, since relatively fewer ribosomes would presumably be required to maintain protein biosynthesis once the differentiation process has been completed.

Estrogen not only causes an increase in ribosome synthesis but also produces a marked change in the distribution of ribosomes analyzed by sucrose gradient centrifugation. Ribosomes were isolated as previously described (19, 20) and applied to a 0.3–1.0 M sucrose gradient. After centrifugation for 2 hr at 62,000 g (R_{av}), the gradients were fractionated and the A_{254nm} was recorded continuously. Figure 1a shows the polysome pattern representative of the unstimulated oviduct. Sedimentation was from left to right, and the first peak in this and subsequent panels represents single ribosomes. It can be seen that in the unstimulated oviduct a large proportion of cell ribosomes are present as monomers. On the other hand, administering DES for 4 days results in a marked change in the polyribosome pattern (Fig. 1b). Ten major peaks of A_{254nm} can now be observed and a large proportion of the particles exist as aggregates of two or more monomers. Further stimulation with estrogen (10 days total) causes still another pattern shift (Fig. 1c). Some of the very large polysomes which were present at 4 days now appear to be absent, and there is a concomitant increase in the proportion of monomers and dimers. Figure 1d demonstrates the hormone specificity of this response, since progesterone, which also induces synthesis of cell-specific proteins in the oviduct but has no effect upon growth, produces no demonstrable effect upon ribosome aggregation. Therefore the conversion of monomers to polysomes may be an early response of estrogen acting on the chick oviduct which allows the synthesis of new proteins necessary for oviduct growth and differentiation.

Ribonucleoprotein preparations were then tested for their ability to synthesize peptide in a cell-free incorporation system. Table 4 shows that estrogen treatment results in a doubling of specific activity within 24 hr after a single injection. By 4 days of hormone administration polysomal protein synthesis reaches a maximum before

Molecular Biology of Estrogen Regulation

beginning to decline at 7 days of estrogen. The marked stimulation of incorporation activity at 4 days is in keeping with the striking increases in ribosome synthesis and conversion of monomers to polysomes noted at this same time (table 3; fig. 1). Again, the decline in protein-synthesizing ability at 10 days occurs coordinately with a decreased synthesis of ribosomes and a further shift in the polysome pattern.

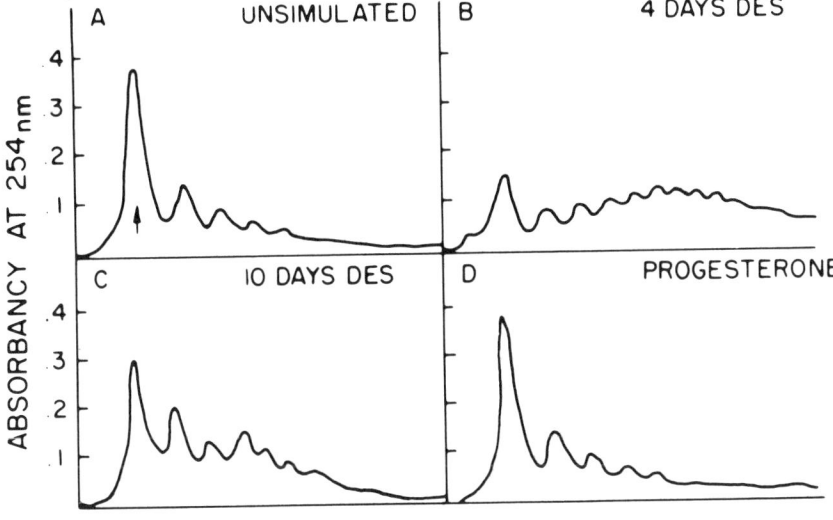

Fig. 1. Sucrose gradient profiles of polyribosomes isolated from chick oviduct. Polyribosomes were isolated as previously described (19, 20). Ten A_{254nm} units of each polyribosomal preparation was applied to each gradient of 27 ml (0.3–1.0 M). Samples were centrifuged at 25,000 rpm for 2 hr at 0° in the SW 25.1 rotor of the Beckman L265B ultracentrifuge. Direction of sedimentation is from left to right and the first peak always represents monomers (arrow in fig. 1a). (a) polysomes from unstimulated oviduct; (b) polysomes from oviducts of 4-day DES-treated chicks; (c) polysomes from oviducts of 10-day DES-treated chicks; (d) polysomes from oviducts of chicks 48 hr after a single injection of progesterone.

We have previously demonstrated that estrogen causes marked changes in the soluble proteins present in a 105,000 g supernatant fluid of oviduct upon analysis by polyacrylamide gel electrophoresis (18, 19). To determine whether these changes in soluble proteins demonstrated in vivo during DES-mediated differentiation were reflected in the cell-free system, we analyzed the peptide products synthesized by oviduct polyribosomes in vitro.

Peptides were released from the polyribosomes after incubation in the cell-free protein-synthesizing system by adding NaF (10 mM) to the incubation. The incubates were centrifuged at 150,000 g to remove ribosomes, and the resulting supernatant fluid was dialyzed overnight against two changes of 0.1M NaHCO$_3$ (pH 7.4). Samples were concentrated by dialysis against 75% sucrose and applied to polyacrylamide gels. To minimize difference due to technique, the

TABLE 4: PROTEIN BIOSYNTHESIS BY ISOLATED CHICK OVIDUCT POLYRIBOSOMES: EFFECT OF ESTROGEN

Days of Estrogen	Pmoles Valine-^{14}C/mg Polysomal Protein
0	18.65
1	39.31
4	77.71
7	61.81
10	39.75

NOTE: Polyribosomes were isolated from oviduct postmitochondrial supernatant fluid at various stages of estrogen-mediated differentiation and assayed in a cell-free system by methods previously described (19, 20). Values have been corrected for zero-time controls and one pmole of valine-^{14}C represents 438 dpm in the acid-precipitable material. Counting efficiency for ^{14}C was 85–88%.

peptides were double labeled; that is, polyribosomes from unstimulated oviducts were incubated with valine-^{3}H, whereas those from chicks treated for 4 days with estrogen were labeled with valine-^{14}C. After incubation these preparations were pooled and carried through the remaining procedures together. Electrophoresis was carried out for 2.3 hr and gels were then fractionated and radioactivity determined by liquid scintillation spectrometry (19, 21). Differences were apparent between 0 and 4 days of DES when corrected cpm were plotted (18, 19). To clarify differences, the ratio of corrected ^{3}H cpm to ^{14}C cpm was plotted, and these data can be seen in figure 2a. The ratio of ^{3}H to ^{14}C at various points on the gels varies considerably, thus demonstrating that striking changes occur

Molecular Biology of Estrogen Regulation

in the population of peptides synthesized in vitro before and after estrogen treatment.

To demonstrate the reliability of the interpretation of the data presented in figure 2a, a similar double-label experiment was performed utilizing only polysomes from 4-day treated chicks (labeling one batch with ^{14}C and one with ^3H). Figure 2b shows that in this case the ratio of ^3H to ^{14}C is nearly constant, varying only between

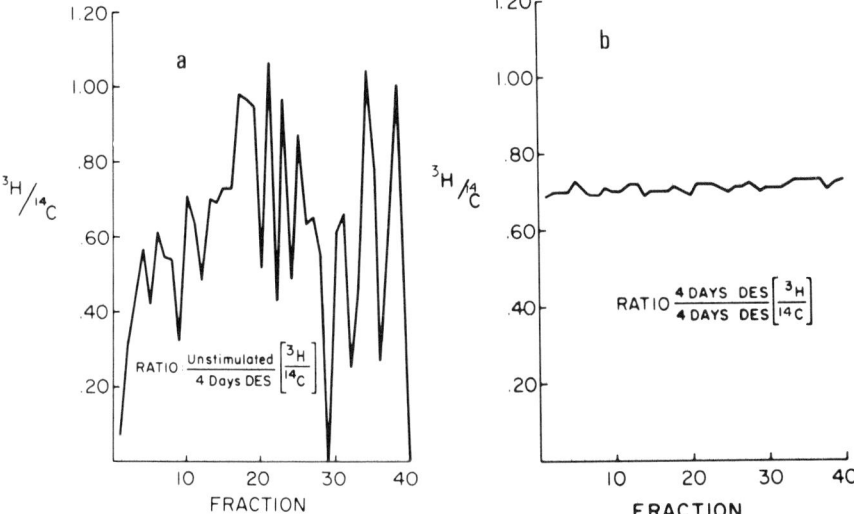

Fig. 2. Analysis by polyacrylamide gel electrophoresis of peptides synthesized by oviduct polysomes in vitro. Samples were prepared as described in text and electrophoresis was continued for 2.3 hr on polyacrylamide gels at a running pH of 10.2 (19, 21). Samples were double labeled and pooled following incubation. Plotted are the ratios of ^3H cpm to ^{14}C cpm; (*a*) unstimulated (^3H) vs. 4-day DES (^{14}C); (*b*) 4-day DES (^3H) vs. 4-day DES (^{14}C).

0.69 and 0.73. Furthermore, concomitant measurements of protease and ribonuclease activity before and after estrogen treatment revealed no demonstrable changes. Therefore we attribute these changes in the peptides synthesized in vitro to earlier changes in hormone-induced synthesis of new populations of target-tissue messenger RNA.

ESTROGENIC CONTROL OF OVIDUCTAL TRANSCRIPTION

Transcriptional events have been shown to precede the synthesis of cell-specific proteins, which are first demonstrable between 3 and 4 days after estrogen treatment. Thus a single injection of estrogen was shown to cause a prolonged stimulation of nuclear RNA polymerase activity, which reached a maximum between 12 and 24 hr (6, 23). This information suggested that estrogenic substances act at the level of gene transcription to promote oviduct protein synthesis and cytodifferentiation. Further support for this was obtained by the demonstration that estrogen elicited an increase in total template activity of isolated chromatin assayed in vitro (6). Moreover, qualitative changes in the composition of the RNA synthesized from chromatin template during estrogen-mediated differentiation were shown by nearest-neighbor base frequency analysis of the RNA products (6). Again these changes preceded the appearance of cell-specific proteins and argue that the steroid must promote the synthesis of new species of nuclear RNA.

Unfortunately, at this time it is not possible to determine directly the synthesis of new specific messenger RNAs. We therefore chose as an alternative to examine total nuclear messenger RNA activity during estrogen-induced growth and differentiation (24). For these experiments chick oviduct nuclear RNA activity was assayed by a modification of the procedure described by Nirenberg (25). This assay assesses the ability of synthetic mRNA or natural DNA-like RNA from animal cells to direct the synthesis of phenylalanine-^{14}C into polyphenylalanine using ribosomes isolated from a mutant of *E. coli* (MRE-600) defective in ribonuclease. Table 5 demonstrates that incorporation was linear up to 15 μg of poly U and a maximal incorporation of 260 pmoles of phe-^{14}C per mg of ribosomal protein was utilized at this level of synthetic messenger. The lower level of assay sensitivity was 0.15 μg poly U. Ribonucleic acid isolated from *E. coli* was effective as messenger in this system but this activity was destroyed by heating the RNA before assay. Likewise, *E. coli* transfer RNA and *E. coli* DNA were inactive. Nuclear RNA extracted from chicken liver was demonstrated to be utilizable as a messenger in the heterologous system and showed linear increases in activity up to 400 μg of RNA (table 5). Finally, it can be seen from table 1 that oviduct nuclear RNA demonstrated messenger activity but that this activity was abolished by adding ribonuclease.

Messenger activity of RNA isolated from oviduct nuclei at various stages of estrogen-mediated differentiation is shown in table 6. A threefold stimulation of activity is revealed within 24 hr after a single injection of DES into previously untreated chicks. Maximal stimulation was obtained at 3 days of hormone treatment, and by

6 days the messenger activity has begun to decline. These data offer one more piece of evidence that early alterations in genetic transcription are prerequisite to the appearance of new cell-specific proteins in response to estrogen. Moreover, they are consistent with other results presented in this chapter which suggest that the major biochemical events necessary for cytodifferentiation of the oviduct

TABLE 5: MESSENGER ACTIVITY OF SYNTHETIC AND NATURAL NUCLEIC ACIDS

Nucleic Acid	Nucleic Acid per Tube (μg)	Pmoles Phe-^{14}C/mg Ribosomal Protein
Poly U	5	87.760
	10	196.440
	15	257.460
	20	263.680
E. coli RNA	200	3.898
Heated E. coli RNA	200	0.325
E. coli+RNA	200	0.311
E. coli DNA	200	—
Chicken liver nuclear RNA	100	0.306
	200	0.762
	300	1.086
	400	1.352
	500	1.412
Oviduct nuclear RNA	200	1.899
Oviduct nuclear RNA plus RNase (20 μg)	200	—

NOTE: Messenger RNA activity was quantitated by the procedure of Nirenberg (25), and incorporated of ^{14}C-amino acid into protein was determined by the method of Mans and Novelli (26). E. coli MRE 600 (27) was the source of the S-30 cell-free extract prepared as described by Nirenberg (25). Finally, nuclear RNA was isolated from liver of oviduct as previously described (15).

All assays were performed in duplicate and contained the following components: 24.6 μmoles Tris-HCL (pH 7.8); 2.1 μmoles Mg acetate; 12 μmoles NH$_4$Cl; 246 nmoles ATP; 7.2 nmoles GTP; 0.1 μl 2-mercaptoethanol; 1.8 μmoles phosphoenolpyruvate; 5 E.U. phosphoenolpyruvate kinase; 49.5 μmoles each of 19 ^{12}C-amino acids; 0.5 μ C phe-^{14}C (350 mc/m mole); 200 μl S-30 extract; and nucleic acid as indicated in a final volume of 300 μl. Activity of complete assay mixture without added nucleic acid has been subtracted from each value (i.e., 0.07 pmoles/mg ribosomal protein).

are complete within the first few days of exposure to hormone (tables 2 and 4, fig. 1).

Increases in nuclear activities of RNA polymerase and messenger RNA clearly precede the initial stimulation of polysomal protein synthesis (fig. 3). This suggests, therefore, that estrogen, upon entering the oviduct cell, rapidly passes into the nucleus and in some manner alters nuclear gene expression. These changes result in the coordinated synthesis of ribosomal and messenger RNAs, which must

TABLE 6: CHANGES IN MESSENGER ACTIVITY OF NUCLEAR RNA ISOLATED DURING VARIOUS STAGES OF ESTROGEN-MEDIATED OVIDUCT DIFFERENTIATION

Days of Estrogen	Pmoles Phe-^{14}C/mg Ribosomal Protein
0	0.109
1	0.311
3	0.526
6	0.392
10	0.210

NOTE: Assays were performed in triplicate as described in the legend to table 5; 200 μg nuclear RNA was used for each determination. Activity of assay mixture in the absence of added RNA has been subtracted from each value.

subsequently be transported into the cytoplasm so that new polyribosomes may be formed to support the synthesis of new protein required for oviduct growth and differentiation.

Thus our experimental evidence suggests that the initial action of estrogen occurs at the level of gene transcription. We therefore predict that the steroid might promote the synthesis of new species of RNA during development which are not present in the undifferentiated gland. To examine populations of nuclear RNA sequences at various stages of estrogen-mediated growth, we have utilized DNA-RNA competition methods. Unlabeled nuclear RNA from immature chicks and subsequent stages of differentiation was used to competitively anneal on DNA binding sites with RNA (rapidly labeled with tritium) from completely differentiated (20 days $\times$ DES) tissue (fig. 4). The RNA from nuclei of the immature

Molecular Biology of Estrogen Regulation

chick oviduct competed poorly with labeled RNA of the differentiated oviduct (20 days × DES), but a progressive increase in competing species of RNA was noted at 2, 5, and 10 days of DES administration. At 20 days of DES we noted full competition of unlabeled RNA with labeled RNA (also from 20-day DES-treated chicks). This experiment demonstrates that the adult species of oviductal RNA can be generated by continuously administering estrogen to the immature chick and is consistent with a marked specific effect of this steroid on nuclear gene transcription. Figure 5 shows the results of a competition experiment in which the ^{3}H-labeled RNA

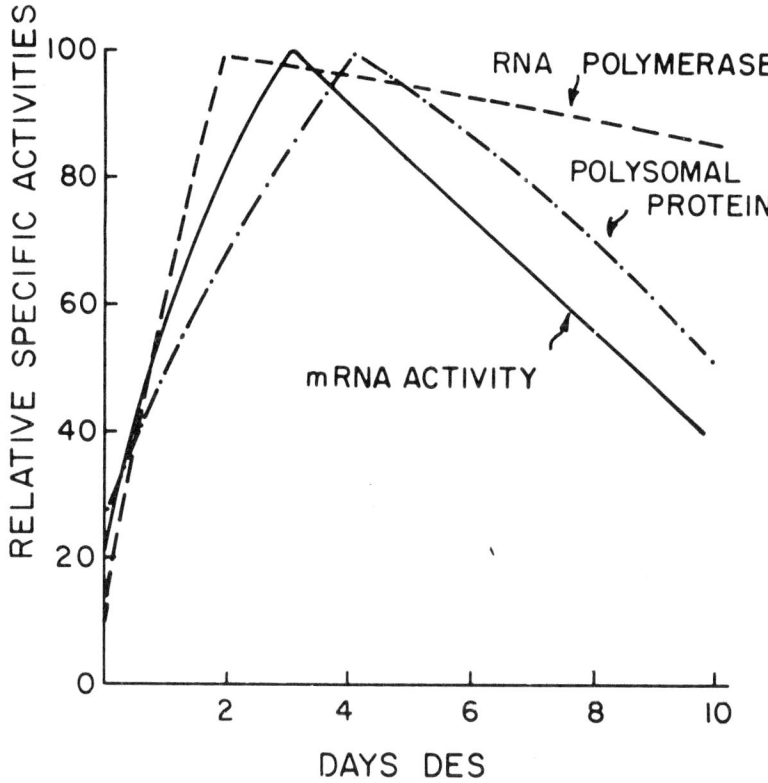

Fig. 3. Summary of the effects of estrogen on relative activities of RNA polymerase, messenger RNA, and polyribosomal protein biosynthesis during hormone-mediated oviduct differentiation. Data are calculated from tables 4 and 6. RNA polymerase values are from O'Malley, McGuire, and Korenman (12).

was prepared from oviduct nuclei of immature chicks. In this experiment, no differences were noted in the species of competing RNA from immature or differentiated oviduct, and both competed well. This implies that no major loss of competing species of RNA occurs during estrogen-mediated growth. The overall interpretation of

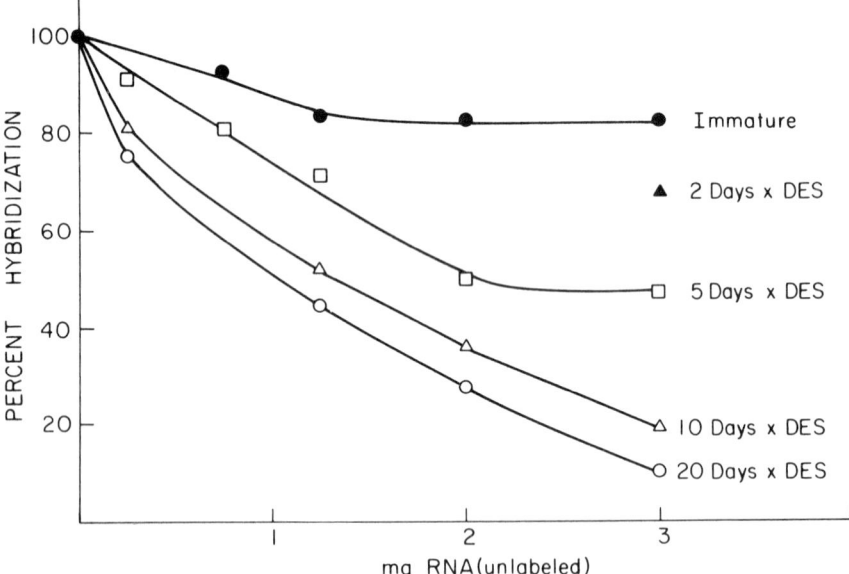

Fig. 4. Population changes in hybridizable nuclear RNA at various stages of DES-mediated differentiation. Tritium-labeled RNA (65 μg) from oviducts treated with DES for 20 days was incubated with increasing amounts of unlabeled RNA from immature, 2 days × DES, 5 days × DES, 10 days × DES, and 20 days × DES. The total ³H-RNA hybridizing to DNA in the absence of unlabeled competitor equals 100% hybridization. Incubation conditions for all hybrids are described in reference 15.

figures 4 and 5 is consistent with the suggestion that estrogen-mediated growth is associated with major activation of "new genes," but that "old genes" transcribed in the undifferentiated state are not "turned off."

MECHANISM OF ESTROGEN ACTION:
THE INITIAL RESPONSE OF GENE ACTIVATION

The appearance of cytological differentiation in the chick oviduct must follow prior biochemical differentiation and changes in patterns of protein synthesis. Estrogen stimulates synthesis of nuclear

Molecular Biology of Estrogen Regulation

rapidly labeled RNA and nuclear RNA polymerase activity. More important, we have identified new species of nuclear RNAs by nearest-neighbor dinucleotide analysis and DNA-RNA hybridization. We have shown that oviductal nuclear "mRNA activity" increased after estrogen coincident with cell differentiation. Similarly, analysis of the mRNA-directed synthesis of oviduct proteins as polysomes in vitro revealed an estrogen-induced qualitative and quantitative change in polysomal bound mRNA. Adult tissue-specific proteins may then be synthesized at the translational level on the ribosomes in response to the appearance of these new chemical signals, resulting in cytological differentiation and the subsequent production of new tissue-specific proteins.

Much of the currently available data on the biochemical mechanism of steroid hormone action would be at least consistent with the

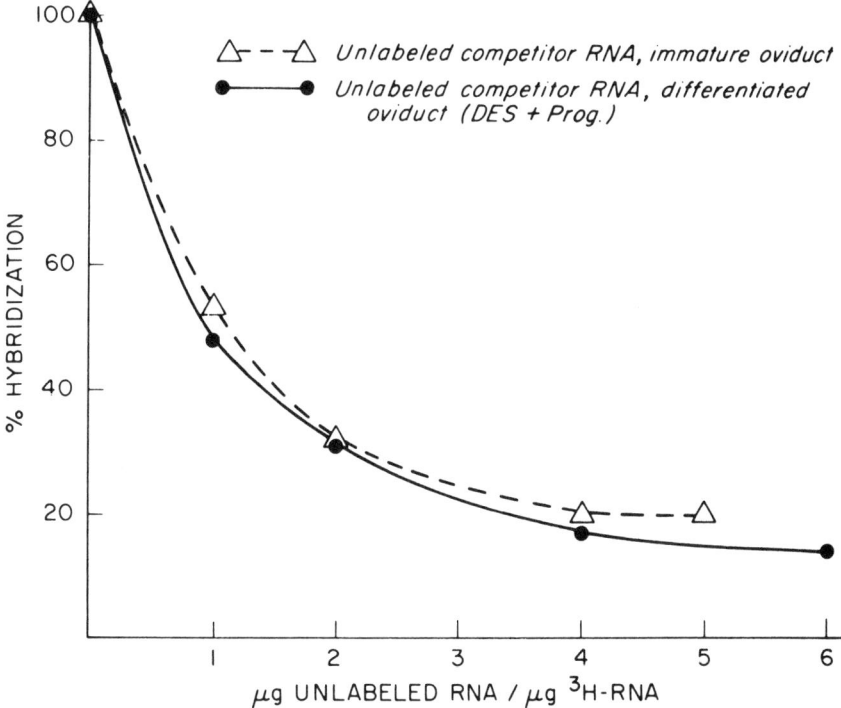

Fig. 5. Hybridizable RNA species lost during differentiation. In these experiments, 70 μg of ³H-RNA extracted from nuclei of immature oviducts is competitively annealed to oviduct DNA in the presence of increasing amounts of unlabeled nuclear RNA from immature chicks (homologous RNA) and differentiated chick oviducts from animals pretreated with 20 days of DES and 1 day of progesterone.

schematic diagram shown in figure 6. This hypothesis implies a coordinated activation of both nuclear structural genes (G_{s1}, G_{s2}), by either a negative or a positive control system, and also nucleolar genes coding for ribosomal RNA (G_r). The mRNAs transcribed from structural genes could then either be degraded within the nucleus or, in combination with specific nuclear proteins (NP), be transported to the cytoplasm. It is still unclear whether there is an obligatory interaction of mRNA-NP particles with rRNA in the

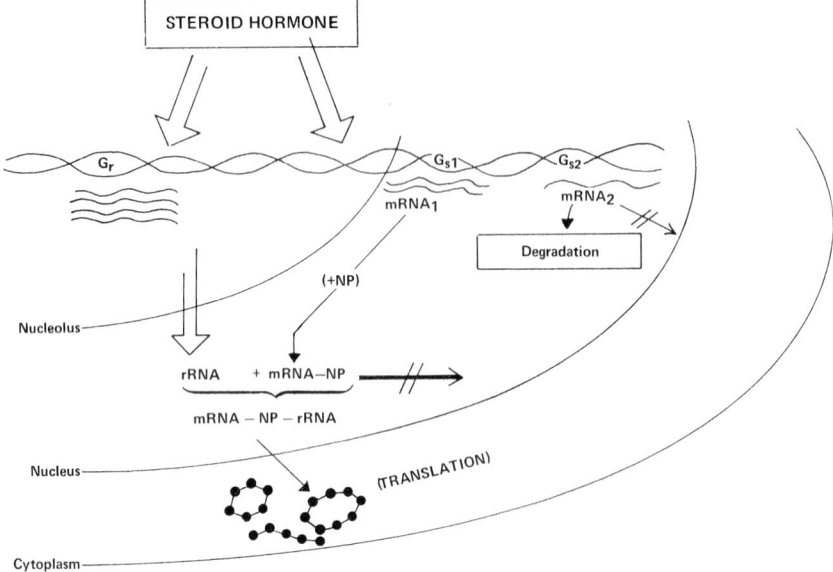

Fig. 6. Mechanism of estrogen action

nucleus or whether the initial interaction takes place only in the cytoplasm during polysome formation. However, we strongly suggest that estrogen mediates differentiation of the chick oviduct by altering nuclear gene expression. The model system is particularly suited to further study of steroid-induced differentiation and biochemical specialization in a defined in vivo animal system.

MECHANISM OF ESTROGEN ACTION:
AMPLIFICATION OF THE INITIAL RESPONSE

As a final consideration of the mechanism of estrogen regulation of growth, we must devise a way that a simple phenolic steroid can stimulate a whole battery of biochemical synthetic reactions. We must

Molecular Biology of Estrogen Regulation

realize that a large growth stimulus often requires an increase in the intracellular concentrations of hundreds of selected proteins. In the chick oviduct model, we necessitate a change in the whole population of intracellular proteins leading to the integrated appearance of completely new morphologic cell types, tissue-specific proteins, and metabolic functions. We must severely stretch our concept of the Jacob-Monod model of gene derepression to explain how a single steroid molecule of molecular weight 272, containing a limited number of reactive groups, could mediate this massive

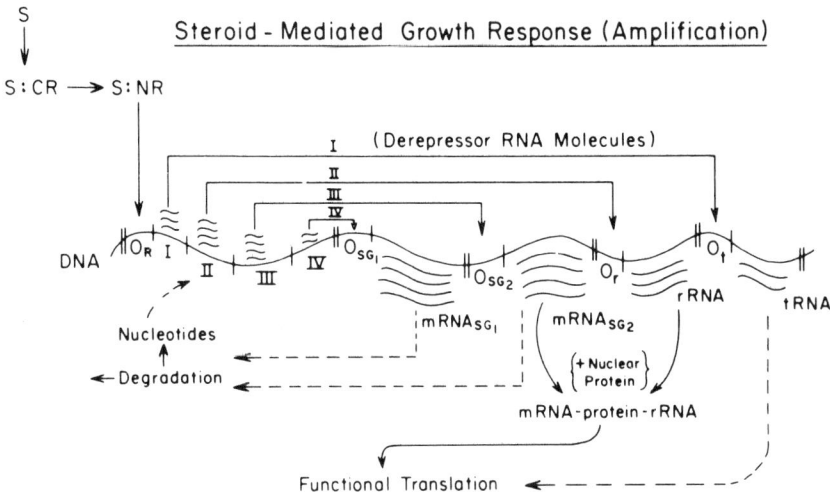

Fig. 7. Mechanism of amplification of target-tissue gene response induced by steroid hormone.

coordinated target-tissue response. Britten and Davidson (28) have recently reviewed a series of facts regarding organization of the genome which provide some clues to possible mechanisms for cells of higher organisms to effect multiple changes in gene activity from a single initiatory event.

Figure 7 contains a possible molecular model for a steroid-mediated growth response which allows amplification of gene response (28). In this model, the steroid (S) reacts with a cytoplasmic receptor (CR) in the target tissue and this complex then is transferred to the nucleus, where the steroid-nuclear protein complex (S:NR) binds to DNA at the estrogen regulator operon. The estrogen regulator operon contains an operator locus (O_R) and a group of functionally linked cistrons which code for intranuclear derepressor

RNA molecules (I, II, III, IV, etc.). The estrogen:receptor complex then activates the regulatory operator locus by positive or negative control and the whole adjacent operon is transcribed. The new functionally linked derepressor RNA molecules then seek out and activate all the genes for structural proteins (SG_1, SG_2, etc.), the ribosomal rRNA genes (r), and tRNA genes (t), which must be coordinately transcribed to result in a maximally efficient and integrated tissue growth response.

Although this model permits an amplification response for the steroid effector molecule which would result in the integrated synthesis of a host of nucleic acid molecules, structural proteins, and metabolic enzymes needed for growth, it is still highly speculative at this time.

Acknowledgments

These investigations were supported in part by research grants HD-04473 and Health Sciences Advancement Award 5-S04-FR06067 from the United States Public Health Service; by grant 630-0141A from the Ford Foundation; and by grant P-576 from the American Cancer Society.

References

1. Pitot, H. C. 1966. Some biochemical aspects of malignancy. *Ann. Rev. Biochem.* 35: 335.
2. Gorski, J.; Noteboom, W. D.; and Nicolette, J. A. 1965. Estrogenic control of the synthesis of RNA in protein in the uterus. *J. Cell Comp. Physiol.* 66, suppl. 1: 91.
3. Segal, S. 1968, Regulatory action of estrogenic hormones. *Dev. Biol.* suppl. 1: 264.
4. Hamilton, T. H. 1968. Control by estrogen of genetic transcription and translation. *Science* 161: 649.
5. Kohler, P. O.; Grimley, P. M.; and O'Malley, B. W. 1967. Estrogen-induced cytodifferentiation of the ovalbumin-secreting gland of the chick oviduct. *J. Cell Biol.* 40: 8.
6. O'Malley, B. W., McGuire, W. L.; Kohler, P. O.; and Korenman, S. G. 1969. Studies on the mechanism of steroid hormones regulation of synthesis of specific proteins. *Recent Prog. Hormone Res.* 25: 105.
7. Brant, J. W. A., and Nalbandov, A. V. 1956. Role of sex hormones in albumin secretions by the oviduct of chickens. *Poultry Sci.* 34: 692.
8. Sjungkvist, H. I. 1967. Light and electron microscopical study of the effect of oestrogen on the chicken oviduct. *Acta Endocr.* 56: 391.
9. Kohler, P. O. Grimley, P. M.; and O'Malley, B. W. 1968. Protein

synthesis differential stimulation of cell-specific proteins in epithelial cells of chick oviduct. *Science* 160: 86.
10. O'Malley, B. W., and McGuire, W. L. 1968. Studies on the mechanism of estrogen-mediated tissue differentiation: Regulation of nuclear transcription and induction of new RNA species. *Proc. Nat. Acad. Sci. U.S.A.* 60: 1527.
11. Oka, T., and Schimke, R. T. 1969. Interaction of estrogen and progesterone in chick oviduct development. I. Antagonistic effect of progesterone on estrogen-induced proliferation and differentation of tubular gland cells. *J. Cell Biol.* 41: 816.
12. O'Malley, B. W.; McGuire, W. L.; and Korenman, S. G. 1967. Estrogen stimulation of synthesis of specific proteins and RNA polymerase activity in the immature chick oviduct. *Biochim. Biophys. Acta* 145: 204.
13. Janne, J., and Raina, A. 1969. On the stimulation of ornithine decarboxylase and RNA polymerase activity in rat liver after treatment with growth hormone. *Biochim. Biophys. Acta* 174: 796.
14. Stastny, M., and Cohen, S. 1970. Epidermal growth factor. IV. The induction of ornithine decarboxylase. *Biochem. Biophys. Acta* 204: 578.
15. Moulton, B. C., and Leonard, S. L. 1969. Hormonal effects on spermidine levels in male and female reproductive organs of the rat. *Endocrinology* 84: 1461.
16. Williams-Ashman, H. G.; Pegg, A. E.; and Lockwood, D. H. 1969. Mechanisms and regulation of polyamine and putrescine biosynthesis in male genital glands and other tissues of mammals. In *Advances in enzyme regulation,* vol. 7, ed. G. Weber, p. 291. Oxford: Pergamon Press.
17. Cohen, S.; O'Malley, B. W.; and Stastny, M. 1970. Estrogenic induction of ornithine decarboxylase *in vivo* and *in vitro. Science* 170: 336.
18. Means, A. R., and O'Malley, B. W. 1970. Estrogen-mediated tissue differentiation: Messenger RNA translation. *Clin. Res.* 18: 33.
19. ———. 1971. Protein biosynthesis on chick oviduct polyribosomes. II. Effects of progesterone. *Biochemistry* 10: 1570.
20. Means, A. R.; Hall, P. F.; Nicol, L. W.; Sawyer, W. H.; and Baker, C. A. 1969. Protein biosynthesis in the testis. IV. Isolation and properties of polyribosomes, *Biochemistry* 8: 1488.
21. O'Malley, B. W.; Means, A. R.; and Sherman, M. R. 1970. Mechanism of action of progesterone: Regulation of gene transcription. In *The sex steroids: Molecular mechanisms,* ed. K. McKerns. New York: Appleton-Century Crofts.
22. Lowry, O. H.; Rosebrough, N. J.; Farr, A. L.; and Randall, R. J. 1951. Protein measurement with the folin phenol reagent, *J. Biol. Chem.* 193: 265.
23. McGuire, W. L., and O'Malley, B. W. 1968. Ribonucleic acid polymerase activity of the chick oviduct during steroid-induced synthesis of a specific protein. *Biochim. Biophys. Acta* 157: 187.

24. Means, A. R.; Abrass, I. B.; and O'Malley, B. W. 1971. Protein biosynthesis on chick oviduct polyribosomes. I. Changes during estrogen-mediated tissue differentiation. *Biochemistry* 10: 1561.
25. Nirenberg, M. W. 1963. Cell-free protein synthesis directed by messenger RNA. In *Methods in enzymology*, ed. S. P. Colowick and N. O. Kaplan, vol. 6. New York: Academic Press.
26. Mans, R. J., and Novelli, G. D. 1961. Measurement of the incorporation of radioactive amino acids into protein by a filter-paper dish method. *Arch. Biochem. Biophys.* 94: 48.
27. Cammack, K. A., and Wade, H. E. 1965. The sedimentation behavior of ribonuclease-active and inactive ribosomes from bacteria. *Biochem. J.* 96: 671.
28. Britten, R. J., and Davidson, E. H. 1969. Gene regulation for higher cells: A theory. *Science* 165: 349.

Elwood V. Jensen, George E. Block, Sylvia Smith,
Kay Kyser, and Eugene R. DeSombre

Estrogen Receptors and Hormone Dependency 2

BINDING OF ESTROGENS IN WHOLE TISSUES

It has long been recognized that certain mammalian tissues, associated with the reproductive process, are unable to grow and function optimally without minute amounts of steroidal compounds known as sex hormones. Although the actual basis of this hormone dependency remains obscure, an important difference between dependent and nondependent tissues was demonstrated by studies of the fate in various tissues of tritiated estrogens administered to hormone-deprived animals. The "target" tissues, such as uterus, vagina, and anterior pituitary, were found to possess a striking affinity for estradiol, indicating that they contained specific estrogen-binding components, now called "estrogen receptors" or "estrophiles."

Extensive investigations[1] of the incorporation and retention of radioactive steroid after the administration of physiologic amounts of various estrogens have established the way in which estrogenic hormones interact with responsive tissues in vivo. In the rat the target tissues show a striking affinity for estradiol, 17α-methylestradiol, 17α-ethynylestradiol, and hexestrol, and a transient affinity for estriol. Each of these substances exerts its hormonal effect without undergoing chemical alteration, even though they are subject to extensive

---

The authors are affiliated with the Ben May Laboratory for Cancer Research and the Department of Surgery at the University of Chicago.

1. More detailed description of these studies of estrogen binding in whole tissues, with specific reference to the contributions of Glascock, Stone, Martin, Baggett, Gorski, Talwar, King, Mahesh, Michael, Eisenfeld, Terenius, Callantine, Villee, and their associates, is given in the review articles, references 1–4.

metabolic transformation elsewhere in the animal. In contrast, neither estrone nor mestranol binds to target tissues; the estrogenic action of these substances appears to depend on their metabolic conversion to estradiol and 17α-ethynylestradiol, respectively, which then accumulate in the target organs.

Specific incorporation of estrogens into hormone-dependent tissues is blocked by certain antiuterotrophic compounds, such as ethamoxytriphetol (MER-25), nafoxidine (Upjohn 11,100), Parke-Davis CI-628, and clomiphene—substances which do not affect the low level of estradiol incorporation into nontarget tissues. The inhibition of estradiol-induced uterine growth by various doses of nafoxidine was found to parallel the reduction in estradiol incorporation, providing evidence that the estrogen-binding phenomenon is closely involved in the biological action of the hormone. In contrast, actinomycin-D and puromycin, each of which blocks overall uterine growth as well as many of the early biochemical responses of the uterus to estrogen, do not interfere with the binding of estradiol to target tissues, indicating that the estrogen-receptor interaction is an early step in the uterotrophic process, preceding the acceleration of biosynthetic reactions sensitive to actinomycin-D or puromycin.

When surviving uterine tissue is exposed to dilute solutions of tritiated estradiol in Krebs-Ringer buffer at 37° C, an interaction of hormone with receptor takes place which shows all the characteristics of the in vivo phenomenon. This interaction in vitro does not require either oxygen or added nutrients. As is illustrated in figure 1, uterine tissue shows a striking incorporation of radioactive steroid compared with diaphragm, where the small amount of hormone appears to be bound in a different manner, inasmuch as it, unlike the steroid in uterus, is rapidly washed out when the tissue is placed in fresh buffer. If a binding inhibitor, such as nafoxidine or Parke-Davis CI-628, is also present, the uptake of estradiol by uterus is reduced essentially to the level in diaphragm. Using the in vitro system, we can demonstrate dependence of estrogen binding on sulfhydryl groups; if *n*-ethyl maleimide or *p*-hydroxymercuribenzoate is present in the incubation system, or if the uterine tissue has been pretreated with these reagents, the uptake by uterus is again reduced to the level in diaphragm, upon which these sulfhydryl reagents have no effect. The uptake of estradiol in the in vitro system and its sensitivity to the action of specific inhibitors provide a simple means of

Estrogen Receptors and Hormone Dependency 25

distinguishing between estrogen-responsive tissues, which contain receptor proteins, and non–estrogen-responsive tissues, which do not.

TWO-STEP INTERACTION MECHANISM

The foregoing studies of the fate of physiologic amounts of estrogenic hormones in vivo and in vitro established the principal characteristics of the specific interaction of estrogenic hormones with estrophilic substances in intact target tissues and provided a basis for

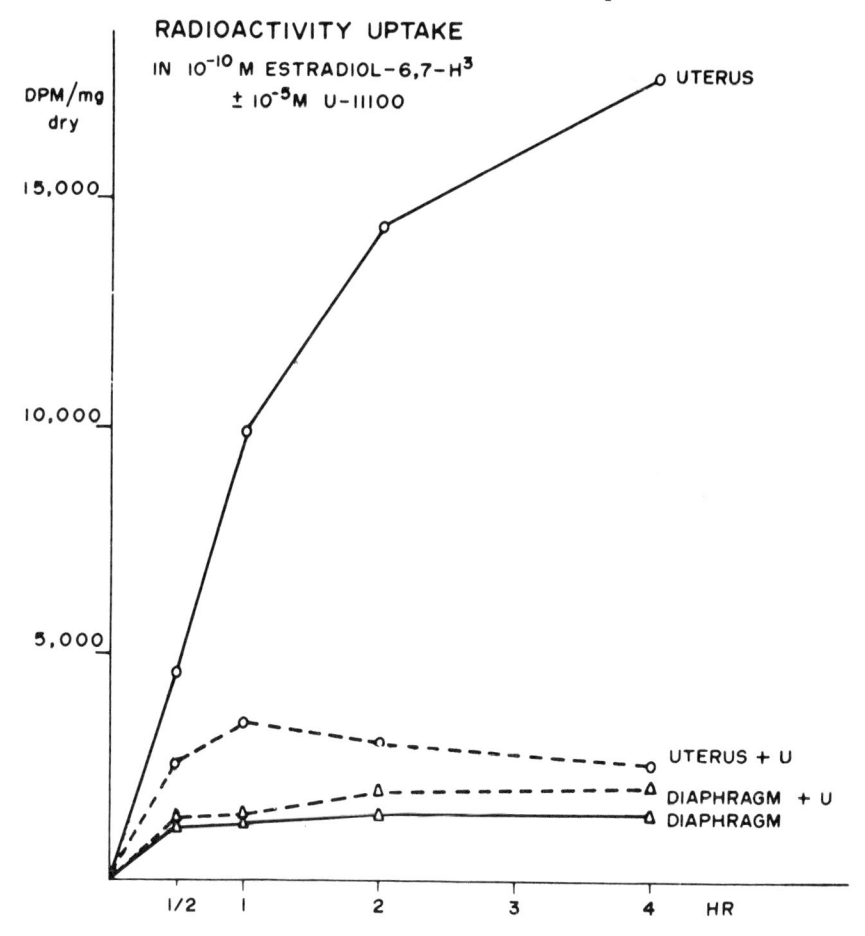

Fig. 1. Concentration of radioactivity in dried, slit uterine horns and hemidiaphragms of immature rats after stirring for various times in 0.1 nM estradiol-6, 7-^{3}H (E-2*) at 38° in KRH-glucose buffer (pH 7.3) in the presence and absence of 10 μM nafoxidine(U). Each point is the median value of 5 horns. (Reproduced by permission from *Arch. Anat. Microscop. Morph. Exp.* 56 [suppl.]: 547, 1967)

evaluating the significance of estrogen-binding phenomena in broken cell systems. As more detailed investigations were carried out,[2] it became apparent from a variety of experimental evidence that the interaction of estradiol with uterine and other target tissues is not a simple association of the hormone with an intracellular binding site, but that it involves some kind of biphasic phenomenon. One such indication is the early observation that as the dose of estradiol administered is increased above the physiologic range, the capacity of uterus, vagina, and pituitary for initial uptake of the hormone far exceeds their ability to retain it. This behavior is in marked contrast to that of the non-target tissues, where the low amounts of steroid incorporated are proportional to the dose at all time points studied, and suggests that the specific binding of estradiol in target tissues consists of two distinct phenomena, uptake and retention, with the latter process saturable at considerably lower hormone concentrations than the former.

A second indication of a dualistic process is that there appear to be two intracellular binding sites for estradiol in uterine tissue, each involving a characteristic hormone-receptor complex. After rat uterus is exposed to tritiated estradiol, either in vivo or at 37° C in vitro, most of the radioactive steroid (75–80%) is localized in the nucleus, as determined both by differential centrifugation of uterine homogenates and by autoradiographic examination of tissue sections, with the remainder of the steroid found in the high-speed supernatant fluid or cytosol fraction. Unlike binding in the cytosol, which occurs in the cold, the fixation of estradiol in the nucleus is temperature-dependent. Exposing uterine tissue to estradiol in vitro at 2° C results primarily in cytoplasmic binding as determined by either centrifugation or autoradiography. Further incubation of such tissues in the cold does not markedly change the distribution pattern, but on brief warming to 37° C redistribution of the radioactive steroid takes place within the tissue to give predominantly nuclear localization as obtained in vivo.

When the cytosol fraction of uteri exposed to tritiated estradiol either in vivo or in vitro is examined by sucrose density gradient ultracentrifugation, the radioactivity is found to sediment as a dis-

2. More complete description of studies of the receptor complexes and their interaction, with specific reference to the contributions of Gorski, Talwar, Erdos, Baulieu, King, Korenman, Wotiz, Maurer, Stumpf, Herrmann, Bresciani, Attramadal, and their associates, is given in references 3–7.

Estrogen Receptors and Hormone Dependency

crete macromolecular band (fig. 2), with a coefficient originally believed to be 9.5S but now known to be about 8S. The major part of the uterine radioactivity, which is bound in the heavy or nuclear-myofibrillar fraction, can be solubilized by extraction with 0.3 to 0.4 M sodium or potassium chloride at pH 7.5 to 8.5, which yields a different macromolecular complex, sedimenting at about 5S. If the 8S complex of the cytosol is exposed to the salt solutions used to extract the nuclear complex, it is reversibly dissociated into a subunit sedimenting at about 4S and clearly distinguishable from the nuclear complex by careful gradient centrifugation. Both the 5S and 8S re-

RAT UTERUS EXTRACTS
0.05 μg ESTRADIOL-6,7-H^3
2 HR.   IN VIVO

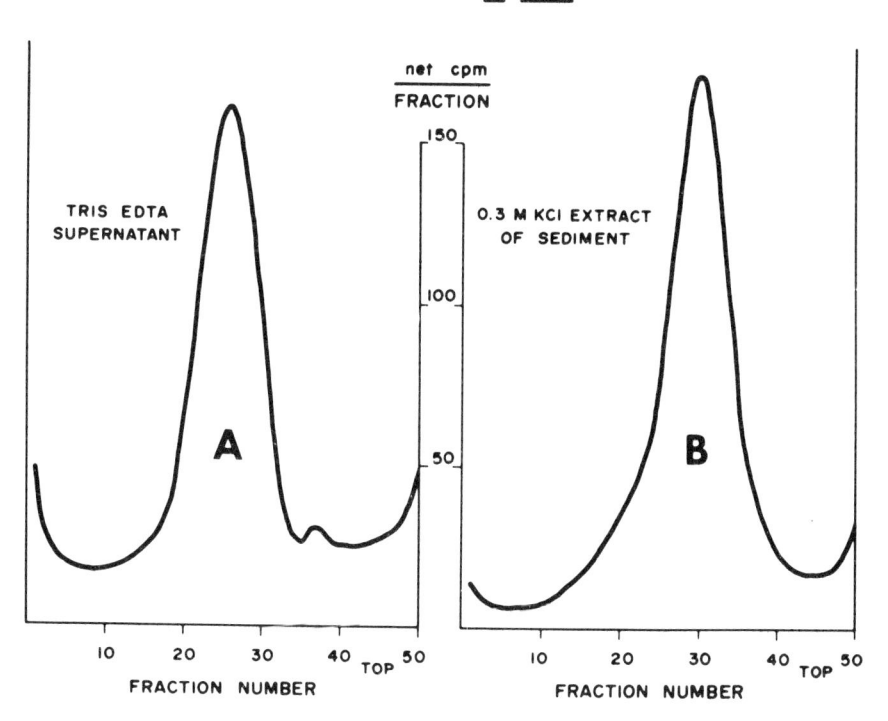

Fig. 2. Sedimentation patterns of two radioactive estradiol-receptor complexes from immature rat uteri excised 2 hr after subcutaneous injection of 45 ng (9.36 μCi) E-2*. (*a*) cytosol fraction, centrifuged 7 hr; (*b*) nuclear extract, centrifuged 10 hr, both at 216,400 g. (Reproduced by permission from *Autoradiography of diffusible substances,* ed. L. J. Roth and W. E. Stumpf, p. 81. New York: Academic Press, 1969)

ceptor substances appear to be proteins, inasmuch as both complexes are decomposed by treatment with proteases but not by nucleases. Both are rather unstable in the crude extracts, and the 8S complex shows a particular tendency to aggregate during storage.

An important difference between the two complexes is that the 8S complex of the cytosol can be formed directly, even in the cold, simply by adding tritiated estradiol to the cytosol fraction from uteri not previously exposed to hormone, whereas the 5S complex is not produced by treating isolated nuclei with the hormone. This direct formation of 8S complex provides a convenient means for estimating the receptor content of a cytosol fraction, simply by determining the total radioactivity in the 8S sedimentation peak when sufficient hormone has been added to saturate the receptor. Saturation is indicated by excess radioactivity appearing either at the top of the gradient (fig. 3a) or, if serum proteins are present, bound nonspecifically to these proteins in the 4.5S region (fig. 3b). By this technique one can demonstrate that many if not all rat tissues possess small amounts of the 8S estrophile; the target tissues are unique in that they contain much higher levels of the binding protein. In fact, the target tissues contain considerably more receptor protein than is utilized by a physiologic dose of the hormone; this reserve capacity of 8S receptor is consistent with its involvement in the nonsaturable uptake process mentioned earlier.

In contrast to the 8S receptor in the cytosol, there is no evidence for the presence of 5S binding protein in uterine nuclei. No 5S complex is formed by adding estradiol either to a nuclear extract or to the nuclei themselves. But if uterine nuclei are incubated with estradiol in the presence of uterine cytosol, so that the hormone is presented to them in the form of 8S complex, the characteristic 5S nuclear complex is produced. This formation of 5S nuclear complex from 8S cytosol complex, or its 4S subunit, is a temperature-dependent process requiring incubation at at least 25° C for the reaction to proceed at a significant rate.

The foregoing indication that the 5S complex of the nucleus is derived from the 8S complex of the cytosol is substantiated by the fact that the 8S receptor disappears from the cytosol as estradiol interacts with uterine tissue to become localized in the nucleus. Not only is the cytosol content of 8S binding protein less after a large dose of estradiol than after a smaller one, but upon administration of a physiologic dose of hormone there is a rapid and progressive decrease in 8S receptor level during a 4 hr period, after which the receptor content is gradually restored, apparently by resynthesis.

The foregoing observations, taken together, are consistent with a two-step interaction mechanism in which the 4S binding unit of the 8S protein, present in excess in the extranuclear regions of uterine cells, serves as the uptake receptor, combining directly with estradiol. This association of hormone with receptor lets the protein enter the nucleus by a temperature-dependent process, accompanied by transformation of the 4S binding unit to a 5S form which becomes bound

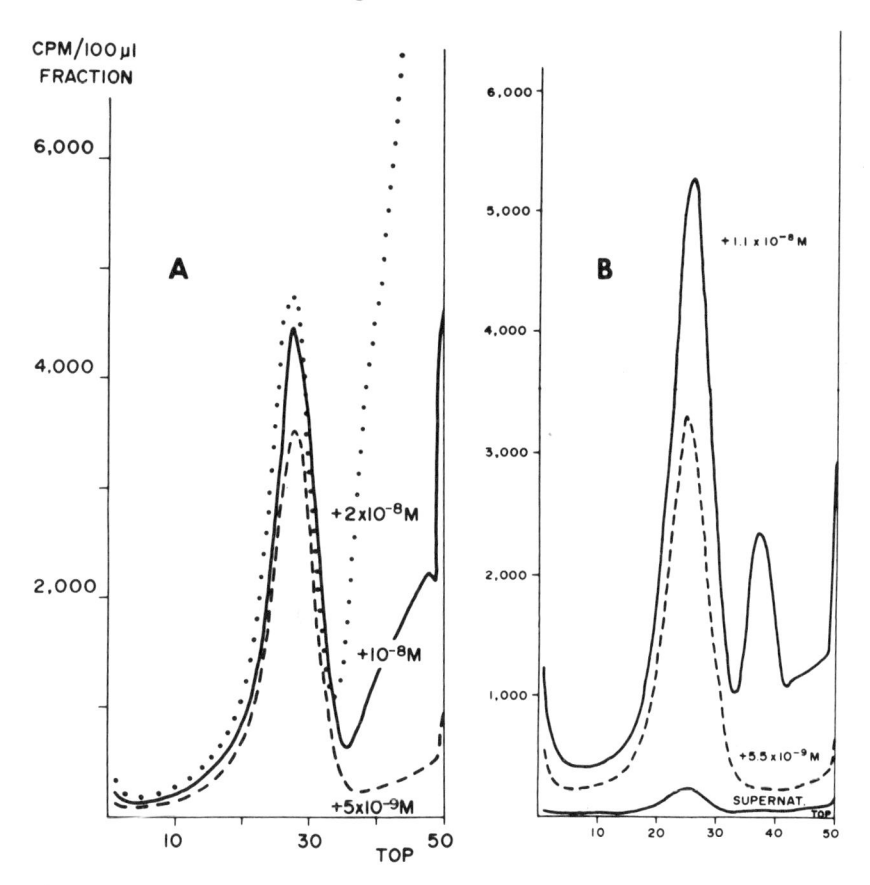

Fig. 3. Saturation of the 8S receptor protein by addition of tritiated estradiol to rat uterine cytosol. (*a*) uteri from untreated rats stirred in KRH buffer, pH 7.3 for 30 min before homogenizing in Tris-EDTA; (*b*) uteri excised 15 min after subcutaneous injection of 50 ng E-2* homogenized directly. Centrifugation 7 hr at 216,000 g. (Curve *a* reproduced by permission from *Develop. Biol.*, suppl. 3: 151, 1969; curve *b* from *Proc. Nat. Acad. Sci. USA* 59: 632, 1968)

in the nuclear chromatin. As the interaction proceeds, the level of extranuclear receptor protein is temporarily depleted, owing to its movement into the nucleus in combination with the hormone.

When the two-step mechanism was first proposed, the transformation to 5S complex was considered to take place within the nucleus itself (fig. 4a). The recent observation (4) that conversion of the 4S subunit to what appears to be the 5S complex can take place when the cytosol is warmed in the presence of estradiol (but not with estrone) raises the possibility that the estrogen-dependent and temperature-dependent transformation of 4S to 5S complex may be a cytoplasmic

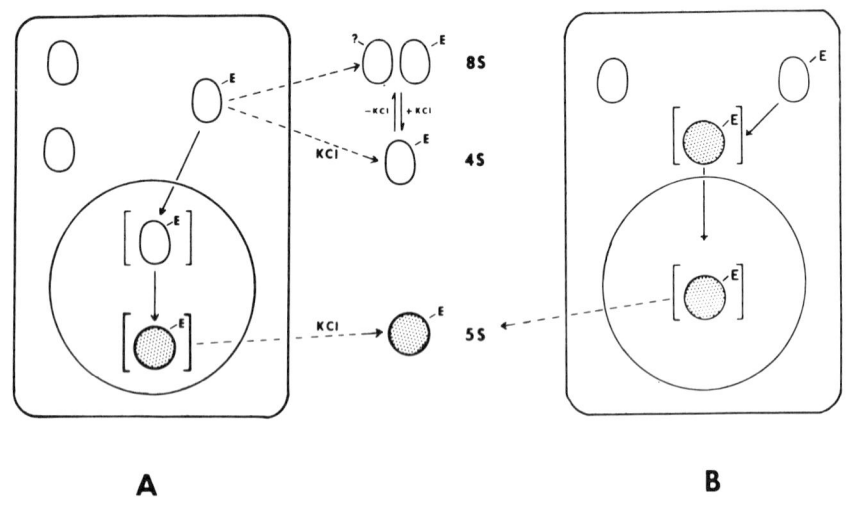

A **B**

Fig. 4. Interaction pathway of estradiol (E) in uterine cells.

process, which is followed by a rapid uptake and fixation of the 5S complex in the nucleus, with or without some further subtle alteration (fig. 4b). The ability of uterine nuclei to take up and bind preformed 5S complex supports this. Experiments so far have failed to distinguish with certainty between these two pathways; for now both possibilities must be considered.

At present, the relation between the transformation sequence of receptor complexes and the stimulation of biosynthetic processes in the hormone-dependent tissue is not clear, although the same general type of two-step mechanism has now been demonstrated for the interaction of several classes of steroid hormones with their target tissues (4). It is possible that the extranuclear protein is only a means of transporting the hormone into the nucleus, where it elicits its response by a mechanism independent of the receptor substance. On the other hand, it is also possible that the receptor protein itself is the active agent, perhaps as participant in some nuclear process analogous to σ factor in microbial systems, and that in dependent tissues this protein requires association with the hormone in order to reach its site of action. In any case, it appears that a principal role of the estrogen is to associate with the extranuclear receptor protein, present in unique amounts in the target tissues, and to render this protein susceptible to a temperature-dependent transformation, which is accompanied by movement of the hormone-receptor complex into the nucleus.

BINDING OF ESTROGENS IN EXPERIMENTAL MAMMARY TUMORS

Although the uptake of estradiol by normal mammary gland is rather low, probably because of the large content of adipose tissue, careful investigations by both biochemical and autoradiographic techniques have demonstrated that specific estradiol binding, similar to that in uterus and vagina, takes place in the mammary glands of the rat (8, 9), the mouse (10), and the human (11). More extensive studies have been carried out with experimental mammary tumors, such as those induced in the Sprague-Dawley rat by feeding or injecting carcinogenic hydrocarbons (12, 13). These hormone-dependent tumors resemble uterus and vagina (fig. 5) in their affinity for estradiol (but not estrone), which is incorporated without chemical transformation, and in the sensitivity of this uptake to nafoxidine and similar binding inhibitors (14–19). A small fraction (10–12%) of these induced tumors appear to be nondependent, inasmuch as they do not regress after ovariectomy; the uptake of estradiol by these nonregressing tumors is considerably smaller than that of the dependent ones (16). Detailed study (20) of the interaction of estradiol with DMBA-induced mammary tumor has demonstrated that this proceeds by a two-step mechanism in which an 8S receptor protein in the cytosol, dissociable into 4S subunits, serves as the precursor of the 5S estradiol-receptor complex extractable from the nucleus. One difference between tumor and uterus is that in tumor a greater proportion (85–90%) of the estradiol incorporated is found in the nuclear fraction.

On exposure to dilute solutions of tritiated estradiol in vitro, slices of hormone-dependent rat mammary tumor show a marked uptake of radioactive hormone which, like that of uterus, is markedly reduced in the presence of binding inhibitors such as nafoxidine (19–21). As is illustrated by figure 6, tumors which do not regress after ovariectomy can be readily distinguished from the "hormone-dependent" tumors both by the magnitude of the estradiol uptake and by the degree of sensitivity to the inhibitor. As with uterus, adding tritiated estradiol to the cytosol fraction of a tumor homogenate gives rise to an estradiol-receptor complex which sediments as a well-defined 8S peak on sucrose density gradient ultracentrifugation and which, in the presence of saturating amounts of estradiol, can serve as a measure of the total 8S receptor content of the tumor cytosol (20).

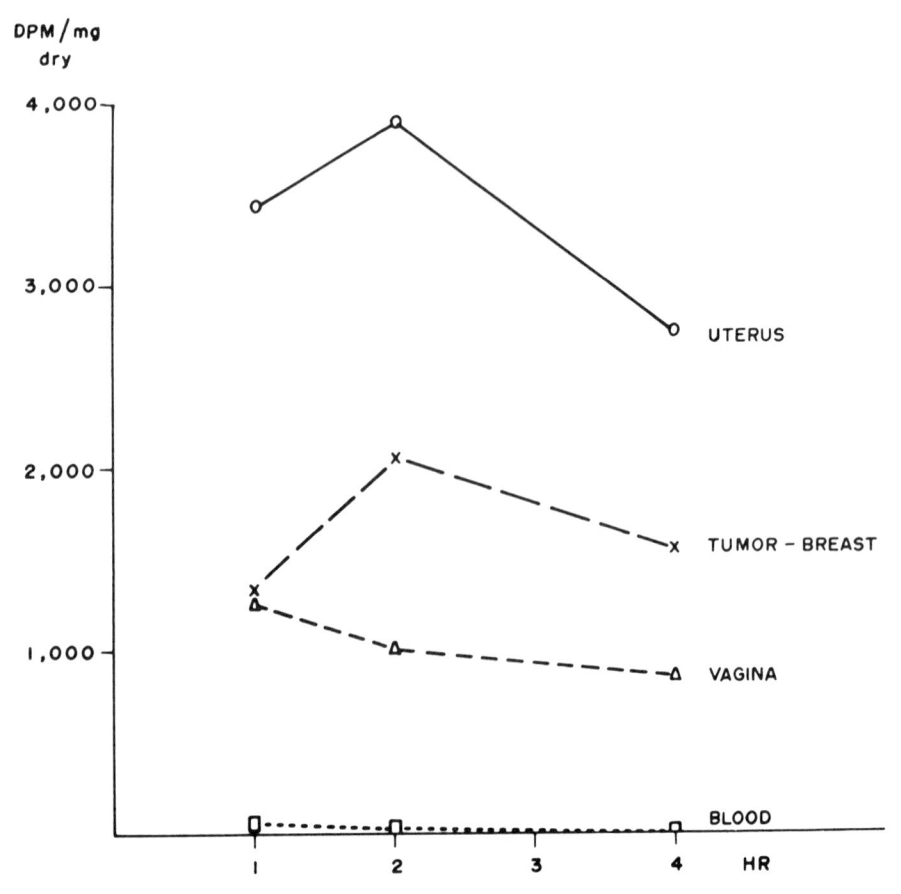

Fig. 5. Concentration of radioactivity in dried tissues of tumor-bearing rats ovariectomized 2 days before intravenous injection of 120 ng (23 μCi) E-2* in saline. (Reproduced by permission from *Endogenous factors influencing host-tumor balance,* ed. R. W. Wissler, T. L. Dao, and S. Wood, Jr., p. 15. Chicago: University of Chicago Press, 1967)

In hormone-dependent tumors, where slices show a large specific estradiol uptake, the 8S sedimentation peak is substantial, whereas those tumors which do not regress on ovariectomy show only small 8S receptor contents.

ESTROGEN RECEPTORS IN HUMAN BREAST CANCER

Since the original demonstration of striking remission of advanced breast cancer after removal of the adrenal glands (22), it has become recognized that hormone deprivation, accomplished by either adrenalectomy or hypophysectomy, is the most effective therapy for advanced breast cancer in the postmenopausal patient, for those who respond to such treatment. However, clinical experience has shown that only a small fraction (30–35%) of postmenopausal breast cancer

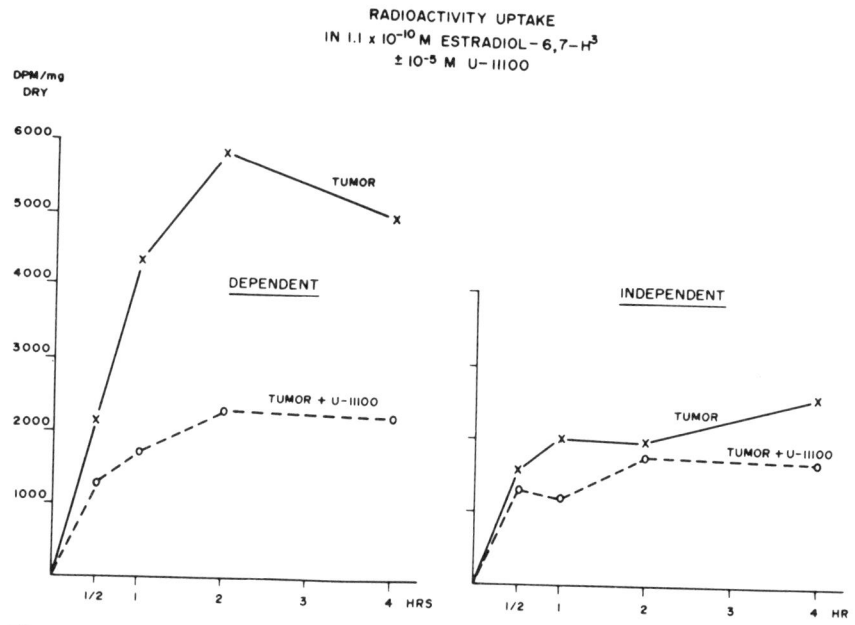

Fig. 6. Comparison of hormone-dependent and hormone-independent rat mammary tumor slices in uptake of radioactivity on exposure to 0.1 nM E-2* in presence and absence of 10 μM nafoxidine. Each point is the median for 5 slices. Dependent tumors were taken from 42-wk-old rats receiving 7, 12-DMBA (3 × 2 mg, i.v.) at age 50 to 56 days and ovariectomized 24 hr before experiment; nondependent tumors were those continuing to grow in similar rats ovariectomized 10 wk before experiment. (Reproduced by permission from *Endogenous factors influencing host-tumor balance,* ed. R. W. Wissler, T. L. Dao, and S. Wood, Jr., p. 68. Chicago: University of Chicago Press, 1967)

patients have tumors which respond to endocrine ablation. A method of predicting which cancers are responsive would greatly enhance the usefulness of ablative therapy by restricting its application to patients in which it has a reasonable chance of success and sparing the majority the trauma of a major surgical procedure which cannot help them.

Soon after the original observations of the striking affinity of estrogens for target tissues, Folca, Glascock, and Irvine (23) injected tritiated hexestrol into breast cancer patients who were about to undergo adrenalectomy and observed that the uptake of radioactive hormone by the tumor, compared with that of skeletal muscle, was greater in four patients who experienced remission than in six patients who did not. These results, together with the accumulation of knowledge concerning the estrogen receptor proteins of normal target tissues and the greater receptor content of dependent compared with nondependent rat mammary tumors, suggested that an estimation of the receptor content of a breast cancer specimen might provide a valuable guide for predicting the response of that patient to ablative therapy. Accordingly we undertook an investigation both of patients with metastatic disease, for correlation with their response to adrenalectomy or hypophysectomy, and of mastectomy patients, in order to characterize the primary tumor for future correlation with the response to endocrine therapy in those patients in which the cancer might recur.

MATERIALS AND METHODS

Tumor specimens were obtained as soon as possible after excision (usually 15 to 30 min) and dissected free of necrotic, adipose, or other extraneous tissue with the advice of a pathologist.[3] For uptake studies, 0.5 mm slices of fresh tumor tissue were cut in a Stadie-Riggs apparatus and kept in cold Krebs-Ringer-Henseleit glucose buffer (KRH), pH 7.3, until all sections had been prepared. Half the slices, selected at random, were transferred to a beaker containing 300 ml of 0.1 nM estradiol-6, 7-^{3}H (specific activity 57 Ci per mmol) in KRH buffer which had been equilibrated in a water bath at 37° C; the remainder of the tissue was placed in a similar solution which also contained an estrogen antagonist, either nafoxidine or Parke-Davis CI-628, in 10

---

3. We are grateful to Drs. T. Sugiyama and R. Fukunishi for their generous assistance in selecting the tissue to be studied.

μM concentration. The two solutions were stirred magnetically in the constant temperature bath. At appropriate intervals, usually 30 min, five or more slices were removed from each solution and blotted, dried from the frozen state, and weighed. The content of tritiated hormone was determined by combustion (earlier by a modified Schöniger technique, more recently in a Packard model 300 oxidizer) to yield tritiated water which was counted in a liquid scintillation spectrometer.

For density gradient studies, the weighed tumor specimens (except for a few which were homogenized fresh) were frozen in liquid nitrogen, and the frozen tissue was shattered under liquid nitrogen in a Thermovac stainless steel pulverizer. The resulting powder was thawed and carefully homogenized in 4 volumes of cold 10 mM Tris buffer, pH 7.5, containing 1.5 mM EDTA, using an all-glass homogenizer and 15-sec homogenization periods each followed by a 45-sec cooling period. The resulting homogenate was centrifuged at 2° C for 30 min at 300,000 g to yield the cytosol fraction. Aliquots (150 μl) of this cytosol were treated with 50 μl of Tris-EDTA buffer either with or without 1 μM PD CI-628; after it had stood 10 min at 0° C, 50 μl of buffer containing tritiated estradiol was added. In more recent experiments, a 2.5 nM solution of estradiol was employed, giving a final concentration of 0.5 nM; in earlier experiments somewhat higher estradiol concentrations were used. A 200 μl portion of each solution was layered carefully on a cold preformed linear sucrose gradient (5–20% or 10–30%) also containing Tris-EDTA buffer, pH 7.5. After centrifugation for an appropriate period (usually 12 to 13 hr for 10–30% gradients or 7 to 8 hr for 5–20% gradients either at 300,000 g in an International SB-405 rotor or at 308,000 g in a Spinco SW-56 rotor), successive 100 μl fractions were drawn off by needle puncture of the bottom of the centrifuge tube using a Hamilton repeating dispenser and paraffin oil to displace the fractions through the needle. The tritium content of each fraction was determined by direct liquid scintillation counting, using a toluene–Triton X-100 scintillation medium.

To determine estradiol binding using the Sephadex G-25 procedure (24), portions of the tumor cytosols were diluted 1:10 with buffer containing various amounts of tritiated estradiol. Each was passed through a 20 ml column of Sephadex to remove the free hormone; the radioactivity present in the void volume (determined by adding the colored macromolecule, blue dextran) was obtained for scintillation counting by ether extraction of each eluate.

RESULTS

When slices of primary breast tumor were examined for estradiol affinity by the uptake inhibition procedure, they fell into two classes—those which show a low uptake not depressed in the presence of nafoxidine or PD CI-628 (negative pattern, fig. 7) and those which exhibit a substantially larger incorporation which is reduced by the inhibitor (positive pattern, fig. 8). In most instances a clear-cut distinction could be made between positive and negative patterns; a few cases showed

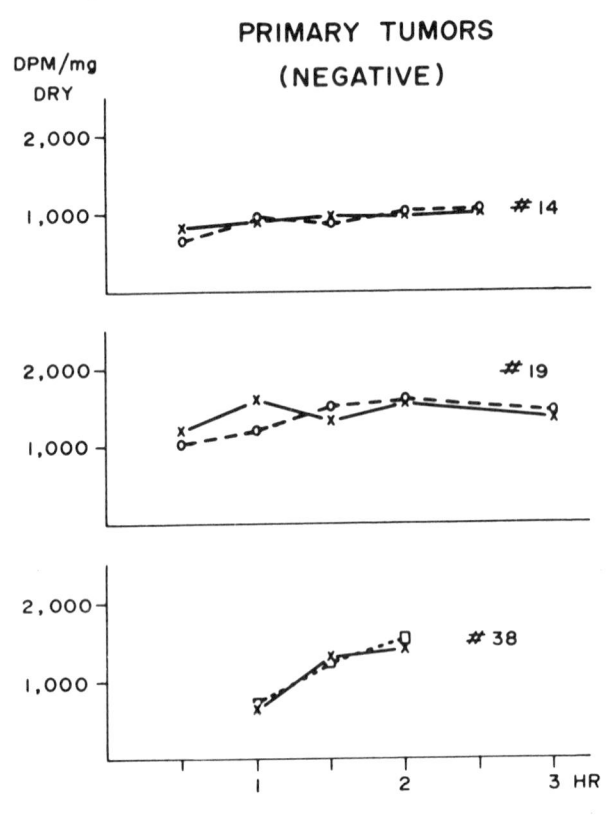

Fig. 7. Negative radioactivity uptake patterns in slices of human primary breast cancers in incubation with 0.1 nM E-2* as described in the text. In this and subsequent figures of this type, x———x indicates uptake in estradiol alone, o-------o in the presence of 10 μM nafoxidine and □---------□ in the presence of 10 μM PD CI-628. Each point is the median value for at least 4 slices, usually 5 or more.

borderline patterns. Metastatic tumors present similar negative (figs. 9, 10) and positive (fig. 11) patterns. For one patient (#24) with multiple skin metastases individual tumors could be examined, and all were negative (fig. 10). Usually, but not always, positive metastatic tumors show a higher total level of estradiol incorporation than primary tumors, possibly because the primary tumors contain adipose tissue, which has little affinity for the hormone.

In earlier experiments, incubation periods of up to 4 hr were employed, but we found that tumor slices, unlike uterus, often lose their binding capacity after longer incubation periods, so that the 4-hr time point (fig. 6), and in some cases even the 2-hr time point (fig. 7), is lower than the one preceding it. In more recent experiments, incu-

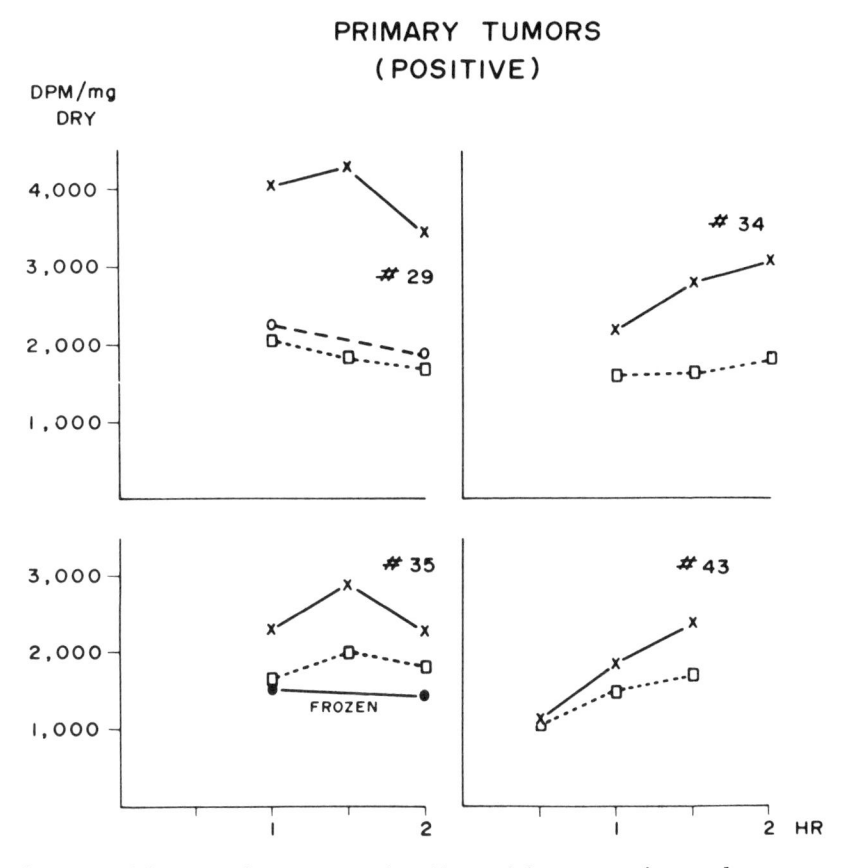

Fig. 8. Positive uptake patterns in slices of human primary breast cancers. In one instance a portion of the specimen had been frozen and thawed before slicing.

bations were usually carried out for a maximum of 90 min and in no case for more than 2 hr.

Thus, the uptake of estradiol by tumor slices permits a convenient characterization of human breast cancers, primary or metastatic, as those which resemble uterus in possessing significant estrogen affinity and those which do not. But this procedure suffers from two limitations. First, the tumor specimen must be large enough (> 0.5 g) to permit the preparation of at least twenty and preferably thirty 0.5 mm slices, so that differences due to heterogeneity of the tumor can be averaged out. Although sample size is usually not a problem with pri-

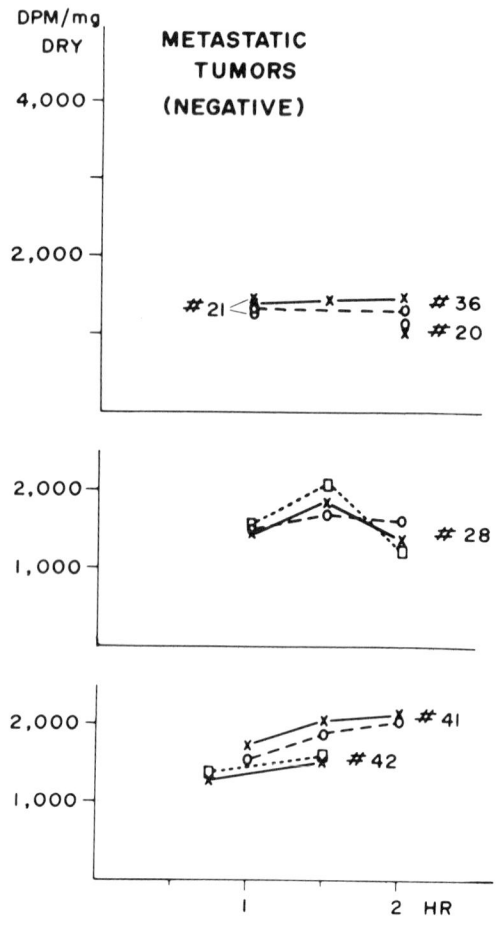

Fig. 9. Negative uptake patterns in slices of metastatic breast cancers. Metastases: #20, 28, 36, 42, skin; #21, adrenal; #41, lymph node. Patients 20 and 21 had only enough tumor specimen for one time point.

Estrogen Receptors and Hormone Dependency

mary tumors, many metastatic cancer specimens are not large enough to permit definitive evaluation by this procedure. Moreover, the determination cannot be carried out on frozen tissue. After freezing, even in liquid nitrogen, the estradiol uptake of positive tumor slices, as well as that of uterine tissue, is markedly reduced, in many instances to the level of nonspecific binding (figs. 8, 11). Freezing the tissue does not destroy the receptor proteins, but it appears to render the cells permeable to the 8S cytosol receptor, which leaks out into the medium during incubation and is not available for uptake of estradiol and fixation in the nucleus.

A method of tumor characterization applicable to small (200 mg)

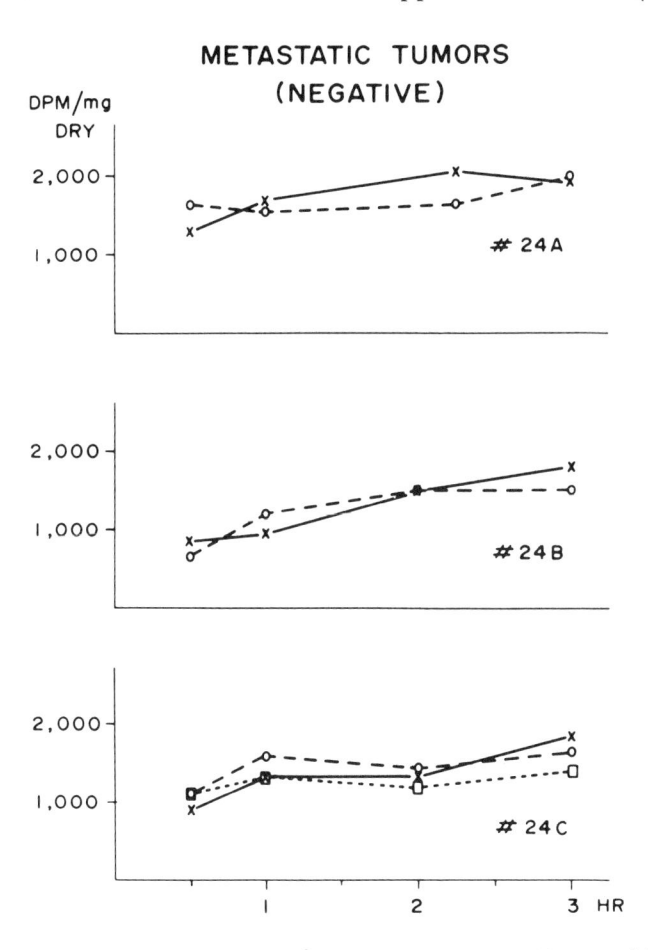

Fig. 10. Negative uptake patterns in slices of three different skin metastases taken from the same patient.

samples of either fresh or frozen tumor is the direct estimation of the cytosol receptor content by sucrose density gradient centrifugation. As was previously described for uterus (fig. 3), adding saturating amounts of estradiol to the cytosol fraction of a tumor homogenate gives rise, in a tumor with a positive uptake pattern, to an 8S complex which can be estimated by the magnitude of its sedimentation peak. As is illustrated in figure 12, the positive metastatic tumor (#32) shows a well-defined 8S peak when either fresh or frozen tissue is examined, in contrast to the negative tumor (#24B), which shows no radioactivity in the 8S region. Similarly, the positive primary tumor (#43) shows an 8S peak, in contrast to the negative tumor (#40), which gives no indication of 8S receptor content (fig. 13).

As was previously described for uterus (fig. 3B), if serum proteins

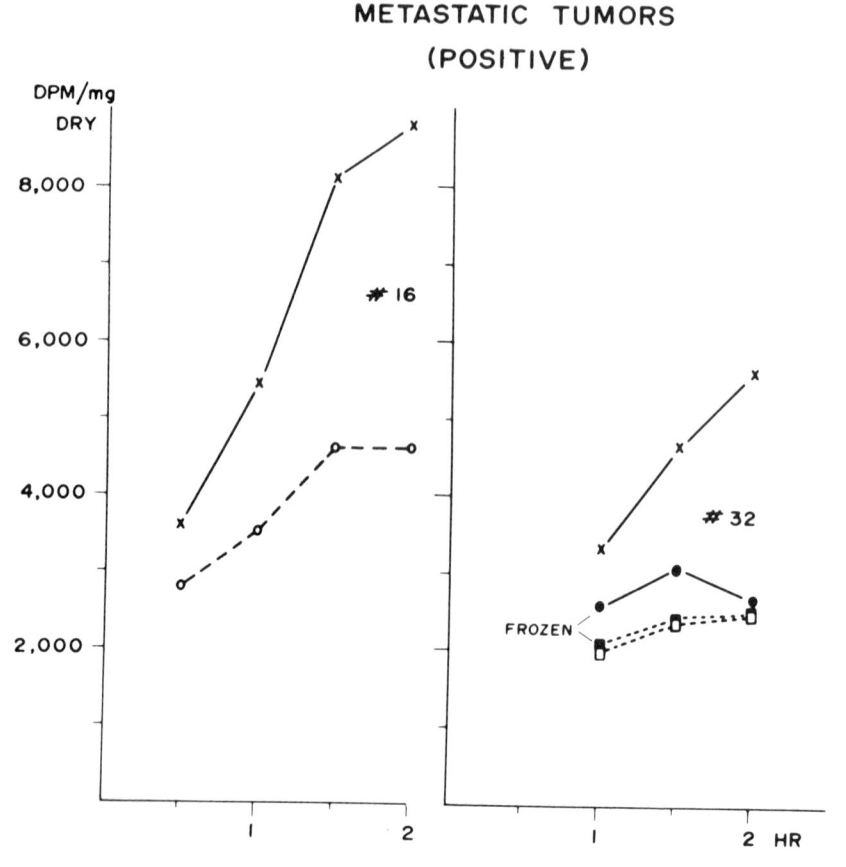

Fig. 11. Positive uptake patterns in slices of adrenal metastases. For #32, a 0.05 rather than 0.1 nM solution of E-2* was used for the incubation.

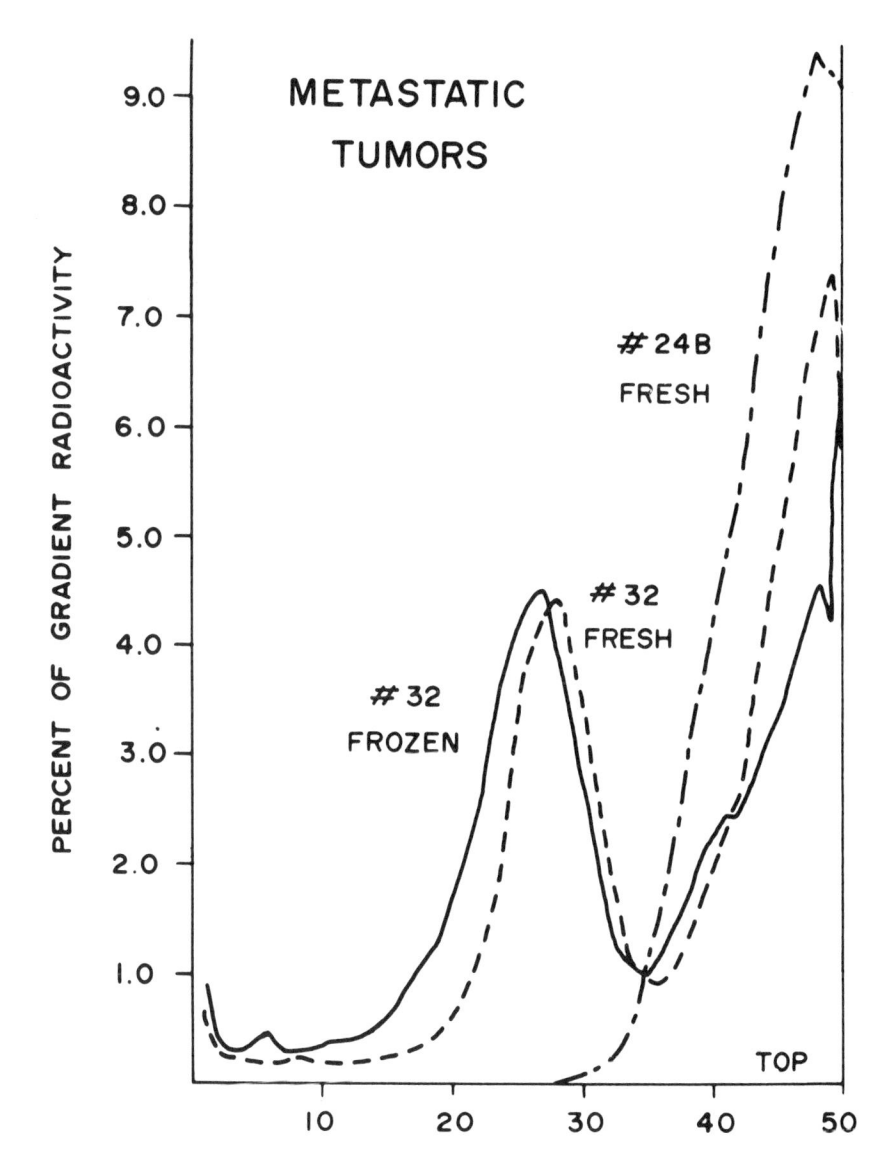

Fig. 12. Sedimentation patterns of cytosol fractions of homogenates of metastatic breast cancers described in Figs. 10 and 11. Estradiol concentrations: #24, 5 nM; #32 fresh, 4 nM; #32 frozen 3 nM. Centrifugation: #24, 8 hr at 186,000 g; #32, 7 hr at 216,000 g (in different runs), in 5–20% sucrose. All gradients also contain 10 mM Tris buffer, pH 7.5, with 1.5 mM EDTA.

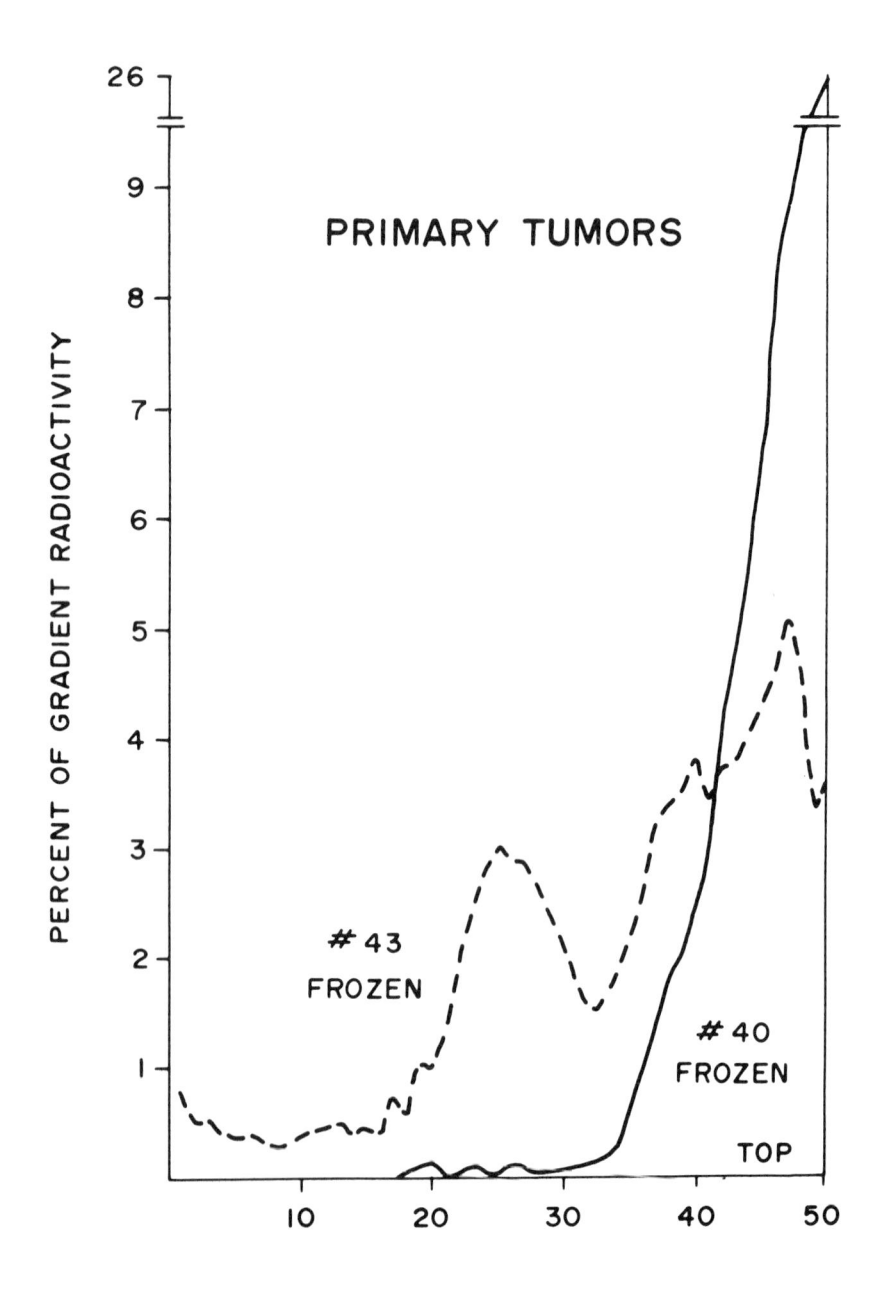

Fig. 13. Sedimentation patterns of cytosol from frozen primary tumors using 1 nM E-2*. Centrifugation: #40, 7 hr at 216,000 g; #43, 8 hr at 204,000 g, in 5–20% sucrose.

Estrogen Receptors and Hormone Dependency 43

are present, as is sometimes but not always the case in human breast cancers, nonspecific binding will be observed in the 4.5S region (fig. 14). This peak is clearly distinguishable from the specific 8S peak, both by its position on the gradient and by its insensitivity to PD CI-628 as described below. This nonspecific binding, when present, is usually in such amounts that it is not saturated by concentrations of

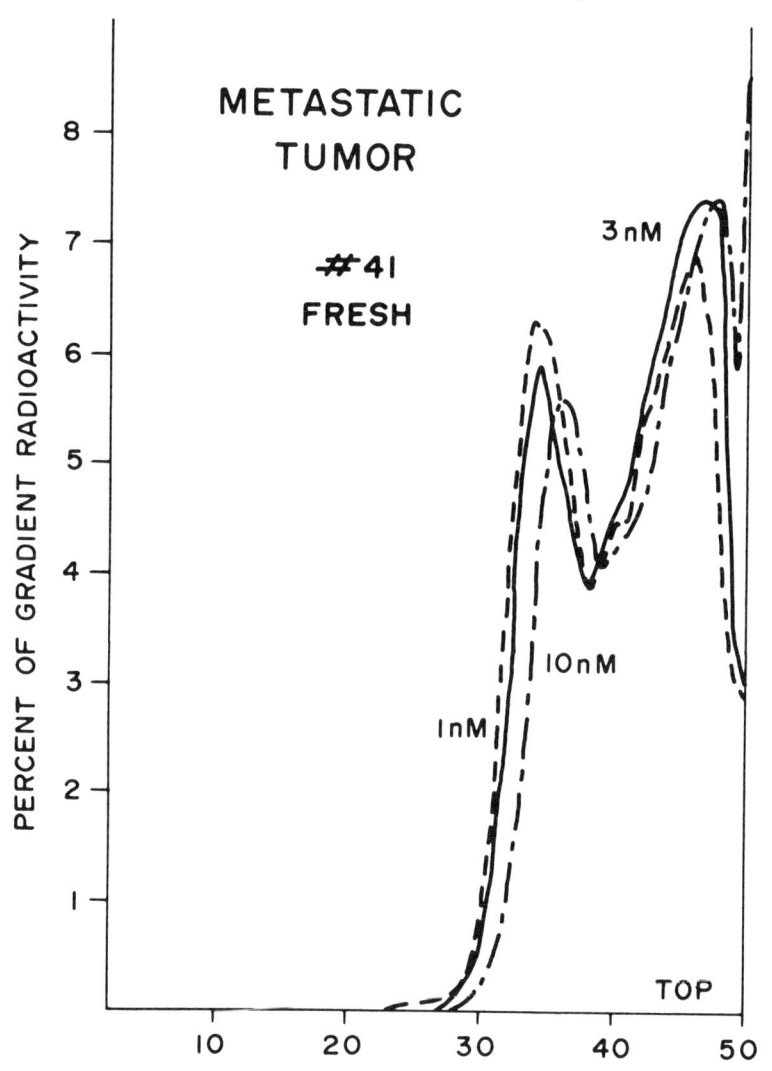

Fig. 14. Sedimentation pattern of cytosol from negative metastatic tumor described in fig. 9 in presence of 1, 3, and 10 nM E-2*. Centrifugation: 7 hr at 258,000 g in 5–20% sucrose. Under these conditions the 8S peak would be expected about fraction 20.

estradiol far greater than those required to saturate even the highest levels of 8S receptor encountered in tumor tissue (fig. 14).

In our earlier sedimentation experiments, sucrose gradients of 5% to 20% and estradiol concentrations of 1 to 2 nM were employed. Under these conditions it was found that the 8S complex from human breast cancers, unlike that of uterus, sometimes tends to decompose partially on the gradient. For example, patient 51 (fig. 15) shows a poorly defined peak, which still permits distinction from the negative pattern of patient 56, in agreement with the comparative uptake patterns of these two patients (fig. 17). Later it was found that this tendency to decompose during centrifugation is much less when a 10% to 30% sucrose gradient is employed. With some tumors the 8S complex tends to aggregate partially; as is illustrated in figure 16, the characterization of patient 66 as having a positive sedimentation pattern is sharpened considerably by carrying out the study both in the presence and in the absence of PD CI-628, which demonstrates clearly that the radioactivity of the aggregated material as well as that in the 8S region represents specific binding sensitive to the inhibitor.

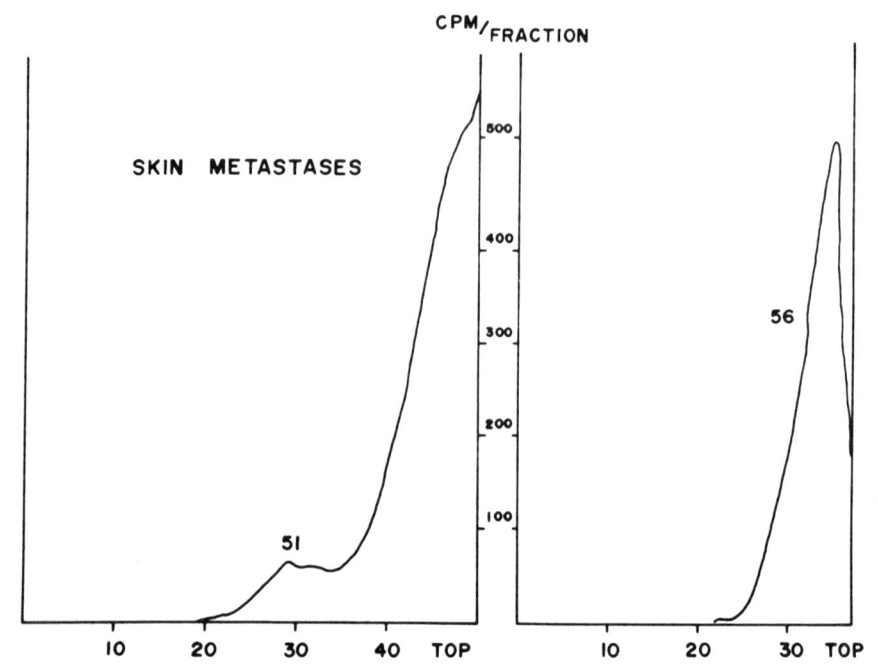

Fig. 15. Sedimentation patterns of cytosol from two specimens of skin metastases, described in fig. 17, using 1 nM E-2* for #51 and 0.5 nM for #56. Centrifugation: #51, 9 hr at 165,000 g; #56, 9 hr at 300,000 g, in 5–20% sucrose.

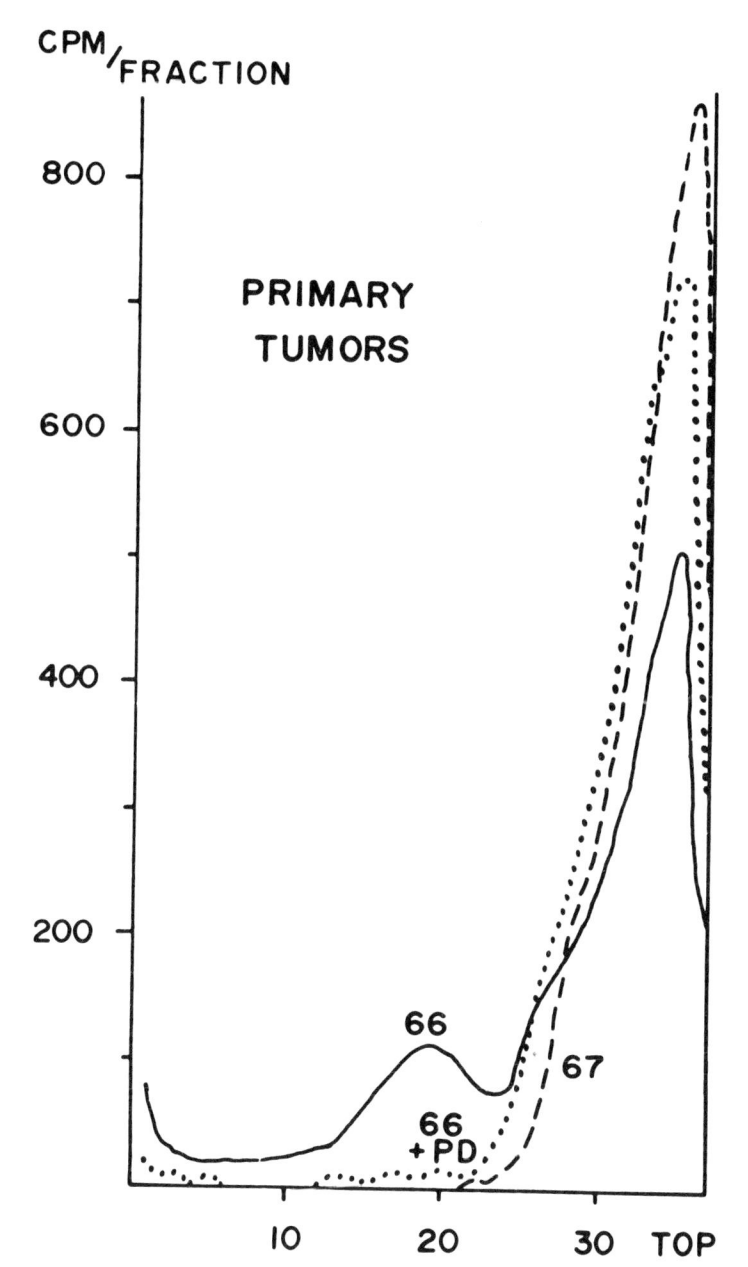

Fig. 16. Sedimentation patterns of cytosol from primary tumors using 1 nM E-2* in the presence or absence of 2 μM PD CI-628. Centrifugation: #66, 7.5 hr at 300,000 g; #67, 10 hr at 200,000 g, in 5–20% sucrose. The curve for #67 + PD was almost identical with that shown.

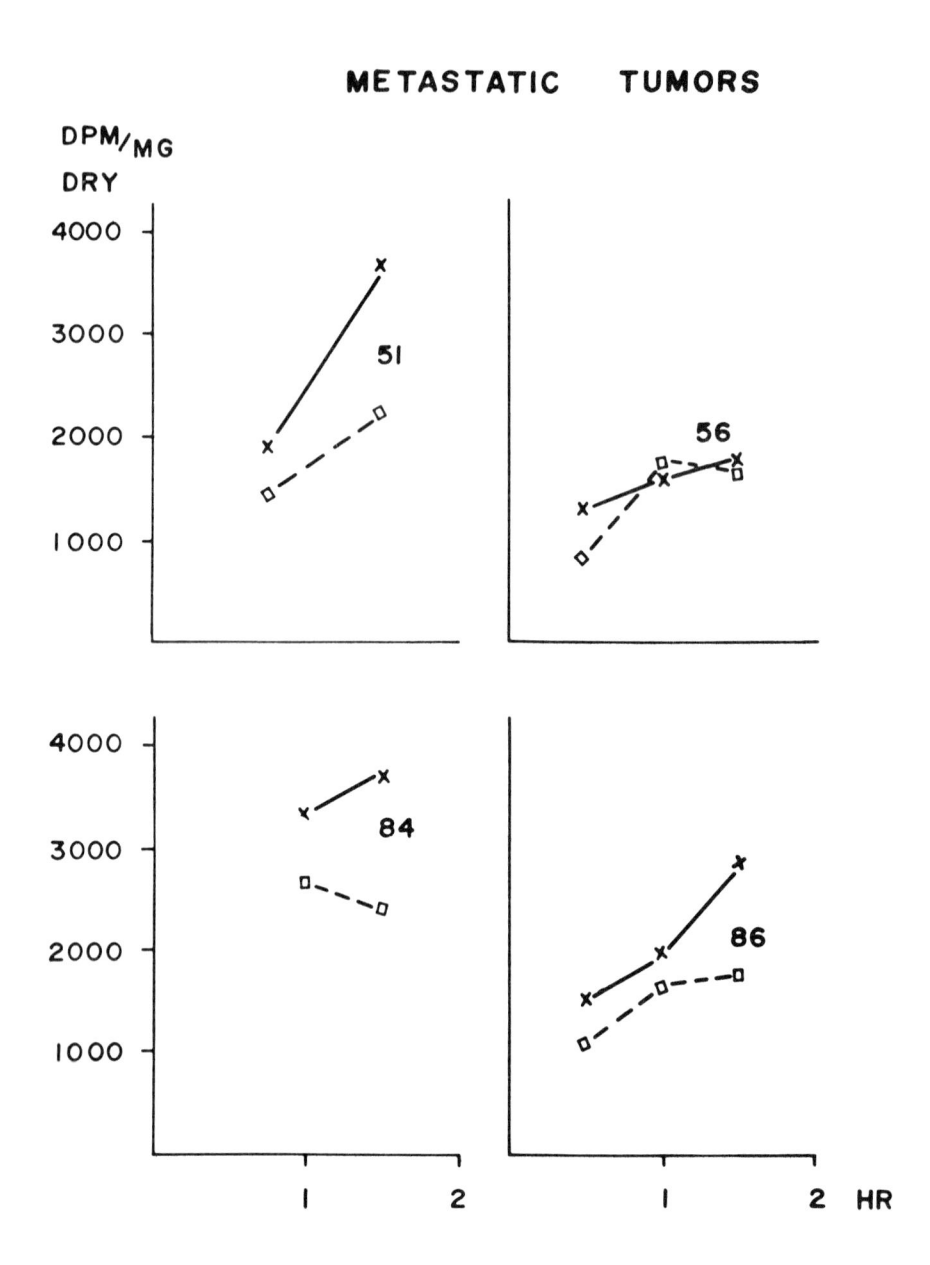

Fig. 17. Three positive and one negative uptake patterns for slices of metastases: #51 and #56, skin, #84, liver; #86, chest wall.

Estrogen Receptors and Hormone Dependency

On the basis of the experience gained as the investigations progressed, a more satisfactory set of experimental conditions for density gradient studies of tumors was adopted. These include the use of 10% to 30% sucrose gradients, which give sharper 8S peaks less subject to decomposition, the use of 0.5 nM rather than 1 or 2 nM estradiol, so that there is less excess radioactivity at the top of the tube, and the comparison of the sedimentation patterns obtained in the presence and absence of the inhibitor, PD CI-628, which permits distinction between specific and nonspecific binding.

Some of the various types of positive sedimentation patterns obtained under these improved conditions with primary and metastatic breast cancers are illustrated in figures 19 to 23; uptake patterns for the same patients are shown in figures 17 and 18. It can be seen that, in addition to the 8S peak, some human breast cancers (#68, #86, #89) show a second peak of specific binding, sensitive to the inhibitor, in the 4S region. This may represent the 4S subunit of the 8S receptor, which has been shown for the adult rat uterus (25), as well as for the adult human uterus (26; G. L. Schertz, personal communication), to differ from that of the immature rat uterus in that the receptor exists partly in the 4S form at low ionic strength. In any case, specific binding in either 8S or the 4S region can be distinguished from the nonspecific 4.5S binding by its sensitivity to the Parke-Davis inhibitor (fig. 21).

The lymph node from patient #90 represents a tumor containing an unusually high concentration of cytosol receptor, as is indicated by its almost complete utilization of the 0.5 nM estradiol. It appears that, because of the large amount of complex formed, a somewhat greater amount of inhibitor is required to completely eliminate the peak. The primary tumor from this patient also showed a large sedimentation peak as well as substantial uptake of estradiol by tumor slices (fig. 18).

In an attempt to obtain a simple procedure for evaluating small amounts of frozen tumor specimen which does not require the use of an ultracentrifuge, many of the tumor cytosols were also studied by the method of Puca and Bresciani (24) in which aliquots of diluted cytosol are treated with different amounts of tritiated estradiol and, after equilibration, the excess free estradiol is removed by filtration through Sephadex G-25. When the bound radioactivity is plotted against the total added (fig. 24), a negative tumor (#67) gives a curve which extrapolates essentially to the origin, in contrast to a tumor

PRIMARY TUMORS (WITH METASTASES)

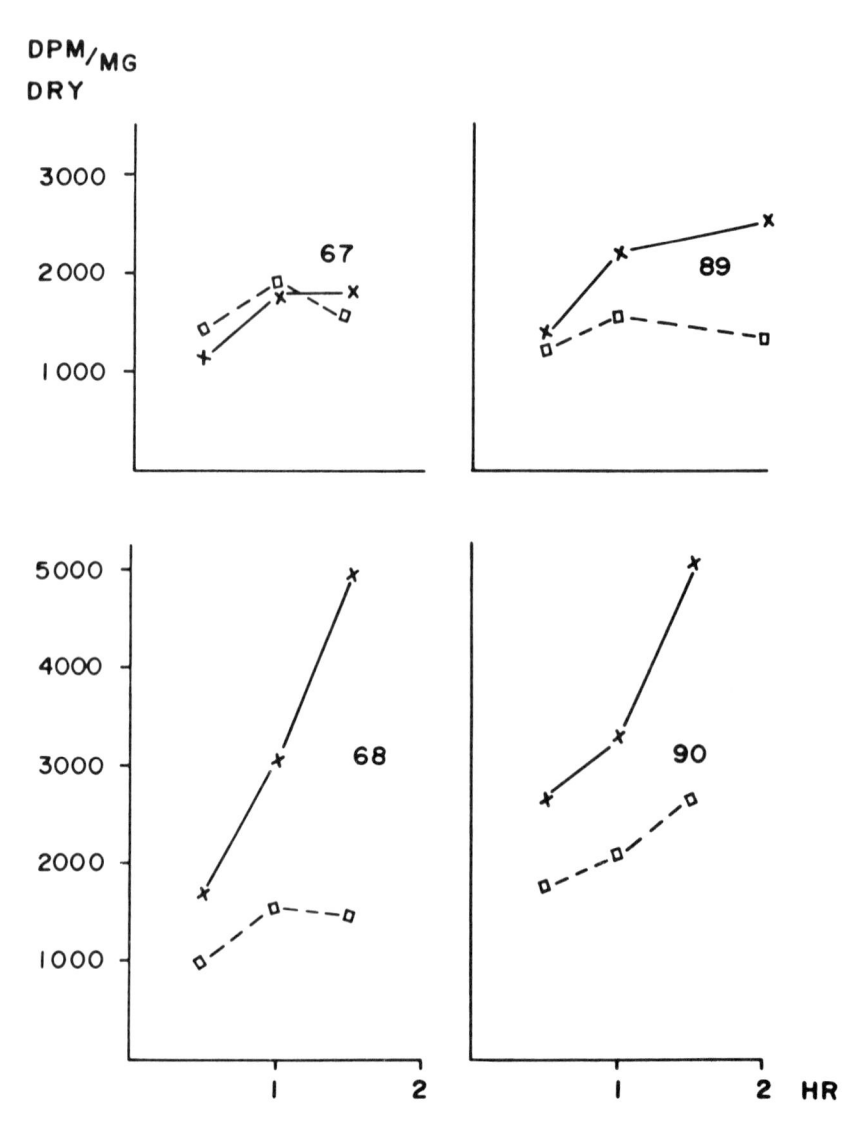

Fig. 18. Three positive and one negative uptake patterns for slices of primary tumors from patients also with metastases.

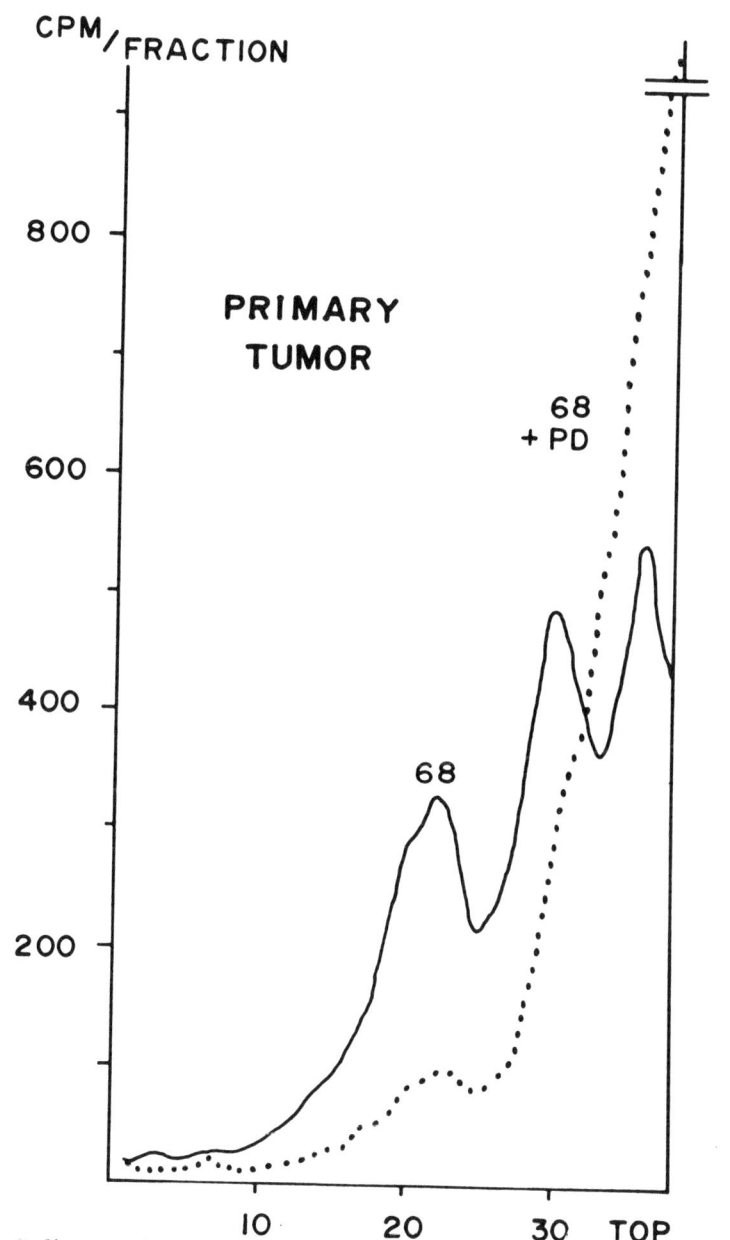

Fig. 19. Sedimentation pattern of cytosol from primary tumor, described in fig. 18, using 2nM E-2* in presence and absence of 0.2 μM PD CI-628. Centrifugation 7.5 hr at 308,000 g in 5–20% sucrose.

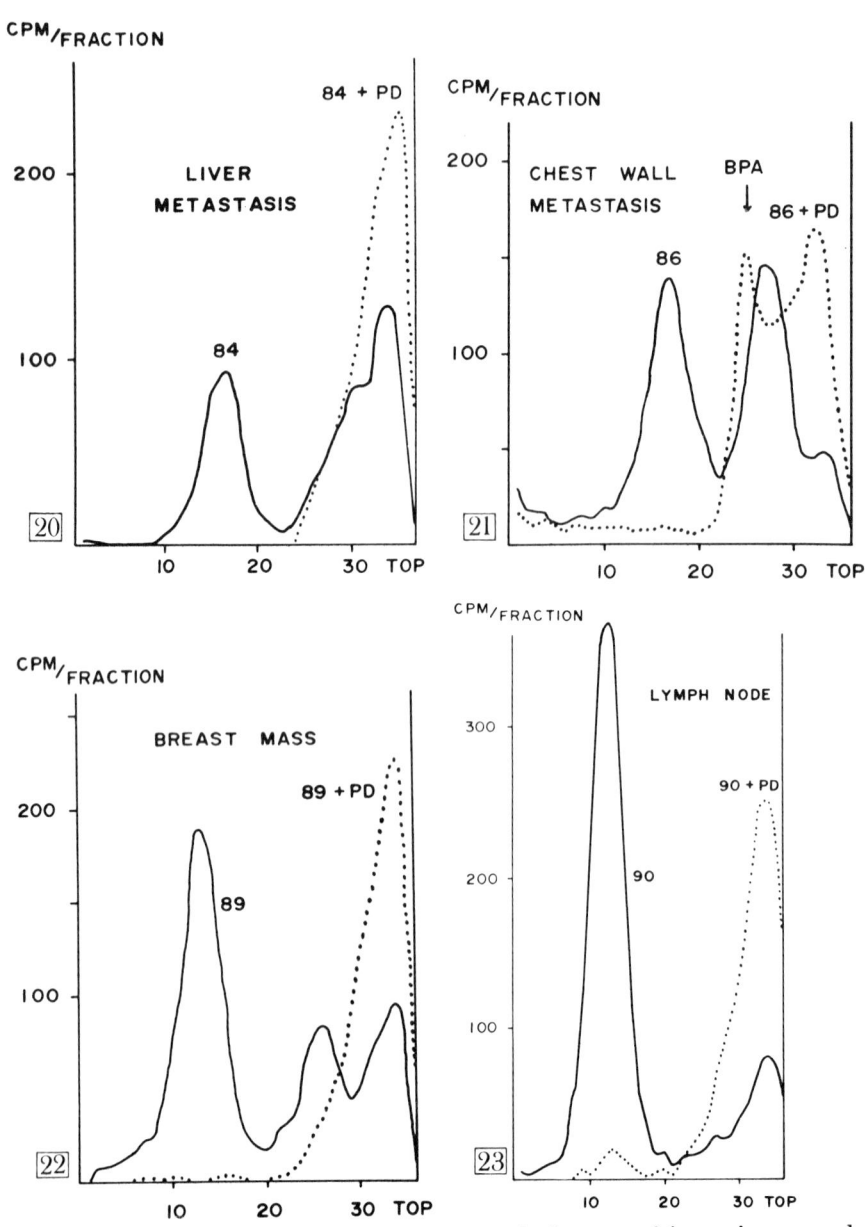

Fig. 20–23. Sedimentation patterns of cytosols from positive primary and metastatic tumors using 0.5 nM E-2* and 0.2 μM PD CI-628. Centrifugation: #84, 12 hr at 308,000 g; #86 and #90, 12 hr at 300,000 g; #89, 13 hr at 300,000 g, in 10–30% sucrose.

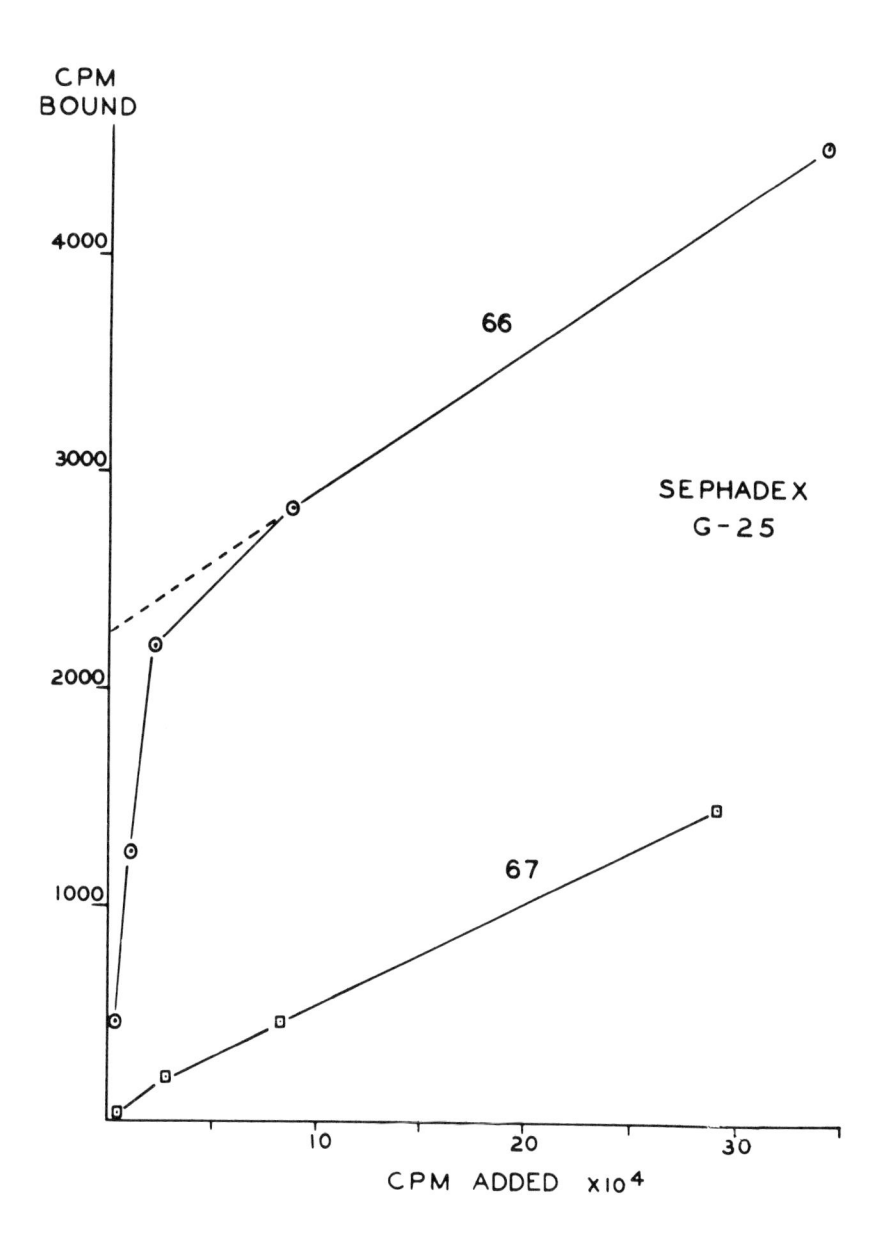

Fig. 24. Estradiol-binding curves of diluted cytosols from two primary breast cancers. #66 shows a combination of specific and nonspecific association; #67 shows only nonspecific binding.

containing receptor (#66), which shows a biphasic curve consisting of a strong, saturable specific binding superimposed on a weaker nonspecific binding, which continues to increase as more hormone is added. Although this technique is a simple means of estimating estradiol binding and of distinguishing specific from nonspecific interaction, on a routine basis it did not prove as reliable and unambiguous as the sucrose gradient sedimentation procedure.

TABLE 1: SUMMARY OF ALL PATIENTS STUDIED

Mastectomy[a,b] (N=51)	Endocrine Therapy (N=33)	
	Pattern	Response
25−	19−	17 Failure
		1 Remission
		1 Surgical casualty[c]
24+	11+	2 Failure
		5 Remission
		4 Surgical casualty
2±	3±	2 Failure
		1 Surgical casualty

[a] In addition to these 51 primary malignancies, one benign breast tumor was found to show a negative pattern, as did one cancer of the male breast.

[b] One mastectomy patient showing a positive pattern underwent prophylactic adrenalectomy 6 wk later.

[c] Surgical casualty signifies that the patient, usually debilitated and in carcinomatosis, did not survive the immediate postoperative period and so the response could not be evaluated.

CLINICAL CORRELATIONS

As table 1 shows, the 51 mastectomy patients studied were divided equally between positive and negative patterns, with two borderline cases. Recurrent disease subsequently was observed in 5 individuals, 1 of whom was subjected to adrenalectomy and failed to respond. This patient's primary tumor had shown a negative pattern in the laboratory test. If tumor recurs in others of this group, especially those with positive patterns, we hope that some of them will undergo endocrine treatment so that their responses can be correlated with their tumor patterns.

Studies have been carried out on 33 patients undergoing endocrine therapy for advanced breast cancer (tables 1 and 2). Of these, 28 had adrenalectomy (7 with accompanying oophorectomy and one with

TABLE 2: RESULTS OF ENDOCRINE THERAPY

Type of Therapy	Remission	Failure	Surgical Casualty
Adrenalectomy[a,b] (N=28)			
+	4	2	4
−	1	13	1
±		2	1
Hypophysectomy (N=3)			
+	1		
−		2	
Radiation Castration (N=1)			
−		1	
Testosterone (N=1)			
−		1	

[a] Of patients undergoing adrenalectomy, 5 with negative patterns and 2 with positive patterns had accompanying (or in 1 case prior) oophorectomy, and another with negative pattern had radiation castration.

[b] In 6 of these adrenalectomy patients, the primary tumor was still present and was used for the study. Of these, 2 positive patterns were associated with remissions, whereas 3 negative patterns and 1 borderline pattern were associated with failure.

subsequent hypophysectomy), 3 had hypophysectomy, 1 had radiation castration, and 1 received depotestosterone. Negative patterns were shown by 19 patients, of whom 17 failed to respond; 1 patient died in the immediate postoperative course, and 1 experienced remission. Of 12 patients showing positive patterns, 5 experienced significant remissions, 2 failed to respond, and 4 died in the immediate postoperative period from overwhelming carcinomatosis. Of 3 patients with borderline patterns, 1 died in the postoperative period and 2 did not show objective remission, although 1 of these did show a subjective remission, living for 18 months despite evidence of progressing disease.

On the basis of the 27 cases which could be evaluated, only 1 of 20 patients whose cancers showed no distinct evidence for the presence of estrogen receptor experienced remission after endocrine therapy. In contrast, 5 of 7 patients with receptor-containing tumors showed objective remission after treatment. Thus it appears that patients whose breast cancers lack the estrogen receptor substance have little chance of responding to endocrine therapy, whereas some, but not all, of those who possess estrogen-binding proteins will benefit from such treatment. The failure of some patients with positive patterns to respond is understandable if one considers that it is possible to have a mixed population of positive and negative metastases. In such cases the pattern observed may be either positive or negative, depending on which metastasis is obtained for study, but the patient will be a failure because the negative metastases will be unresponsive.

The existence of some "false positives" does not represent a serious problem, because in the absence of any selective criterion these patients would undergo treatment. It is important that there be no significant number of "false negatives," because it is on the basis of a negative test that a decision would be made not to carry out treatment. So far, the correlation between lack of receptors and lack of response has been good, and one can hope that this relation will continue to hold as a substantial number of cases are accumulated.

ADDENDUM

Since the original presentation of this report, additional patients have been included in the study. Of a total of 84 primary tumors investigated, 39 showed the presence of estrogen receptor, 38 were negative, and 7 were borderline. The median age of patients with positive primary tumors was 64 (range 34–83) and with negative tumors 52 (range 32–86). Of 40 metastatic tumors examined, 12 were positive, 25 negative, and 2 borderline, and 1 patient with multiple metastases showed both positive and negative specimens.

Of 58 patients with metastatic disease studied, 42 received some type of endocrine therapy under conditions permitting evaluation of clinical response. Table 3 summarizes results demonstrating the correlation of receptor presence with clinical response to endocrine therapy.

TABLE 3: CORRELATION OF RECEPTOR PRESENCE WITH CLINICAL RESPONSE TO ENDOCRINE THERAPY

Receptor Test		Positive		Borderline		Negative	
Therapy[a]	Specimen Examined	R	F	R	F	R	F
Adrenalectomy[b]	Primary	3		2			4
	Metastasis	3	3[c]		1	1	11
Hypophysectomy	Primary						2
	Metastasis	1					3
Oophorectomy[d]	Primary	1					
	Metastasis						4
Androgen	Primary						1
	Metastasis	1					
Estrogen plus progestin	Primary	1					
Total		10	3	0	3	1	25

NOTE: R = objective remission; F = failure.

[a] With one positive, one borderline, and three negative adrenalectomy patients, as well as one negative hypophysectomy and one negative androgen therapy, treatment was carried out 4 to 12 mo after the tumor specimen was examined. With one borderline adrenalectomy, one negative hypophysectomy, and two negative oophorectomy-plus-androgen patients, the tumor specimen was examined 4 to 12 mo after unsuccessful therapy was instituted.

[b] Three positive, two borderline, and seven negative adrenalectomy patients had accompanying oophorectomy or, in one case, radiation castration.

[c] One of these "false-positive" patients had experienced remission after oophorectomy 6 mo earlier and showed subjective but not objective remission to adrenalectomy. Another had remission to oophorectomy 19 mo earlier.

[d] One positive and three negative oophorectomy patients also received androgen.

Acknowledgments

The authors gratefully acknowledge the technical assistance of Marsha Gage, Suzie Adler, and Lois Kahn and the cooperation of Drs. Donald Ferguson, Paul Harper, Hilger Jenkins, René Menguy, Edward Paloyan, and John Prohaska of the University of Chicago Clinics and Dr. Frances Knock of Augustana Hospital in supplying some of the clinical specimens. The human tumor studies were supported by United States Public Health Service contract PH 43-66-945 from the National Cancer Institute, and the rat uterus investigation was supported by United States Public Health Service grant CA-02897 from the National Cancer Institute, grant P-422 from the American Cancer Society, and grant 690-0109 from the Ford Foundation.

References

1. Hechter, O., and Halkerston, I. D. K. 1964. On the action of mammalian hormones. In *The hormones,* ed. G. Pincus, K. V. Thimann, and E. B. Astwood, 5: 697. New York: Academic Press.
2. Jensen, E. V.; Jacobson, H. I.; Flesher, J.; Saha, N. N.; Gupta, G.; Smith, S.; Colucci, V.; Shiplacoff, D.; Neumann, H. G.; DeSombre, E. R.; and Jungblut, P. W. 1966. Estrogen receptors in target tissues. In *Steroid dynamics,* ed. G. Pincus, T. Nakao, and J. F. Tait, p. 133. New York: Academic Press.
3. Jensen, E. V.; DeSombre, E. R.; Hurst, D. J.; Kawashima, T.; and Jungblut, P. W. 1967. Estrogen-receptor interactions in target tissues. *Arch. Anat. Microscop. Morphol. Exp.* 56 (suppl.): 547.
4. Jensen, E. V.; Numata, M.; Brecher, P. I.; and DeSombre, E. R. 1971. Hormone-receptor interaction as a guide to biochemical mechanism. In *The biochemistry of steroid hormone action,* ed. R. M. S. Smellie. p. 133. London: Academic Press.
5. Jensen, E. V.; Suzuki, T.; Kawashima, T.; Stumpf, W. E.; Jungblut, P. W.; and DeSombre, E. R. 1968. A two-step mechanism for the interaction of estradiol with rat uterus. *Proc. Nat. Acad. Sci. USA* 59: 632.
6. Gorski, J.; Toft, D.; Smith, D.; and Notides, A. 1968. Hormone receptors: Studies on the interaction of estrogen with the uterus. *Recent Progr. Hormone Res.* 24: 45.
7. Shyamala, G., and Gorski, J. 1969. Estrogen receptors in the rat uterus. *J. Biol. Chem.* 244: 1097.
8. Sander, S. 1968. The uptake of 17β-oestradiol in breast tissue of female rats. *Acta Endocr.* 58: 49.
9. Sander, S., and Attramadal, A. 1968. An autoradiographic study of oestradiol incorporation into the breast tissue of female rats. *Acta Endocr.* 58: 235.
10. Puca, G. A., and Bresciani, F. 1969. Interactions of 6, 7-^{3}H-17β-estradiol with mammary gland and other organs of the C3H mouse *in vivo. Endocrinology* 85: 1.
11. Deshpande, N.; Jensen, E. V.; Bulbrook, R. D.; Berne, T.; and Ellis, F. 1967. Accumulation of tritiated oestradiol by human breast tissue. *Steroids* 10: 219.
12. Huggins. C.; Grand, L. C.; and Brillantes, F. P. 1961. Mammary cancer induced by a single feeding of polynuclear hydrocarbons and its suppression. *Nature* 189: 204.

13. Huggins, C.; Grand, L.; and Fukunishi, R. 1964. Aromatic influences on the yields of mammary cancers following administration of 7, 12-dimethylbenz(a)anthracene. *Proc. Nat. Acad. Sci. USA* 51: 737.
14. King, R. J. B.; Cowan, D. M.; and Inman, D. R. 1965. The uptake of [6, 7-^{3}H] oestradiol by dimethylbenzanthracene-induced rat mammary tumours. *J. Endocr.* 32: 83.
15. King, R. J. B.; Gordon, J.; Cowan, D. M.; and Inman, D. R. 1966. The intranuclear localization of [6, 7-^{3}H]-oestradiol-17β in dimethylbenzanthracene-induced rat mammary adenocarcinoma and other tissues. *J. Endocr.* 36: 139.
16. Mobbs, B. G. 1966. The uptake of tritiated oestradiol by dimethylbenzanthracene-induced mammary tumors of the rat. *J. Endocr.* 36: 409.
17. ———. 1968. The uptake of simultaneously administered ^{3}H-oestradiol and ^{14}C-progesterone by dimethylbenzanthracene-induced rat mammary tumours. *J. Endocr.* 41: 339.
18. Jungblut, P. W.; DeSombre, E. R.; and Jensen, E. V. 1967. Estrogen receptors in induced rat mammary tumor. In *Hormone in Genese und Therapie des Mammacarcinoms,* ed. H. Gummel, H. Kraatz, and G. Bacigalupo, p. 109. Berlin: Akademie-Verlag.
19. Jensen, E. V.; DeSombre, E. R.; and Jungblut, P. W. 1967. Estrogen receptors in hormone-responsive tissues and tumors. In *Endogenous factors influencing host-tumor balance,* ed. R. W. Wissler, T. L. Dao, and S. Wood, Jr., pp. 15, 68. Chicago: University of Chicago Press.
20. Kyser, K. A. 1970. The tissue, subcellular and molecular binding of estradiol to dimethylbenzanthracene-induced rat mammary tumor. Ph.D. diss., University of Chicago, Dept. of Physiology.
21. Sander, S. 1969. The *in vitro* uptake of oestradiol in DMBA-induced breast tumours of the rat. *Acta Path. Microbiol. Scand.* 75: 520.
22. Huggins, C., and Bergenstal, D. M. 1952. Inhibition of human mammary and prostatic cancer by adrenalectomy. *Cancer Res.* 12: 134.
23. Folca, P. J.; Glascock, R. F.; and Irvine, W. T. 1961. Studies with tritium labeled hexoestrol in advanced breast cancer. *Lancet* 2: 796.
24. Puca, G. A., and Bresciani, F. 1968. Receptor molecule for oestrogens from rat uterus. *Nature (Lond.)* 218: 967.
25. Steggles, A. W., and King, R. J. B. 1969. Sedimentation studies on oestrogen receptors. *Acta Endocr.*, suppl. 138: 36.
26. Wyss, R. H.; Heinrichs, W. L.; and Hermann, W. L. 1968. Some species differences of uterine estradiol receptors. *J. Clin. Endocr. Metab.* 28: 1227.

Stanley G. Korenman

Human Breast Cancer as a Steroid Hormone Target 3

INTRODUCTION

While studying the mechanisms of estrogen action on target tissues, Jensen and Jacobson (1) showed that administered tritiated 17β-estradiol ($E_2{}^3H$) accumulated in the uterus, vagina, and pituitary of the rat and was retained in these organs long after the plasma was cleared of hormone. The retained ^3H persisted as E_2 in the rat uterus. It has been shown subsequently that the hormone was bound to specific protein components of the high-speed ultracentrifugal supernatant fluid (cytosol) and of the nuclear pellet of the uterus (2). Although the relationship between cytoplasmic and nuclear binders has not yet been established, evidence has accumulated that the estrogen moves from cytoplasm to nucleus over time at 37° C (3, 4). The chemical characteristics of the binding moieties and their role in the series of events culminating in growth and differentiation of the uterus have not been fully agreed upon (5, 7). There is some evidence that the estrogen-binder complex in the nucleus stimulates transcription (8). The physiological importance of binding is further supported by data showing that high levels of active steroid accumulation are found predominantly in target tissues (1, 9) and by binding studies of various estrogenic and nonestrogenic substances for rabbit uterine cytosol (10). Only estrogens bind to a significant degree, and the relative activity as binders of various estrogens was, in general, parallel to their uterotropic activity. Furthermore, a group of putative estrogen

The author is affiliated with the Department of Medicine, College of Medicine, at the University of Iowa.

inhibitors have been shown to compete for binding sites in rabbit and human uterine cytosol (11) in relation to their potency.

On the basis of tritiated estrogen accumulation and retention data, rat, goat, and sheep mammary glands were shown to be estrogen targets (12, 13). The estrogen-dependent dimethylbenz(a)anthracene-induced rat mammary carcinoma was also shown to bind estrogens, and a relation between extent of binding and response to oophorectomy apparently has been established (14-17).

There have been a number of studies of estrogen accumulation by human mammary carcinoma and other tissues after intravenous injection (18-22). Each reported an increment in recovered counts in the tumor compared with blood or other tissues. I doubt that these studies are physiologically important, because an amount of estrogen far greater than the entire circulating pool was injected and specificity of the uptake process was not studied. But there has been a report (18) of an impressive correlation between tumor uptake and response to adrenalectomy as well as a study characterizing breast tumor slices for high and low uptake of $E_2{}^3H$ (23).

The importance of appropriate specificity studies cannot be overestimated. The concept of a target organ receptor implies a limited number of extremely selective binding sites, preferably with a high affinity for the appropriate hormone, its active congeners, and its competitive inhibitors.

This chapter extends a previous report (24) on the steroid binding properties of human breast carcinomas.

Methods

Cytosol was prepared by high-speed centrifugation of homogenates as previously described (24). I determined the presence or absence of steroid binding activity and quantified the relative binding activity of other substances in comparison with $E_2{}^3H$ by incubating to equilibrium and by using activated charcoal to separate bound from free $E_2{}^3H$ (24, 25). To compare binding activities I employed a precise mathematical estimate of the ratio of association constants (RAC) based on relative binding activity (RA) (11) as follows:

We assume that formation of the hormone-binder complex is second order and its dissociation is first order. To determine K_p, the equilibrium constant of association of a single ligand P to a single type of binding site Q, where (PQ) is the concentration of ligand-binder complex, I employed the formulation of Ekins (25).

(1) $\quad K = \dfrac{(PQ)}{(P)(Q)}$

Let $R = \dfrac{(P)}{(PQ)}$

p = the initial concentration of unradioactive ligand
p^* = the initial concentration of radioactive ligand
q = the concentration of binding sites.

Then:

(2) $\quad R^2 + R\left(1 - \dfrac{p + p^*}{q} - \dfrac{1}{K_p q}\right) - \dfrac{1}{K_p q} = 0$ (equation 8 of Ekins).

Since q can be estimated by a saturation curve, K_p can be calculated directly.

When a substance H is allowed to compete with p^* for q binding sites, K_h may be calculated if K_p is known.

Let h = the initial concentration of competing substance required to bring R to the same point used for K_p estimation.

(3) $\quad R^2 + R\left(1 - \dfrac{p^*}{q} - \dfrac{1}{K_p q}\right) - \dfrac{1}{K_p q} - \dfrac{h/q(R + 1)R}{K_p/K_h(R + 1)} = 0$ (equation 30 of Ekins).

Then subtracting 2 from 3:

$$p\left(\dfrac{p}{q}\right) = \dfrac{h/q(R + 1)R}{(K_p/K_h)R + 1}.$$

Rearranging and eliminating:

(4a) $\quad p/h = \dfrac{R + 1}{(K_p/K_h)R + 1}\quad$ or $\quad$ (4b) $\quad \dfrac{K_h}{K_p} = \dfrac{R(p/h)}{R + 1 - p/h} = RAC$.

If K is calculated at the R value used for RA estimation, then $p/h = RA$ and the relation between the RA and RAC may be calculated directly.

(5) If $k_h \ll K_p$, $\quad RAC \simeq \dfrac{R}{R + 1} RA$.

Equations 4a and 4b are general; the results are dependent upon a number of assumptions.

1. Equilibrium has been attained. I have tested a variety of times of binding at 4° C, and equilibrium is achieved by 5 hr.

2. The method of separating bound and free is complete and does not interfere with the equilibrium. I have shown that over a wide range of times the amount of hormone bound to charcoal changes very slowly, so that influence on this equilibrium is small. Tests in the absence of cytosol have shown that the counts remaining unbound are 2% or less of those added, whether in the presence or absence of large amounts of unlabeled estrogen or inhibitor.

3. The substances tested are all pure and properly identified.

4. There is only one type of binding site.

Scatchard plots of binding of a group of breast cancer cytosols indicated that there was a single type of binding site permitting calculation of the equilibrium constants of association K_p for tumor cytosols with E_2 for the RAC; neither K need be shown.

TABLE 1: CLINICAL STATUS

				Status	
Activity	Number	Age Range	Died	Recurrence	NED[a]
+	6	55–83	1	2	3
±	3	51–67	1		2
−	13	37–82	1	3	9

[a] No evidence of disease.

RESULTS AND DISCUSSION

Thus far 22 breast neoplasms have been evaluated—20 primaries and 2 specimens of metastatic lesions. Pertinent clinical data are presented in table 1. Six tumors had clear-cut substantial specific estrogen binding activity. Of these 1 patient died before endocrine manipulation and 2 patients are being considered for ablative procedures. There were 3 cases with specific estrogen binding activity at low concentration. One patient died after response to a course of 5-fluorouracil. Of the 13 patients with inactive tumors one premenopausal woman died after failing to respond to oophorectomy. Three of the inactive tumors had nonspecific binding activity as previously described (24).

No specimen of mammary gland or mammary adipose tissue had E_2 binding activity.

The *RAC* values available for the 6 active tumors are presented in table 2. Severe limitations of material in some cases made it impossible to carry out a complete battery of tests. Dimethylstilbestrol, Erythro MEA cis-clomiphene and Parke-Davis CI-628 are estrogen "inhibitors." In general the binding proteins showed comparable *RAC* values for each substance. These values differed little from those presented previously for rabbit and human uterus (11). The important possibility of molecular heterogeneity of estrogen binding proteins which could be evaluated by examination of *RAC*s is not supported by these data.

TABLE 2: EFFECT OF ESTROGEN "INHIBITORS" ON RAC VALUES IN SIX ACTIVE TUMORS

Estrogen "Inhibitors"	RAC						
	R. L.	F. V.	M. G.	M. L.	H. C.	H. M.
Estrone	0.085			0.21		0.06
Estriol	0.043	0.13		0.074	0.051	
Epiestriol	0.15	0.30				
17α-Estradiol	0.035	0.12	0.14	0.094	0.07	<0.04
Dimethylstilbestrol	0.041	0.17	0.094		0.089	
Erythro-MEA	0.36			0.37	0.31	
Cis-clomiphene	0.001	0.004	0.007	0.002	0.001	0.002
CI-628	<0.0006	0.008	0.004	0.002	0.003	0.004

Testosterone, cortisol, and progesterone did not compete for E_2 binding sites; 5α-dihydrotestosterone (DHT) in high concentration had an *RAC* of about 0.0003.

Employing the E_2 binding curves I obtained linear scatchard plots, from which the concentration of binding sites per mg cytosol and a value for K_{E_2} were determined as shown in table 3. These data, giving a mean value for several rabbit uterine preparations and individual determinations for the others, show substantial heterogeneity and suggest significant individual variation. However, the uterine binding protein is very sensitive to temperature and ion concentration and these differences may simply reflect variability in the endogenous concentration of these or other important factors. The tumor of R. L., however, had the most efficient binder I have seen.

I have previously shown that one patient's tumor had a high concentration of relatively unsaturable estrogen binding sites (24). Two other such tumor cytosols have been found, which prompted me to examine a group of tumor cytosols for binding sites for other tritiated steroids, using the same approach I employed in estrogen binding studies.

Table 4 shows the amounts of triated E_2, progesterone, dihydrotestosterone (DHT), and testosterone bound by 5 tumor cytosols. Progesterone is bound very poorly, suggesting that little CBG[1] was

TABLE 3: PARAMETERS OF CYTOSOL BINDING

Breast Tumor	Binding Sites (M/mg protein $\times 10^{14}$)	K_{E_2}
R. L.	36	8×10^{10}
F. V.	17	3×10^{10}
M. G.	14	6×10^{9}
M. L.	9	5×10^{9}
H. C.	8	8×10^{9}
Human uterus	14	2×10^{9}
Rabbit uterus		3×10^{10}

TABLE 4: AMOUNTS OF HORMONES BOUND BY TUMOR CYTOSOLS

| E_2 Binding | Volume (μl) | Moles Bound $\times 10^{14}$ | | | | |
		E_2	Progesterone	DHT[a]	Testosterone	DHT/Testosterone
NS[b]	200	3.1	0.4	5.2	1.6	3.2
S[b]	200	3.6	0.5	2.9	1.1	2.6
S	50	9.2	1.0	4.6	1.8	2.5
—	200	0.7	0.9	8.0	2.8	2.8
NS	200	1.6	0.3	5.8	2.2	2.6

NOTE: Aliquots of cytosol were incubated at 0° for 16 hr with equimolar concentrations of tritiated steroid except for progesterone, where 1.6 $\times$ the concentration was used. Bound and free steroid were separated by incubation for 15 min at 0° C with activated charcoal and centrifugation.

[a] DHT = 5α-dihydrotestosterone.

[b] NS = nonspecific binding; S = specific binding.

[1] Cortisol binding globulin.

present in the cytosol fractions. Of great interest is the rather substantial binding of DHT. We know that DHT, progesterone, and testosterone were not competing for E_2 binding sites, and so another receptor protein must be present. Binding of testosterone at about 40% the concentration of DHT suggested that the sex hormone binding globulin of plasma might be involved, but the absence of significant binding of progesterone to CBG suggested that this may not be so. Because DHT is important as the intracellular androgenic effector (27–29), further study of this binding phenomenon is in order.

Current views concerning mechanisms of steroid hormone action for both androgens and estrogens emphasize the presence of specific binding proteins in high concentration in target tissues. If mammary gland and mammary tumor are estrogen and androgen targets, one might anticipate the presence of specific receptors. I hope that when the fundamental question about the biochemical role of binding in initiating hormonal responses is resolved I can rationalize my expectation that determining the presence or absence of *specific* binding proteins will allow us to predict therapeutic response in breast cancer.

Acknowledgments

This work was supported by grants from the American Cancer Society (grant #P456) and the California Cancer Research Coordinating Committee.

References

1. Jensen, E. V., and Jacobson, H. I. 1960. Fate of steroid estrogens in target tissues. In *Biological activities of steroids in relationship to cancer,* ed. G. Pincus and E. P. Vollmer, p. 161. New York: Academic Press.
2. Notebroom, W. D., and Gorski, J. 1965. Stereospecific binding of estrogens in the rat uterus. *Arch. Biochem. Biophys.* 111: 559.
3. Jensen, E. V.; Suzuki, T., Kawashima, T.; Stumpf, W. E.; Jungblut, P. W.; and DeSombre, E. R. 1968. A two-step mechanism for the interaction of estradiol with rat uterus. *Proc. Nat. Acad. Sci. USA* 59: 632.
4. Shyamala, G., and Gorski, J. 1969. Estrogen receptors in the rat uterus. *J. Biol. Chem.* 244: 1097.
5. Korenman, S. G., and Rao, B. R. 1968. Reversible disaggregation of

the cytosol-estrogen binding protein of uterine cytosol. *Proc. Nat. Acad. Sci. USA* 61: 1028.
6. Rochefort, H., and Baulieu, E. 1969. New *in vitro* studies of estradiol binding castrated rat uterus. *Endocrinology* 84: 108.
7. Jensen, E. V.; Suzuki, T.; Numata, M.; Smith, S.; and DeSombre, E. 1969. Estrogen-binding substance of target tissues. *Steroids* 13: 417.
8. Raynaud-Jammet, C., and Baulieu, E. E. 1969. Action de l'oestradiol *in vitro:* Augmentation de la biosynthèse d'acide ribonucléique dans les noyaux urtérins. *C. R. Acad. Sci. Paris, series D* 268:3211.
9. Stumpf, W. E. 1969. Nuclear concentration of ^{3}H-estradiol in target tissues: Dry-mount autoradiography of vagina, oviduct, ovary, testis, mammary tumor, liver and adrenal. *Endocrinology* 85: 31.
10. Korenman, S. G. 1969. Comparative binding affinity of estrogens and its relation to estrogenic potency. *Steroids* 13: 163.
11. ———. 1970. Relation between estrogen inhibitory activity and binding to cytosol of rabbit and human uterus. *Endocrinology* 87: 1119.
12. Glascock, R. F., and Hoekstra, W. G., 1959. Selective accumulation of tritium-labeled hexoestrol by the reproductive organs of immature female goats and sheep. *Biochem. J.* 72: 673.
13. Sander, S. 1968. The uptake of 17β-oestradiol in breast tissue of female rats. *Acta Endocr.* 58: 49.
14. King, R. J. B.; Cowan, D. M.; and Inman, D. 1965. The uptake of [6, 7-^{3}H] oestradiol by dimethylbenzanthracene-induced rat mammary tumors. *J. Endocr.* 32: 83.
15. Mobbs, B. G. 1966. The uptake of tritiated oestradiol by dimethylbenzanthracene induced mammary tumors of the rat. *J. Endocr.* 36: 409.
16. Jensen, E. V.; DeSombre, E. R.; and Jungblut, P. W. 1967. Estrogen receptors in hormone-responsive tissues and tumors. In *Endogenous factors influencing host-tumor balance,* ed. R. W. Wissler, T. L. Dao, and S. Wood, Jr., p. 15. Chicago: University of Chicago Press.
17. Sander, S., and Attramadal, A. 1968. The *in vivo* uptake of oestradiol 17β by hormone responsive and unresponsive breast tumors of the rat. *Acta Path. Microbiol. Scand.* 74: 169.
18. Folca, P. J.; Glascock, R. F.; and Irvine, W. T. 1961. Studies with tritium labeled hexoestrol in advanced breast cancer. *Lancet* 2: 796.
19. Denetriou, J. A.; Crowley, L. G.; Kushinsky, S.; Donovan, A. J.; Kotin, P.; and MacDonald, I. 1964. Radioactive estrogens in tissues of postmenopausal women with breast neoplasms. *Cancer Res.* 24: 926.
20. Deshpande, N.; Jensen, V.; and Bulbrook, R. D. 1967. Accumulation of tritiated oestradiol by human breast tissue. *Steroids* 10: 219.
21. Pearlman, W. H.; DeHertogh, R.; Laumas, K. R.; and Pearlman, M. R. J. 1969. Metabolism and tissue uptake of estrogen in women with advanced carcinoma of the breast. *J. Clin. Endocr.* 29: 707.
22. Braunsberg, H.; Irvine, W. T.; and James, V. H. T. 1967. A com-

parison of steroid hormone concentrations in human tissues including breast cancer. *Brit. J. Cancer* 21: 714.
23. Sander, S. 1968. The *in vitro* uptake of oestradiol in biopsies from 25 breast cancer patients. *Acta Path. Microbiol. Scand.* 74: 301.
24. Korenman, S. G., and Dukes, B. A. 1970. Specific estrogen binding by the cytoplasm of human breast carcinoma. *J. Clin. Endocr.* 30: 639.
25. Korenman, S. G. 1968. Ratio-ligand binding assay of specific estrogens using a soluble uterine macromolecule. *J. Clin. Endocr.* 28: 127.
26. Ekins, R. P.; Newman, G. B.; and O'Riodan, J. L. H. 1968. In *Radioisotopes in medicine,* ed. L. H. Raymond, F. A. Goswitz, and B. E. P. Murphy, p. 59. *In Vitro* Studies, U.S. Atomic Energy Commission/Division of Technical Information Extension, Oak Ridge, Tennessee.
27. Bruchovsky, N., and Wilson, J. D. 1968. The conversion of testosterone to 5α-androstan-17β-ol-3-one by rat prostate *in vivo* and *in vitro*. *J. Biol. Chem.* 243: 2012.
28. ———. 1968. The intranuclear binding of testosterone and 5α-androstan-17β-ol-3-one by rat prostate. *J. Biol. Chem.* 243: 5953.
29. Fang, S.; Anderson, K. M.; and Liao, S. 1969. Receptor proteins for androgens. *J. Biol. Chem.* 244: 6584.

Roger W. Turkington

Hormonal Regulation of Histone Phosphorylation 4

There is increasing evidence that an early action of many hormones upon their target cells is represented by increased activity at the transcriptional level (1). The possibility that hormonal regulation of RNA synthesis and of gene expression may involve alterations in histones has led to a renewed interest in these nuclear proteins.

CHARACTERIZATION OF HISTONES

A major problem in determining the functional role of the histones has been the technical difficulty of obtaining purified proteins which could be characterized free from artifact. Earlier studies on the purification of histones demonstrated a marked heterogeneity, partly based upon the formation of association products between different classes of histones (2). The search for "minor components" which would demonstrate the requisite structural specificity for action as the repressors of specific genes led to the examination of histones under a variety of conditions in different laboratories and with various results. However, a major conclusion derived from a number of more critical analytical approaches is that the heterogeneity of the histones is very limited. Panyim and Chalkley (3, 4), for example, have quantitatively determined the number of electrophoretic species of calf histones and their relative concentrations in several tissues. This electrophoretic analysis of histones has demonstrated five classes of molecules composed of perhaps no more than twelve molecular species. However, the histones appear to be grouped into five

The author is affiliated with the Departments of Medicine, the University of Wisconsin Medical Center, Madison, Wisconsin.

major classes rather than twelve or more independent species, since each group of proteins behaves in a manner characteristically distinct from the others over a wide range of conditions for isolation and electrophoresis. In all mammalian cells studied so far, the F2b fraction appears to be present in the greatest amount and is homogeneous and without electrophoretic variation among species. The band of lowest electrophoretic mobility in the lysine-rich (F1) histones has been found only in calf tissues characterized by a high rate of cell division, whereas the fastest-moving band in this class is characteristically present in calf tissues with a low rate of cell division (4). Cells that are rapidly dividing appear to contain increased amounts of the acetylated form of the F2a1 histone, whereas very slowly dividing cells have a predominance of the unacetylated form of the molecule (4). Recently, a new, very lysine-rich histone which is present in small amounts in nonreplicating or intermittently replicating cells has been described (5). Cancer cells in general appear to retain the same complement of histones found in normal cells, although this recently demonstrated species of histone which is present in somatic, nonreplicating cells is not detectable in mammary carcinoma ascites cells (6). Smith, De Lange, and Bonner (7) have utilized ion-exchange chromatography to fractionate histones, and have demonstrated in several cases precisely eight species of histones. This group has also elucidated the entire amino acid sequence of the glycine-arginine-rich (GAR) calf histone, (8), thus demonstrating its homogeneity. That it differs from the GAR histone of pea seedling by only two amino acids strongly suggests that a vital function performed by this structure has preserved it essentially unchanged throughout phylogeny. The amino acid sequence of the GAR histone from Novikoff hepatoma has recently been determined by Starbuck et al (9). The sequence information has been used in molecular model building, which demonstrates that the basic residues of the histone pair perfectly with the negatively charged phosphate groups of the DNA helix. The histone is inserted into the large groove, and DNA in this model demonstrates a requirement for an amino acid sequence which permits little or no variation. Recently Bustin and Cole (10) demonstrated that the chromatographic fraction of rabbit thymus lysine-rich histone is molecularly homogeneous. The carboxy-terminal portion of the molecule is rich in lysine and proline residues, whereas the amino-terminal segment has a higher content of hydrophobic, and dicarboxylic residues capable of forming ionic bonds with DNA. The other end of the molecule may interact with other molecules and may be the site for addition of substituents.

Such substituent modification of the basic polypeptide sequence may partly explain the microheterogeneity encountered within major histone classes. For example, in the GAR histone the lysine 20 residue may be in the mono- or dimethyl form, lysine 16 residue may be in the acetylated or unacetylated form, and possible phosphorylation of serine or threonine residues could lead to a variety of forms of the single peptide.

PHOSPHORYLATION OF HISTONES

The reported estimates of the extent of phosphorylation of purified histone fractions vary according to the procedures for purification, the method of phosphorus incorporation used, and the various biological sources studied. Phosphorus-containing contaminants have been demonstrated to be bound to histones through a large number of purification steps, and phospholipids (11, 12), RNA (13, 14), DNA (15), mono- and oligonucleotides (16, 17), nonhistone nuclear phosphoproteins (18), and RNA-acidic protein and RNA-histone complexes (19, 20) have been identified among partially purified preparations of histones. Evaluation of the metabolic significance of histone phosphorylation has thus depended upon the development of powerful methods of resolution to eliminate any contribution from nonhistone contaminants.

There is now abundant and convincing evidence that histone polypeptides become phosphorylated. Ord and Stocken (21, 22) have demonstrated the incorporation of (^{32}P) phosphate into rat liver histones, and Kleinsmith and his colleagues (23-26) have demonstrated similar incorporation into calf thymus histones. The presence of O-phosphoserine has been demonstrated in specific histone polypeptides as well as in highly purified histone fractions. Specific kinases which catalyze the phosphorylation of histones have been discovered in a wide range of species (27-29), lending further support to the concept that histones become phosphorylated. Langan (30) has demonstrated that the partially purified histone kinase from rat liver phosphorylates F1 histone in vitro with a high degree of specificity. The distribution of phosphate in tryptic peptides of the enzymatically phosphorylated F1 histone has been studied, and one major ^{32}P-phosphopeptide has been analyzed. Partial sequence analysis of the isolated peptide has shown a single ^{32}P-phosphoserine residue. This observation that the histone kinase acts upon a specific histone serine and not on many sites in a minor contaminant of the histone preparation is conclusive evidence for histone phosphorylation.

FUNCTIONAL SIGNIFICANCE OF HISTONE PHOSPHORYLATION

The function of the histones appears to relate to the repression of genetic activity (31) and to the primary coiling of the DNA which occurs in interphase and metaphase chromosomes (32). But these functions remain to be more fully elucidated, as does the function of histone phosphorylation. The idea that phosphorylation of the histones may alter their interaction with the DNA and thus alter its template activity for transcription is attractive, and a number of experiments have been designed in an attempt to correlate histone phosphorylation with gene activation. It seems likely that introducing a phosphate group with its high density of negative charge might alter the basic properties of the histone and perhaps modify the electrostatic forces between histones and DNA. Phosphorylation could also alter the interaction of the histones with nuclear acidic (nonbasic) chromosomal proteins and with possible repressor or activator molecules. The data presented by Langan (30) on the extent of phosphorylation of histones show that only one or two phosphate groups per molecule of F1 and F2b histone can be introduced by the histone kinase. Certainly such a low number would be expected from the limited number of serine and threonine residues available for phosphate esterification in the known histone amino acid compositions. However, the effect of a low extent of phosphorylation and a small change in net charge on the reactivity of the histone molecule cannot be predicted, and could represent a very significant alteration in its properties.

A possible physiological role of histone phosphorylation has been suggested by the experiments of Stevely and Stocken (33). These investigators increased the phosphorylation of histone F1 by enzymatic treatment in vitro. A 50% increase in the phosphorylation of this histone increased the priming ability of a DNA-histone F1 complex in the DNA-dependent RNA polymerase reaction. This increase in phosphorylation of histone F1 was also associated with an increased priming activity of the complex in the DNA polymerase reaction. This latter effect may be of less functional significance, since it has been demonstrated that the complexing of the basic histones with the DNA renders it incapable of being transcribed by RNA polymerase while permitting it to be replicated by the DNA polmerase (34). Although these results suggest that phosphorylation may modify the repressor activity of histones, this possible interpretation must be approached with caution. Many of the inhibitory effects of added histones upon RNA polymerase activity can be mimicked by other basic proteins and by synthetic polycations such as polylysine. Histones complicate the already complex enzymology of RNA-synthesizing systems, since nucleohistone aggregates tend to precipitate from aqueous solutions. Phosphorylation of histones in such a system may simply decrease the effect of histones to promote nucleohistone aggregation and a physical state of the DNA which is inaccessible to interaction with the polymerase enzyme.

An alternate interpretation of the functional significance of histone phosphorylation is that phosphorylation in itself is not sufficient to alter histone-DNA binding and to derepress the DNA. It is possible that phosphorylation of the histones modifies their molecular conformations and their interactions with DNA and with other nucleoproteins so that the phosphorylated histones can be removed from the nucleohistone complex. Phosphorylation of histones occurs concomitantly with an activation of the RNA synthesis which precedes the initiation of DNA synthesis in phytohemagglutinin-stimulated lymphocytes (23, 24), in regenerating liver (21, 22, 35), and in insulin-stimulated mammary epithelial cells in vitro (36). The phosphorylated histones may represent an intermediate stage in the "molecular remodeling" of the nucleohistone complex for the activation of previously repressed genes, the expression of which may be required for the replication of the DNA. The presence of phosphate near the N-terminal end of the histone (30) could serve as an initiation point for the subsequent unraveling of the histone from around the DNA helix. Phosphorylation of the histone component of the chromatin might thus serve as a requisite intermediate form with which cytoplasmic repressors or other factors (37) react to activate genes. A third possibility is that activation of the genome by various activator molecules might be associated with the exposure of serine and threonine residues which could serve as "passive" substrates for phosphokinases. Such an alteration could possibly be "repaired" by histone phosphatases (30). However, the existence of specific histone kinases activated by cyclic AMP suggests that histone phosphorylation is of greater significance than such an "accidental" process.

Hormonal Regulation of Histone Phosphorylation

The possible role of histone phosphorylation in regulating transcription has been investigated in some detail in several hormone-dependent systems. Following the early demonstration by Kleinsmith, Allfrey, and Mirsky (23, 24) that RNA synthesis is activated in lymphocytes by the exogenous agent phytohemagglutinin, Marushige, Ling, and Dixon (38) demonstrated that the gonadotrophin-dependent process of spermatogenesis in the trout is associated with phosphorylation of preformed histones and protamine polypeptides. All major histone fractions were found to be phosphorylated at the terminal stages of spermatogenesis.

The observations that the phosphorylation of histones is catalyzed by a specific, cyclic AMP-activated protein kinase in liver and that cyclic AMP acts as the mediator of many hormone responses in liver have led Langan (39, 40) to investigate the action of various hormones on liver histone phosphorylation. Administering glucagon to rats in doses that are effective in inducing specific hepatic enzymes caused a fifteen- to twenty-five-fold increase in the incorporation of $^{32}P_i$ into a specific serine residue of the liver F1 histone within 15 min. Administering insulin, which also induces specific enzymes in liver, caused a marked increase in the rate of hepatic histone phosphorylation. The primary site of glucagon action appears to be the hepatic enzyme adenyl cyclase (41-43). It has been proposed that activation of this enzyme generates increased amounts of intracellular cyclic AMP, which may activate histone kinases and thereby stimulate phosphorylation of histones. But it remains to be demonstrated that it is this chain of events which leads to increased histone phosphorylation. For example, information is lacking about whether the intracellular concentration of cyclic AMP in the unstimulated cell is sufficiently below the K_m of the histone kinase that a hormone-induced increase would lead to activation of the enzyme. Although the action of insulin administered to rats is associated with a stimulation of liver histone phosphorylation, it is clear that insulin does not act through the proposed chain of events. Insulin does not activate adenyl cyclase in liver. It also remains to be demonstrated that its effect on hepatic histone phosphorylation represents a direct interaction of the hormone with this cell. Hydrocortisone, which induces the synthesis of specific enzymes in liver by a mechanism which does not involve cyclic AMP (44), has no effect on the phosphorylation of F1 histone tryptic peptide in the livers of intact animals (30). However, Murthy, Pradhan, and Sreenivasan (45) have demonstrated increased rates of incorporation of $^{32}P_i$ into histone preparations from the livers of adrenalectomized rats after administration of hydrocortisone. Lysine-rich histone preparations were phosphorylated to a greater extent than the arginine-rich fractions. The increased rate of histone phosphorylation was accompanied by an increased rate of incorporation of $^{32}P_i$ into nuclear DNA-like RNA. These effects could not be explained by an increase in the intracellular pool of $^{32}P_i$ or an increase in the specific activity of liver ATP. Since hydrocortisone induces enzyme synthesis in the livers of intact and adrenalectomized animals by a mechanism which does not involve cyclic AMP, other mechanisms may exist for the hormonal regulation of histone phosphorylation.

In studies on a more precisely defined system, the mouse mammary gland in organ culture (46), the hormonal regulation of histone synthesis (47), and phosphorylation (36) have been considered together with the synthesis of other classes of macromolecules during specific periods of the cell cycle. In mouse midpregnancy mammary explants, insulin induces a rapid increase in the rate of synthesis of rapidly labeled (20-min labeling period with ^{3}H-uridine) nuclear RNA (48), as shown in figure 1. This RNA is predominantly preribosomal RNA, but the formation of high molecular weight, DNA-like RNA is also stimulated. Four-hour labeling periods have shown that increased amounts of 28S and 18S ribosomal RNA are consequently formed, and this increase is associated with increased activity of chromatin-associated and nucleolar RNA polymerase (49). Associated with these increases in transcriptive activity in the G_1 period is a marked increase in the rate of phosphorylation of histones and nonhistone nuclear phosphoproteins. Cytoplasmic protein synthesis subsequently increases (47). The phosphorylation of histone synthesis indicates that the markedly increased incorporation of $^{32}P_i$ into these proteins is not a consequence of an increased pool of histone substrate. As in numerous other cell types (50–52), histone synthesis in mammary epithelial cells is initiated at the beginning of the DNA-synthetic (S) period, and the synthesis of all histone fractions occurs concomitantly with replication of the DNA (47). The passage of the majority of the epithelial cells from G_1 into the S period (53) is associated with the induction of DNA polymerase (1, 54).

Figure 2 shows a polyacrylamide gel electrophoretogram of ^{32}P-histones labeled in organ cultures of mouse mammary gland with $^{32}P_i$. All the histone fractions except the F2a1 histones become phosphorylated, and insulin stimulates the rate of phosphorylation of each of these specific histones. In the experiment shown in figure 3, mammary explants were incubated with insulin and hydrocortisone for 72 hr before the addition of prolactin. Prolactin induced a further stimulation of RNA synthesis before specific milk proteins were formed by the epithelial cells, and this hormone also stimulated the rate of phosphorylation of specific histone fractions. The histones undergoing increased rates of phosphorylation were primarily the F2b

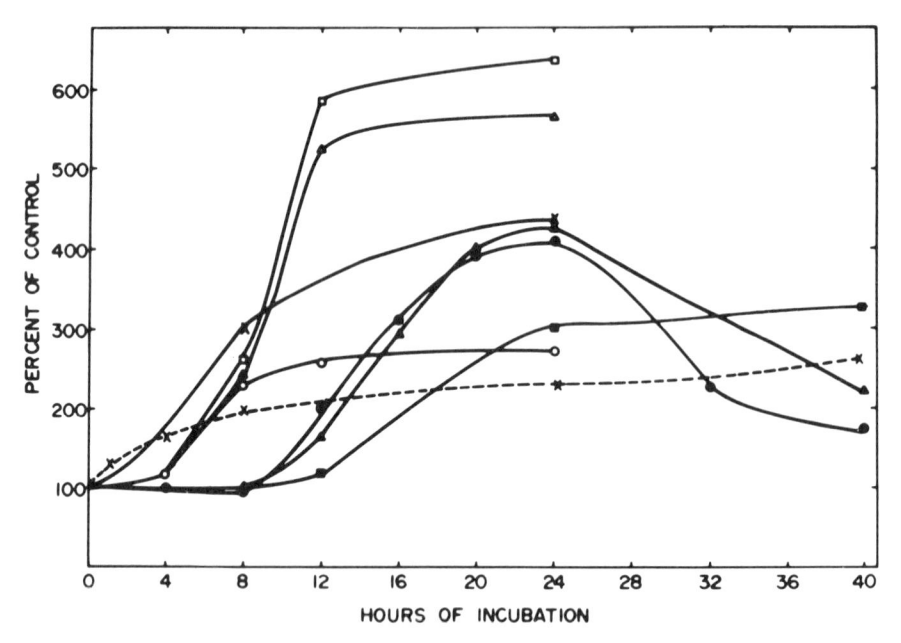

Fig. 1. Time course of macromolecular synthesis in mammary epithelial cells explanted onto synthetic medium containing insulin, 5 μg/ml. x-------x, rate of incorporation of ^{3}H-uridine into RNA during a 20-min labeling period. x————x, RNA polymerase activity. The rate of incorporation of $^{32}P_i$ into histones (□————□) or nonhistone nuclear proteins (△————△) or of ^{14}C-amino acids into cytoplasmic protein (○————○) is plotted as the amount of precursor incorporated during the preceding 4-hr labeling period. ●————●, DNA synthesis, as measured by the incorporation of ^{3}H-thymidine into DNA. ▲————▲, histone synthesis. ■————■, DNA polymerase activity.

and the F2a2 histones. Some minor components with low electrophoretic mobilities also appeared to contain increased amounts of ^{32}P. These proteins are not casein and are isolated in the histone fraction. Whether they are authentic histones has not been determined. Otherwise, the increased incorporation of ^{32}P into the histone polypeptides was not associated with a significant change in their relative electrophoretic mobilities. Experiments with inhibitors of protein synthesis demonstrated that the preformed histone polypeptides are phospho-

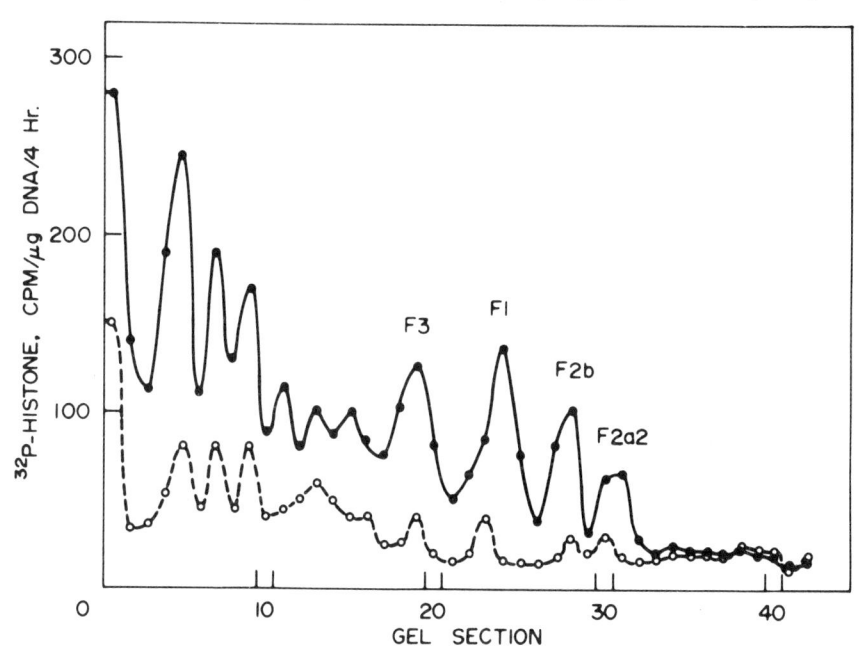

Fig. 2. Electrophoretogram radioactivity profile showing the effect of insulin on the rate of phosphorylation of specific histone fractions. Mammary gland explants were incubated in control (O-------O) or insulin-containing (●————●) medium for 20 hr, and were then exposed to medium containing ^{32}P$_i$ for 4 hr. (Reproduced from *J. Biol. Chem.* 244: 6040, 1969, by permission of the publishers)

rylated in these experiments, and "chase" studies failed to detect any exchange of phosphate groups on the phosphorylated histones during the experimental period. *O*-phosphoserine and *O*-phosphothreonine were the sole phosphorylated amino acids found in the phosphohistone products. Failure to observe changes in the electrophoretic mobilities of histones as a consequence of phosphorylation has also been reported (55) for histones phosphorylated enzymatically in vitro.

However, Sherod et al. (6) recently described conditions of urea concentration and pH under which an increase in the electrophoretic microheterogeneity of histones following phosphorylation has been demonstrated.

The studies on the hormonal activation of gene expression in mammary epithelial cells in vitro have provided a correlation between the phosphorylation of nuclear proteins and the activation of transcription. Although these two types of macromolecular formation appear to be closely associated temporally and in a variety of experimental circumstances, the observations made to date in this system merely offer an initial clue to the molecular mechanisms in which histone phosphorylation may be involved.

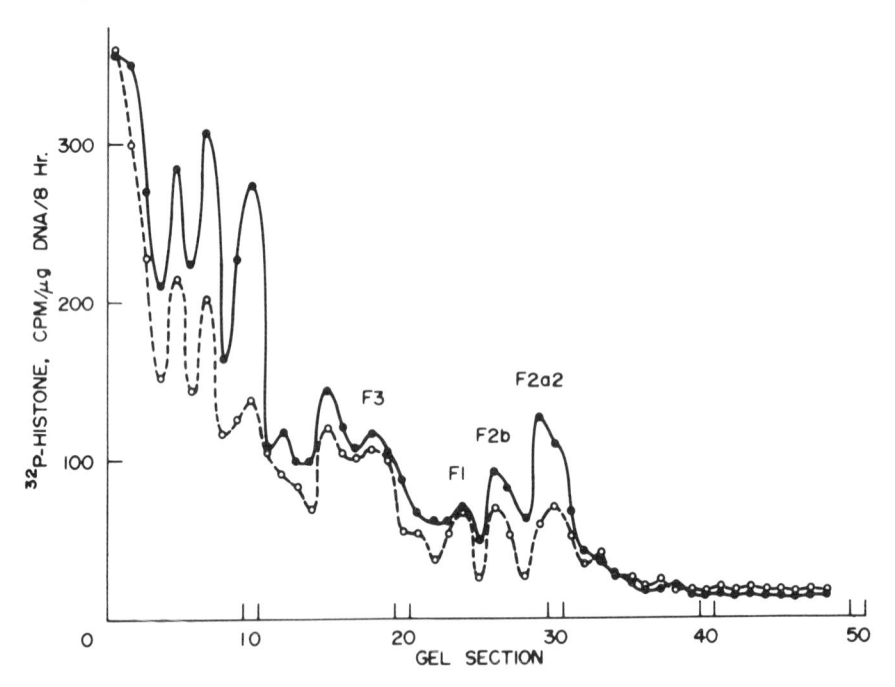

Fig. 3. Electrophoretogram radioactivity profile showing the effect of prolactin on the rate of phosphorylation of specific histone fractions. Mammary gland explants were incubated for 72 hr in medium containing insulin and hydrocortisone. Prolactin was then added to some dishes, and the incubation was continued for 16 hr before an 8-hr period of labeling with $^{32}P_i$. O-------O, insulin and hydrocortisone; ●———●, insulin, hydrocortisone, and prolactin. (Reproduced from *J. Biol. Chem.* 244: 6040, 1969, by permission of the publishers)

Phosphorylation of Nuclear Proteins in Mouse Mammary Cancer Cells

The possible association between gene transcription and histone phosphorylation in normal mammary cells cannot be extrapolated with certainty to mammary carcinoma cells, but certain preliminary experimental observations on mammary carcinoma cells suggest a possible relationship which may warrant investigation in the future. Studies on the nuclear, hybridizable, rapidly labeled RNA of normal and neoplastic mammary cells (56) have demonstrated the presence in the carcinoma cells of DNA-like RNA sequences which are not detectable in the nonneoplastic mammary cells. A typical experimental result using RNA-DNA hybridization-competition reactions to compare the RNA populations derived from normal and neoplastic cells is shown in figure 4. Although the extent of the competition in the homologous reaction (carcinoma nonisotopic RNA vs. carcinoma ^{3}H-RNA) approaches 95% of the theoretical value predicted for identical sequences competing with saturation-dependent kinetics, the RNA from the normal cells competes to only approximately 60% of this value. These studies could not detect the loss of any hybridizable RNA sequences from the carcinoma cell nuclei in comparison with the normal cells. These experimental results thus support the concept that a greater diversity of genes is being transcribed in the neoplastic cell. Comparisons of the rates of phosphorylation of nuclear proteins in the normal and neoplastic mammary cells also demonstrated a greater rate of phosphorylation of histones and nonhistone phosphoproteins in association with the formation of this greater diversity of nuclear RNA sequences in the carcinoma cells (table 1). The formation of a greater diversity of nuclear, hybridizable RNA sequences as a result of hormone-dependent mammary epithelial cell differentiation (57) is also associated with increased histone and nonhistone nuclear protein phosphorylation (fig. 3) (36). These results tentatively suggest that increased rates of histone phosphorylation reflect primarily a greater number of sites on the genome which are active or are being activated. A greater diversity of active genes has been demonstrated by RNA-DNA hybridization-competition criteria not only in mammary carcinoma cells, but also in hepatoma cells (58, 59) and in human chronic lymphocytic leukemia cells (60), suggesting that altered regulation of gene transcription may be a general property of malignant cells. Changes in the phosphorylation of histones may offer a clue to mechanisms which are important in the regulation of transcription. The possibility that defective regulation of transcription is a fundamental characteristic of the cancer cells makes this a vital area for future research.

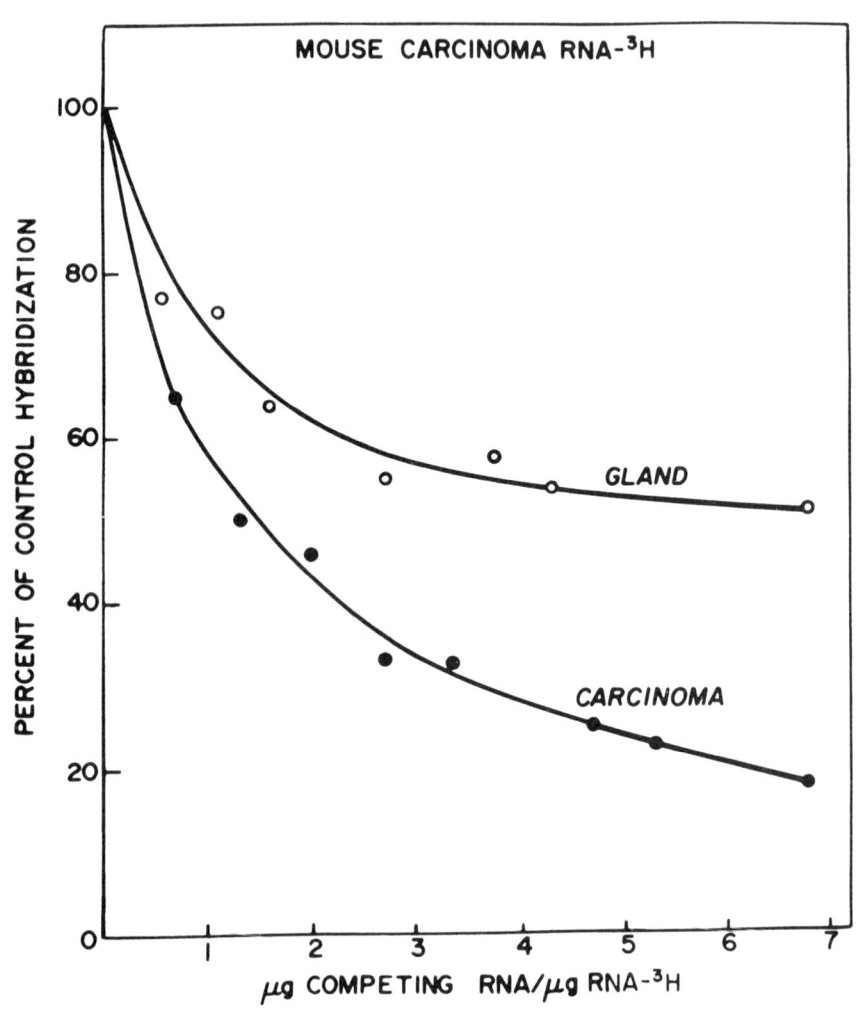

Fig. 4. Comparison of nuclear RNA populations by RNA-DNA hybridization-competition reactions. Increasing amounts of unlabeled nuclear RNA from mouse mammary gland (O———O) or mouse mammary carcinoma (●———●) were allowed to compete in the hybridization of mouse carcinoma ^{3}H-RNA with mouse DNA. The control hybridization was 1,258 counts per min. (Reproduced from *Cancer Res.* 30: 1833, 1970, by permission of the publishers)

TABLE 1: RATES OF PHOSPHORYLATION OF HISTONES AND NONHISTONE NUCLEAR PROTEINS AND HYBRIDIZATION-COMPETITION COMPARISONS OF NUCLEAR RNA IN NORMAL AND NEOPLASTIC MAMMARY CELLS OF THE C₃H MOUSE

Tissue	Nuclear ^{32}P-Protein (cpm/μg DNA) Histones	Nonhistone Protein	RNA-DNA Hybridization (% of theoretical competition with carcinoma ^{3}H-RNA)
Mammary gland	225	13,800	60
Mammary carcinoma	317	22,300	94

NOTE: Tissues from spontaneous mammary carcinoma or lactational mammary gland were explanted onto Medium 199 containing ^{32}P$_i$, 70 μC/ml, for 3 hr. Highly purified cell nuclei were then prepared, and the F1, F3, F2b, and F2a2 histones and the nonhistone nuclear proteins were isolated and counted as previously described (36). Nonisotopic nuclear RNA was isolated from separate tissue samples and was compared by hybridization-competition reactions. The percentages listed represent the extent to which each RNA population approached theoretical values for identical RNA populations in competing with carcinoma ^{3}H-RNA.

Acknowledgments

This work was supported in part by grant T-525 from the American Cancer Society.

References

1. Turkington, R. W. 1971. Hormonal regulation of cell proliferation and differentiation. In *Developmental aspects of the cell cycle*, ed. I. L. Cameron, G. M. Padilla, and A. M. Zimmerman, p. 315. New York: Academic Press.
2. Murray, K. 1966. The acid extraction of histones from calf thymus deoxyribonucleoprotein. *J. Molec. Biol.* 15: 409.
3. Panyim, S., and Chalkley, R. 1969. High resolution acrylamide gel electrophoresis of histones *Arch. Biochem. Biophys.* 130: 337.
4. ———. 1969. The heterogeneity of histones. I. A quantitative analysis of calf histones in very long polyacrylamide gels. *Biochemistry* 8: 3972.
5. ———. 1969. A new histone found only in mammalian tissue with little cell division. *Biochem. Biophys. Res. Commun.* 37: 1042.
6. Sherod, D.; Panyim, S.; Balhorn, R.; and Chalkley, R. 1970. A comparison of histones from tumor cells and normal somatic tissue. *Fed. Proc.* 29: 730A.
7. Smith, E. L.; DeLange, R. J.; and Bonner, J. 1970. Chemistry and biology of the histones. *Physiol. Rev.* 50: 159.

8. DeLange, R. J.; Fambrough, D. M.; Smith, E. L.; and Bonner, J. 1969. Calf and pea histone IV. *J. Biol. Chem.* 244: 5669.
9. Starbuck, W. C.; Taylor, C. W.; Wilson, K.; and Busch, H. 1970. Structural studies on the glycine-rich, arginine-rich (GAR) histone from Novikoff hepatoma. *Proceedings of the Tenth International Cancer Congress,* 442A.
10. Bustin, M., and Cole, R. D. 1970. Regions of high and low cationic charge in a lysine-rich histone. *J. Biol. Chem.* 245: 1458.
11. Cruft, H. J.; Mauritzen, C. M.; and Stedman, E. 1958. The isolation of β-histone from calf thymus thymocytes and the factors affecting its aggregation. *Proc. Roy. Soc. London,* ser. B 149: 21.
12. Hirschbein, L., and Rozencwajg, R. 1960. Action diisopropylphosphofluorure et du pH dans l'association et la dissociation des histones du placenta humain. *C. R. Acad. Sci. (Paris)* 251: 1309.
13. Huang, R. C., and Bonner, J. 1965. Histone bound RNA, a component of native nucleohistone. *Proc. Nat. Acad. Sci. USA* 54: 960.
14. Benjamin, W.; Levander, O. A.; Gellhorn, A.; and Debellis, R. H. 1966. An RNA-complex in mammalian cells: The isolation and characterization of a new RNA species. *Proc. Nat. Acad. Sci. USA* 55: 858.
15. Marks, D. B., and Schumaker, V. N. 1968. Some physical and chemical properties of trypsin-digested nucleoprotein. *Biochem. J.* 109: 625.
16. Ord, M. G., and Stocken, L. A. 1965. Histones from rat liver and thymus. *Biochem. J.* 98: 5P.
17. ———. 1967. Phosphate and thiol groups in histone F3 from rat liver and thymus nuclei. *Biochem. J.* 102: 631.
18. Benjamin, W., and Gellhorn, A. 1968. Acidic properties of mammalian nuclei: Isolation and characterization. *Proc. Nat. Acad. Sci. USA* 59: 262.
19. Huang, R. C., and Huang, P. C. 1969. Effect of protein-bound RNA associated with chick embryo chromatin on template specificity of the chromatin. *J. Molec. Biol.* 39: 365.
20. Shepherd, G. R.; Noland, B. J.; and Roberts, C. N. 1970. Phosphorus in histones. *Biochim. Biophys. Acta* 199: 265.
21. Ord, M. G., and Stocken, L. A. 1966. Metabolic properties of histones from rat liver and thymus gland. *Biochem. J.* 98: 888.
22. ———. 1968. Variations in the phosphate content and thiol disulphide ratio of histones during the cell cycle. *Biochem. J.* 107: 403.
23. Kleinsmith, L. J.; Allfrey, V. G.; and Mirsky, A. E. 1966. Phosphorylation of nuclear protein early in the course of gene activation in lymphocytes. *Science* 154: 780.
24. ———. 1966. Phosphoprotein metabolism in isolated lymphocyte nuclei. *Proc. Nat. Acad. Sci. USA* 55: 1182.
25. Kleinsmith, L. J., and Allfrey, V. G. 1969. Nuclear phosphoproteins. I. Isolation and characterization of a phosphoprotein fraction from calf thymus nuclei. *Biochim. Biophys. Acta* 175: 123.
26. ———. 1969. Nuclear phosphoproteins. II. Metabolism of exogenous phosphoprotein by intact nuclei. *Biochim. Biophys. Acta* 175: 136.

27. Kuo, J. F., and Greengard, P. 1969. Cyclic nucleotide-dependent protein kinase. IV. Widespread occurrence of adenosine 3', 5'-monophosphate-dependent protein kinase in various tissues and phyla of the animal kingdom. *Proc. Nat. Acad. Sci. USA* 64: 1349.
28. Miyamoto, E.; Kuo, J. F.; and Greengard, P. 1969. Adenosine 3', 5'-monophosphate-dependent protein kinase from brain. *Science* 165: 63.
29. Kuo, J. F., and Greengard, J. 1969. An adenosine 3', 5'-monophosphate-dependent protein kinase from *Escherichia coli*. *J. Biol. Chem.* 244: 3417.
30. Langan, T. A. 1968. Phosphorylation of proteins of the cell nucleus. In *Regulatory mechanisms for protein synthesis*, ed. A. San Pietro, M. R. Lamborg, and F. T. Kenney, p. 101. New York: Academic Press.
31. Allfrey, V. G. 1966. Control mechanisms in ribonucleic acid synthesis. *Cancer Res.* 26: 2026.
32. Sadgopal, A., and Bonner, J. 1970. Proteins of interphase and metaphase chromosomes compared. *Biochim. Biophys. Acta* 207: 227.
33. Stevely, W. S., and Stocken, L. A. 1968. Variations in the phosphate content of histone FI in normal and irradiated tissues. *Biochem. J.* 110: 187.
34. Schwimmer, S., and Bonner, J. 1965. Nucleohistone as template for the replication of DNA. *Biochim. Biophys. Acta* 108: 67.
35. Stevely, W. S., and Stocken, L. A. 1969. Variations in the phosphate content of histone FI in normal and irradiated tissues. *Biochem. J.* 110: 24P.
36. Turkington, R. W., and Riddle, M. 1969. Hormone-dependent phosphorylation of nuclear proteins during mammary gland differentiation *in vitro*. *J. Biol. Chem.* 244: 6040.
37. Mueller, G. C. 1969. Biochemical events in the animal cell cycle. *Fed. Proc.* 28: 1780.
38. Marushige, K.; Ling, V.; and Dixon, G. H. 1969. Phosphorylation of chromosomal basic proteins in maturing trout testis. *J. Biol. Chem.* 244: 5953.
39. Langan, T. A. 1968. Histone phosphorylation: Stimulation by adenosin 3', 5'-monophosphate. *Science* 162: 579.
40. ———. 1969. Phosphorylation of liver histone following the administration of glucagon and insulin. *Proc. Nat. Acad. Sci. USA* 64: 1276.
41. Sutherland, E. W., and Rall, T. W. 1960. The relation of adenosine 3', 5'-phosphate and phosphorylase to the actions of catecholamines and other hormones. *Pharmacol. Rev.* 12: 265.
42. Exton, J. H., and Park, C. R. 1966. The stimulation of gluconeogenesis from lactate by epinephrine, glucagon and cyclic 3', 5'-adenylate in the perfused rat liver. *Pharmacol. Rev.* 18: 181.
43. Robinson, G. A.; Butcher, R. W.; and Sutherland, E. W. 1968. Cyclic AMP. *Ann. Rev. Biochem.* 37: 149.
44. Wicks, W. D.; Kenney, F. T.; and Lee, K. L. 1969. Induction of

hepatic enzyme synthesis *in vivo* by adenosine 3′, 5′-monophosphate. *J. Biol. Chem.* 244: 6008.
45. Murthy, L. D.; Pradhan, D. S.; and Sreenivasan, A. 1970. Effects of hydrocortisone upon metabolism of histones in rat liver. *Biochim. Biophys. Acta* 199: 500.
46. Turkington, R. W. 1968. Hormone-dependent differentiation of mammary gland *in vitro*. In *Current topics in developmental biology*, ed. A. A. Moscona and A. Monroy, 3: 199. New York: Academic Press.
47. Marzluff, W. F., Jr.; McCarty, K. S.; and Turkington, R. W. 1969. Insulin-dependent synthesis of histones in relation to the mammary epithelial cell cycle. *Biochim. Biophys. Acta* 190: 517.
48. Turkington, R. W. 1970. Hormonal regulation of rapidly-labeled nuclear RNA in mammary cells *in vitro*. *J. Biol. Chem.* 245: 6690.
49. Turkington, R. W., and Ward, O. T. 1969. Hormonal stimulation of RNA polymerase in mammary gland *in vivo*. *Biochim. Biophys. Acta* 174: 291.
50. Robbins, E., and Borun, T. W. 1967. The cytoplasmic synthesis of histones in hela cells and its temporal relationship to DNA replication. *Proc. Nat. Acad. Sci. USA* 57: 409.
51. Gurley, L. R., and Hardin, J. M. 1968. The metabolism of histone fractions. I. Synthesis of histone fractions during the left cycle of mammalian cells. *Arch. Biochem. Biophys.* 128: 285.
52. Takai, S., Borun, T. W.; Muchmore, J.; and Leiberman, I. 1968. Concurrent synthesis of histone and deoxyribonucleic acid in liver after partial hepatectomy. *Nature (Lond.)* 219: 860.
53. Turkington, R. W. 1968. Hormone-induced synthesis of DNA by mammary gland *in vitro*. *Endocrinology* 82: 540.
54. Lockwood, D. H.; Voytovich, A. E.; Stockdale, F. E.; and Topper, Y. J. 1967. Insulin-dependent DNA polymerase and DNA synthesis in mammary epithelial cells *in vitro*. *Proc. Nat. Acad. Sci. USA* 58: 658.
55. Buckingham, R. H., and Stocken, L. A. 1970. Histone F1 from rat thymus. *Biochem. J.* 117: 509.
56. Turkington, R. W., and Self, D. J. 1970. New species of hybridizable nuclear RNA in breast cancer cells. *Cancer Res.* 30: 1833.
57. ———. 1970. Changes in hybridizable nuclear RNA during differentiation of mammary cells. *Biochim. Biophys. Acta* 213: 484.
58. Drews, J.; Brawerman, G.; and Morris, H. P. 1968. Nucleotide and sequence homologies in nuclear and cytoplasmic RNA from rat liver and hepatomas. *Europ. J. Biochem.* 3: 284.
59. Church, R. B.; Luther, S. W.; and McCarthy, B. J. 1969. RNA synthesis in taper hepatoma and mouse-liver cells. *Biochim. Biophys. Acta* 190: 30.
60. Neiman, P. E., and Henry, P. H. 1969. Ribonucleic acid-deoxyribonucleic acid hybridization and hybridization-competition studies of the rapidly labeled ribonucleic acid from normal and chronic lymphocytic leukemia lymphocytes. *Biochemistry* 8: 275.

Paul R. Libby

Effect of Hormones on Histone Acetylation 5

The early biochemical events which occur in the rat uterus following treatment with estradiol have been studied extensively in several laboratories (1–3). We now know that administering estrogen initiates new RNA and protein synthesis, and that these effects on the uterus precede the morphological changes and imbibition of water that occur in the estrogen-stimulated uterus. Studies by Jensen and his associates (4) and by Toft and Gorski (5) have demonstrated that estradiol interacts with a macromolecular species in the uterus, most likely a protein.

These different approaches to the problem of hormone action have given much insight into the molecular processes involved in estrogen action. But how estrogens stimulate the synthesis of macromolecules in the uterus and the possible physiological significance of the estrogen receptor complex remain to be determined. One approach to the first problem is to ascertain whether estradiol influences histone acetylation, since it has been postulated that such an effect may alter DNA (chromatin) template activity and thus indirectly affect RNA and protein synthesis. Pogo, Allfrey, and Mirsky (6) demonstrated an effect of phytohemagglutinin on histone acetylation in human lymphocytes before any effect was seen on the stimulation of RNA synthesis in these cells. Means and Hamilton (7) observed a lag period in the stimulation by estradiol of the synthesis of uterine nuclear RNA, similar to the lag period found by Pogo, Allfrey, and Mirsky (6). Barker and Warren (8) found that an increased capacity of uterine

The author is affiliated with the Department of Breast Surgery at the Roswell Park Memorial Institute of the New York State Department of Health in Buffalo.

chromatin acted as template for exogenous RNA polymerase after estradiol treatment. Similar responses of chromatin to hormone action have been reported by O'Malley (the action of estrogen on the chick oviduct chromatin) (9) and by Dahmas and Bonner (the action of cortisol on rat liver chromatin) (10).

This chapter reports a study of the effects of estrogen on the acetylation of histones in rat uterus and mammary tissue. In the uterus, estrogen both in vitro and in vivo markedly stimulated the acetylation of the arginine-rich histone fraction, whereas in the mammary gland evidence was obtained for an estrogen-mediated increase in histone acetokinase activity. In a related study, aldosterone and other steroids with mineralocorticoid activity were observed to produce a significant increase in the acetylation of kidney histones (11).

STUDIES ON UTERINE HISTONE ACETOKINASE

The demonstration of histone acetokinase activity in rat uterus depended on the presence of a sulfhydryl compound (I found that dithiothreitol was the most satisfactory) and high concentrations of glycerol (25%) (12) in the homogenization medium.

Under these conditions either a uterine homogenate, a 10,000 g supernatant fraction, or a 780 g precipitate was found to incorporate $1-^{14}C$ acetate into histones in the presence of the added cofactors ATP, Mg^{2+}, and coenzyme A. This suggested that the acetate first was converted to acetyl CoA by the action of an aceto-CoA-kinase, and the acetyl moiety was then transferred to histone by the action of a histone acetokinase. Under the conditions of my assay system, assays were linear with time and enzyme concentration, and were absolutely dependent upon ATP and CoA.

I found that the enzyme system was distributed throughout the subcellular components of the uterine homogenate. Most of the measurable activity occurred in the supernatant fraction (81%), with smaller amounts in the nuclear (12%) and the mitochondrial pellets (5%). The microsomal pellet was essentially devoid of activity. However, it was not possible under these conditions to determine the distribution of the histone acetokinase, since the availability of the generating system, (or the lack) would certainly affect the apparent distribution of activity.

After the characteristics of the enzyme were established, I studied the effect of 17β-estradiol on histone acetokinase activity. When ei-

Effect of Hormones on Histone Acetylation

ther the 10,000 g supernatant fraction or the nucleus was the source of the enzyme, the presence of low concentrations (10^{-7} M) of estradiol caused a striking increase in the rate of incorporation of acetate into added histones. Pogo, Allfrey, and Mirsky (6) had reported that not all histones are equally acetylated. Their electrophoretic system separates the lysine-rich histones (F1) from other histones, the "arginine-rich" histones, although the one band contains F2 and F3 histones. They reported in human leukocytes that PHA stimulated histone acetylation only in arginine-rich histones, but not in the

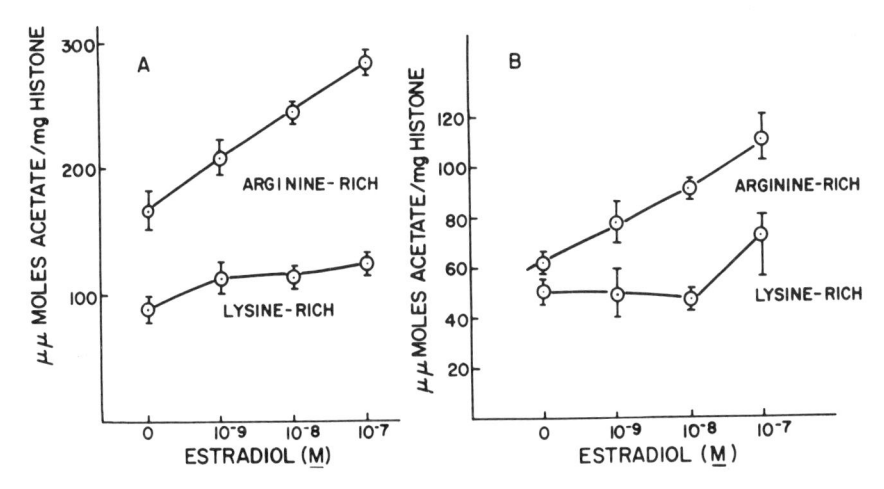

Fig. 1. Effect of 17β-estradiol on histone acetylation: (*a*) Effect of estradiol on an enzyme preparation from the 10,000 g supernatant fluid; (*b*) Effect of estradiol on an enzyme preparation from the nuclear pellet.

lysine-rich histone fraction of the lymphoid cells. I also noted this specificity of histone labeling. Figure 1 shows the results of incubating the standard system in the presence of low concentrations of estradiol. Whereas the lysine-rich histones are only slightly, if at all, stimulated by 10^{-7} M estradiol, the incorporation of acetate into the arginine-rich histones is stimulated by as low as 10^{-9} M estradiol. This differential effect occurs with both the supernatant enzyme (fig. 1*a*) and the nuclear enzyme (fig. 1*b*). One interpretation of these data is that the hormone directly stimulates histone acetokinase activity in vitro. Estrogen could also be acting in this regard by (1) enhancing the production of acetyl CoA; (2) inhibiting the breakdown of acetyl-CoA; or (3) inhibiting the deacetylation of the acetylated histones.

In Vivo Effect of Estradiol on Acetate Incorporation into Histones

To test the effect of estrogens in vivo on the nuclear histone acetylation, I performed the following experiments on immature rats. The rats were injected subcutaneously with ^{3}H-sodium acetate (1 mc/rat) in saline, and half of the group also received 10 µg of estradiol. At various time intervals after injection, the animals were killed and the uteri removed. The histones were isolated, purified by electrophoresis, and counted. Figure 2 shows the results of one such experi-

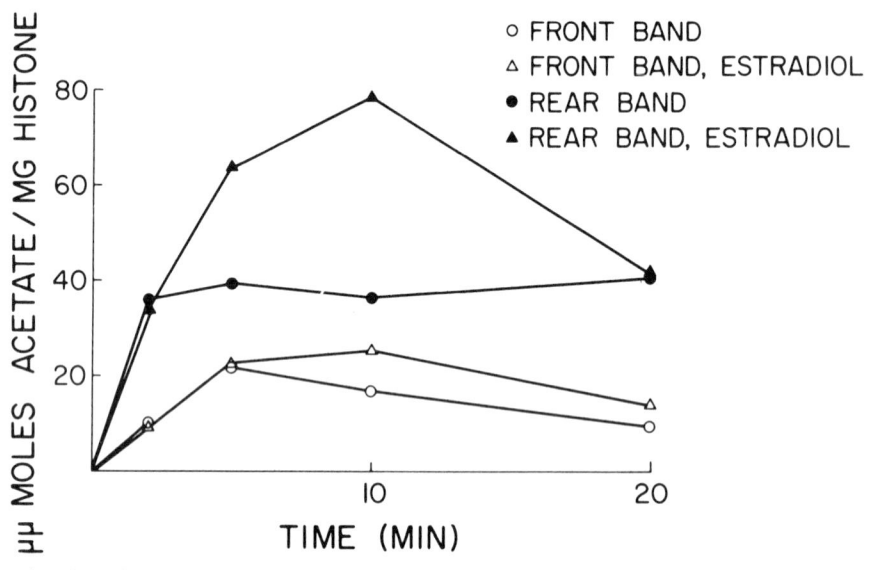

Fig. 2. Time course of incorporation of acetate into uterine histones. Effect of estradiol. Three uteri were pooled for one determination. Each point represents the average of four such pools.

ment. The open circles and triangles show the incorporation of acetate into the lysine-rich or fast histones. The triangles show the results from the estradiol-treated animals, and it is obvious that the hormone has no effect on this fraction at any time. The solid symbols show the incorporation into the arginine-rich, slow moving histones. Five minutes after injection of the hormone, there is a large stimulation of acetylation of the histones derived from the uterus of the hormone-treated animals. At 10 min, the stimulation is double the control. By 20 min, experimental levels have come down to the control levels.

The in vitro data suggest that this effect of the hormone in vivo may be explained by an activation by the hormone of the enzyme histone acetokinase. Other explanations might also be found; for instance, that the hormone affects either acetyl CoA generation or the passage of cytoplasmic acetyl CoA through the nuclear membrane. Two experimental findings, however, seem to contradict these possibilities. First, the hormone does not affect the acetylation of the lysine-rich histones (fig. 2). Second, the hormone has no effect on the labeling of other chromatin proteins. Table 1 presents results of a study on the radioactivity of the acid-insoluble, alkali-soluble proteins of the chromatin from both control animals and animals injected with estradiol. It is quite clear that at time periods after injection when the acetylation of the arginine-rich histones is stimulated to its maximum, the hormone has no effect on these other chromatin proteins.

TABLE 1: ACETATE INCORPORATION INTO ACID-INSOLUBLE CHROMATIN PROTEINS

Time	Incorporation ($\mu\mu$moles/mg protein)	
	Control	Estradiol
5	16.7 ± 8.8	18.5 ± 4.9
10	40.2 ± 11.9	46.6 ± 26.7
20	90 ± 27.5	115.5 ± 12.0

If histone acetylation is a direct consequence of hormone action, antiestrogenic drugs should inhibit this effect. Nafoxidine, or Upjohn 11,100, is antiestrogenic (13) and has been shown by Jensen et al. (14) to block the uptake of estradiol by the uterus. One would expect that nafoxidine would also block the increased acetylation of the arginine-rich histones caused by estradiol, if this effect of the hormone were indeed a direct effect on the uterus and not in some way mediated through an effect on some other organ. Figure 3 shows how pretreating the animals with nafoxidine affects incorporation of acetate into the histones, compared with animals which were not so pretreated. The open bars on the left represent data from the 5-min point of figure 2, and the bars on the right represent the data from animals pretreated with nafoxidine. Nafoxidine had little or no effect on the incorporation of acetate into the lysine-rich histones, but it did somewhat inhibit the incorporation of the acetate into the arginine-rich histones, and it completely abolished the stimulation caused by estradiol.

In Vivo Effect of Estradiol on Mammary Gland Enzyme

I attempted to study the incorporation of acetate into mammary gland histones but found that under the experimental conditions

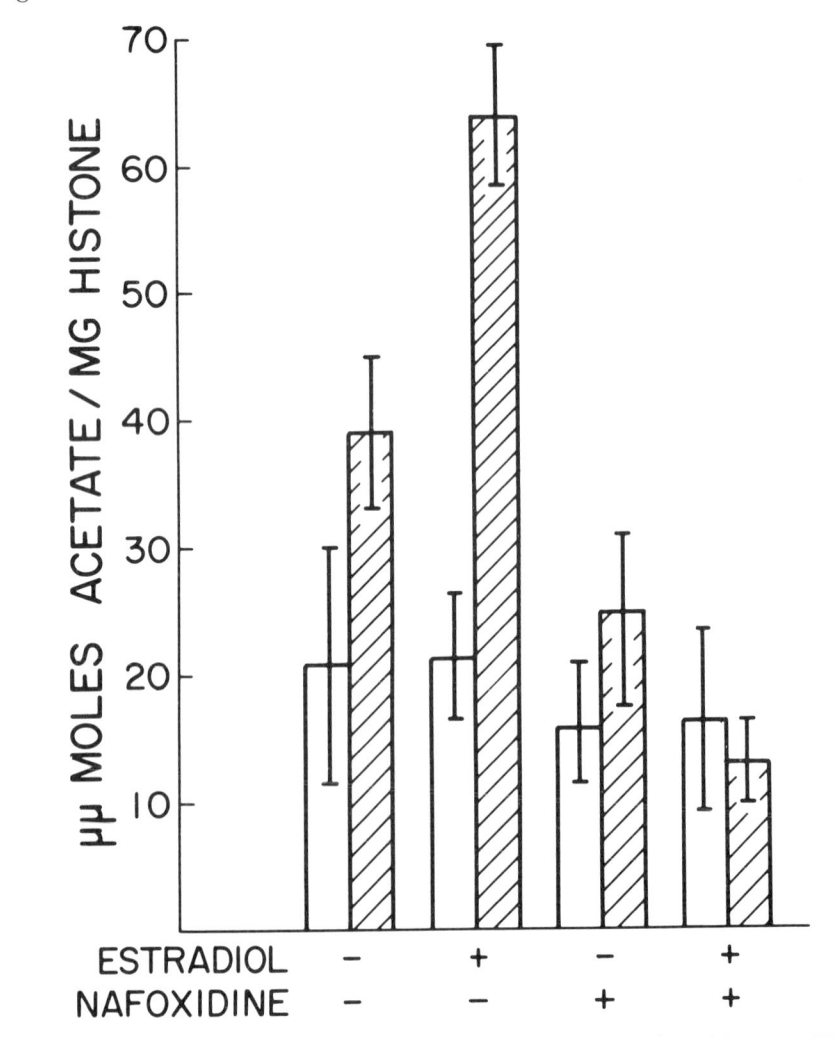

Fig. 3. Effect of nafoxidine on incorporation of acetate into histones. The open bars refer to the lysine-rich histones. The crossbars refer to the arginine-rich histone. Nafoxidine, 50 μg in 0.1 ml of glycerol, was given 30 min before the injection of acetate.

Effect of Hormones on Histone Acetylation

used—about 1.5 mc of ^{3}H-acetate/100 g of rat—the incorporation was too low to be properly assessed.

To get some information on this process in the mammary gland, I decided to study the enzyme histone acetokinase in the gland to see the effect of estradiol in vivo. Preliminary experiments showed such an enzyme activity in the nuclear pellet, being assayed with calf thymus histones and labeled acetyl CoA. Under the conditions employed, the enzyme activity was linear with time and enzyme concentration, had a pH optimum at 8.3, and was inhibited by *p*-chloromercuribenzoic acid (15).

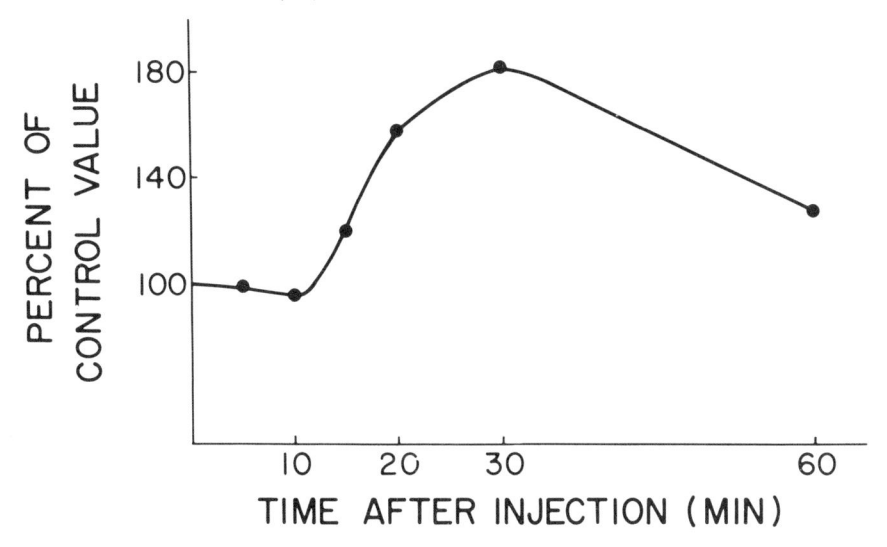

Fig. 4. Effect of estradiol on activity of mammary gland histone acetokinase. Experimental animals were injected with 10 μg of estradiol at the times shown before death. Control animals received saline. The source of enzyme was the nuclear pellet.

I then studied the effect of estradiol pretreatment on enzyme activity in the mammary gland nuclei of castrate rats. I injected rats intraperitoneally with either 10 μg of estradiol or with the vehicle alone and killed them at various time intervals. The mammary glands were excised and a nuclear preparation was used as the source of enzyme. Activities were calculated per μg of DNA, and the experimental values were expressed as percentages of the control values.

The results of such experiments are shown in figure 4. During the first 10 to 15 min after the hormone is injected, there is no effect on the enzyme activity, although there is a suggestion of a rise at 15 min. At 20 and 30 min, however, there are significant rises from the control values, the 20-min value being some 60% higher and the 30-min value 85% higher than controls. Interestingly, the 1 hr values seem to be coming back down to the levels of the controls.

Although it was unlikely that the in vitro action of estrogen on histone acetokinase in uterus was due to new protein synthesis, I wished to determine if the in vivo effect of estrogen on the mammary gland could be blocked by the protein inhibitor cycloheximide. Figure 5 shows the results of experiments in which the animals were exposed to estradiol for 30 min before death. The right two bars show

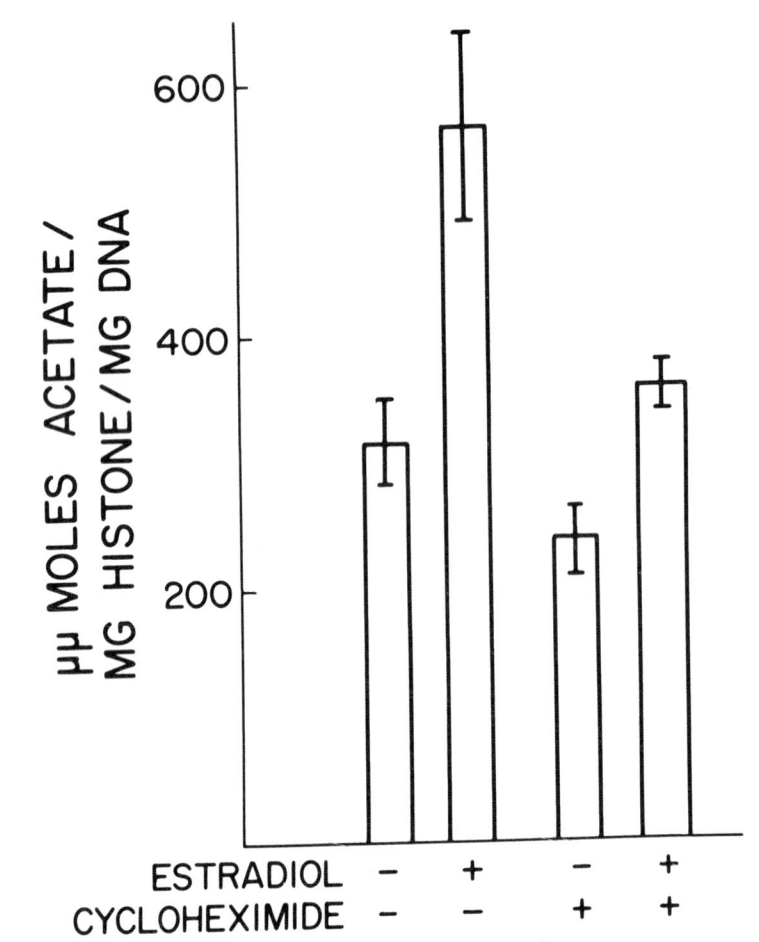

Fig. 5. Effect of cycloheximide on the stimulation of mammary gland enzyme by estradiol. Cycloheximide (5 mg/kg) was given 3 hr before estradiol (10 μg) or vehicle alone and rats were killed 30 min after estradiol treatment. The source of enzyme was the nuclear pellet.

the experiments carried out on animals which had received cycloheximide 3 hr before. In both sets of animals, estradiol administration caused a significant increase in the specific activity of the enzyme, indicating that protein synthesis is not necessary for the increase in enzyme activity caused by estradiol. I cannot yet assess whether the difference in stimulation between cycloheximide-treated and untreated animals (52% vs. 80% stimulation) is due to experimental variation, a partial effect of inhibition of protein synthesis on an estradiol-mediated effect, or the presence of two enzymes, one of which is stimulated by estradiol, with differential rates of breakdown. (The effect of cycloheximide on mammary gland protein synthesis was assessed in this experiment by including 5 μc of ^{14}C-L-leucine in the vehicle with which all animals were injected. Non–cycloheximide-treated animals incorporated 400 cpm/mg protein, and cycloheximide-treated animals incorporated 26 cpm/mg, indicating inhibition of protein synthesis of greater than 90%.)

EFFECTS OF ALDOSTERONE ON KIDNEY HISTONE ACETOKINASE

The actions of aldosterone on the kidney of adrenalectomized animals are similar in many respects to the actions of estradiol on the uterus. Specifically, the kidney contains mineralocorticoid receptors which bind aldosterone, and the early action of aldosterone seems to be concerned with the induction of new RNA synthesis, which leads to new protein synthesis, which leads to increased salt-retention capacity (16).

Examining the kidney of the adrenalectomized rat revealed an enzyme system very similar to that of the uterus of the immature rat (17). The action of aldosterone was studied and its effect on enzyme activity is shown in figure 6, where it is obvious that a striking increase is caused by increasing the aldosterone concentration from 10^{-10} M to 10^{-9} M. It is within this range that Sharp and Leaf (18) found the lowest concentration of aldosterone (3×10^{-10} M) which would stimulate the short-circuit current of the toad bladder, another measure of mineralocorticoid activity. This figure also shows a similar experiment in which crystalline acetate kinase and phosphotransacetylase were added to create an exogenous acetyl CoA generating system. This experiment, in which the activity of the enzyme is stimulated in a way very similar to the first experiment, shows that the action of aldosterone is not an effect of the hormone on the generation of acetyl CoA.

In addition to aldosterone, large numbers of other steroids, both synthetic and natural, are known to have mineralocorticoid activity. Among those with high activity are deoxycorticosterone (DOC), cortisol and 9α-fluorocortisol. The effect of these steroids, along with aldosterone, on the enzyme activity of the kidney preparations was examined, and the results are shown in figure 7. In this experiment, the stimulations caused by the steroids ranged from 30% (DOC) to 60% (aldosterone). Included in figure 7, and shown in the stippled bars, is a parallel experiment in which the incubations were carried out in the presence of aldactone, a potent inhibitor of mineralocorticoid activity (19). In these experiments, aldactone has no effect on the control rate of acetylation of the histones, but it completely abolishes the stimulation caused by adding mineralocorticoids, and

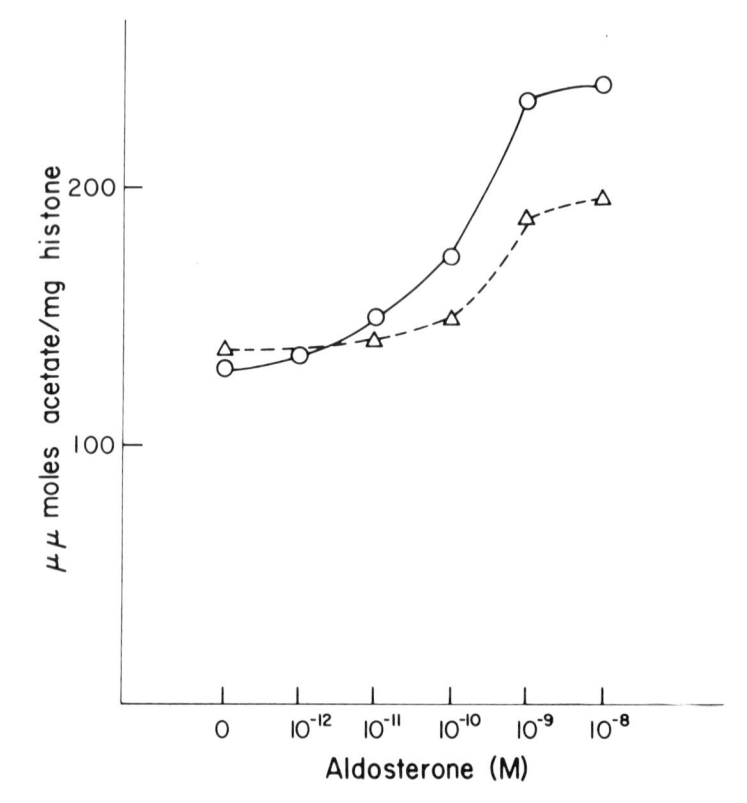

Fig. 6. Effect of aldosterone on the incorporation of acetate into histones by a kidney supernatant enzyme from adrenalectomized rats (△-------△) in the presence of kidney preparation alone. (O————O) in the presence of 2 units of acetate kinase and 5 units of phosphotransacetylase.

Effect of Hormones on Histone Acetylation

the incorporation in these experiments is brought back to the control levels.

Conclusions

The data suggest that some steroid hormones have as one primary action the stimulation of histone acetylation through a direct effect of hormone on the enzyme histone acetokinase. In both uterus and

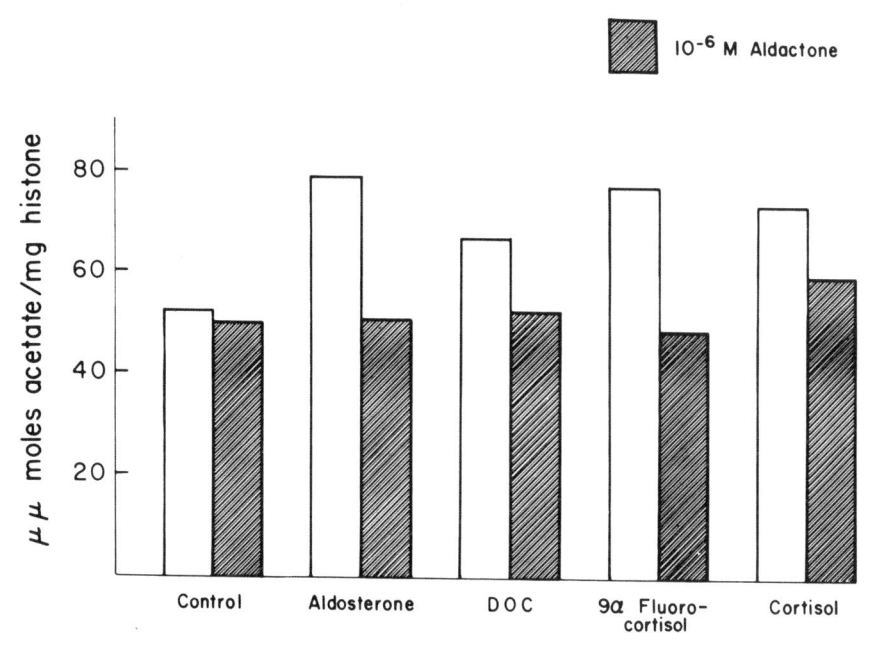

Fig. 7. Effect of mineralocorticoids on kidney histone acetokinase reaction. Concentrations: aldosterone, 10^{-9} M, 9α-fluorocortisol, 10^{-8} M, DOC 10^{-7} M, and cortisol, 10^{-7} M. Open bars in the absence of, and stippled bars in the presence of 10^{-6} M aldactone.

kidney, enzymes are present which are stimulated in vitro by the steroid hormones which act on the tissue. The studies on the kidney enzyme are of special interest because they show that the enzyme is stimulated by several mineralocorticoids, and the stimulation, but not the basal value, can be obliterated by the antimineralocorticoid aldactone. The effect of estradiol on the mammary gland enzyme suggests that in the mammary gland also there is an enzyme which may be directly stimulated by the hormone. This idea arises from the finding that the increase in the enzyme caused by the hormone is not blocked by the protein synthesis inhibitor cycloheximide.

The in vitro work on the activation of the enzymes, from which I originally suggested that this reaction might be involved with the response of the tissue to the hormone, is supported by some in vivo data. I have shown that treatment with estradiol will stimulate the incorporation of acetate into the uterine nuclear histones, and this effect is apparent within 5 min after the hormone is given. This is a very early effect of the hormone, and apparently precedes the stimulation of nuclear RNA synthesis reported by Means and Hamilton (7).

There is an interesting parallel between these studies and recent studies on cyclic AMP (cAMP). Many hormones seem to act, at least in part, by stimulating the cell membrane enzyme adenyl cyclase (20). This increases the intracellular concentration of cAMP, which then acts as a second messenger to bring about the effects attributed to the hormone. Cyclic AMP is known to stimulate enzymes which catalyze the phosphorylation of various proteins. Three protein kinases, from skeletal muscle (21), brain (22), and liver (23), have been partially purified, and the preferred substrate in each of these cases seems to be histones or histone fractions. It is interesting that cAMP does not activate the liver enzyme if protamine is used as a substrate (23). Langan has studied the effect of glucagon, a hormone which appears to act by means of cAMP, on liver histone phosphorylation in vivo (24). He was able to show a ten- to twenty-fold stimulation of the incorporation of phosphate into the liver histones. This implies, as do the data on mammary cells presented by Turkington (chapter 4), that histone phosphorylation may be another response to hormone stimulation.

One would expect the acetylation or phosphorylation of histones to neutralize some of the net positive charges found in these proteins. These processes may be highly selective in terms of the histone molecule. Ogawa et al., in reporting the structure of the GAR histone, say that apparently only lysine residue 16 is N-acetylated in the epsilon position (25). Langan (24) has found that only one serine residue is phosphorylated in the lysine-rich histones. These specificities imply some precise function of the modification of the histones.

In bacteria, repressors are protein molecules which bind directly to DNA and control the portion of the genome which is read by RNA polymerase. Since the time of the Stedmans (26), attempts have been made to consider the histones as fulfilling the same functions in eukaryotic cells. However, it has become apparent that there are too few different histone molecules to fulfill this function, and there seems to be identity of some of these across species lines (27). However, the data presented above, the data of Pogo, Allfrey, and Mirsky (6), Pogo, Pogo, and Allfrey (28), Takaku et al (29), and Langan (24) all seem to indicate that the histones may be importantly concerned with the control of readout of portions of the genome.

If this is so, then some factor(s) external to the histones themselves must control the specificity, or selectivity, of readout. At present there are three such possibilities: the acidic chromosomal proteins, the chromosomal RNA, and the sequence of bases in the DNA itself. Several laboratories have reported (30–32) that the acidic chromosomal proteins can modify the inhibition of template activity of DNA caused by histones. It may be that chromosomal proteins can control the interaction of histone in complex with DNA and either histone kinase or histone acetokinase and thus determine the ease with which polymerase can interact with various portions of the genome.

Both Bekhor, Kung, and Bonner (33) and Huang and Huang (34) have reported that for complete reassociation of components of chromatin into "natural" chromatin, chromosomal RNA is necessary. Thus, chromosomal RNA may fulfill the function suggested above for the chromosomal proteins.

The third possibility is that the DNA may itself control the exposure of the side groups of the histones. Lewin (35) has suggested that since histones lie along the wide groove of the helix, and since there is the possibility of hydrogen bonding between the histone side groups and the amino groups of adenine and cytosine, the sequence of nucleotides along the helix may control the binding of different histones; and it is possible that sequences of nucleotides may control the exposure of lysine amino groups to the histone acetokinase.

At present our knowledge is such that none of these possibilities excludes the others. The final understanding of the control of genome repression and activation of eukaryotic cells must await further work.

The mechanism by which steroid hormones cause the stimulation of the histonekinase is as yet unknown. The possibility that the steroid hormone might in some way affect the supply of acetyl CoA is obviated by the data presented above. In addition, preliminary evidence has been obtained in our laboratory that the uterine enzyme shows the stimulatory effect of estrogens using added acetyl CoA rather than a generating system (16). Another possibility is that the steroid hormone may in some way affect a histone deacetylase enzyme. I have presented evidence (36) to suggest that the level of such an enzyme may be important in controlling acetyl group turnover in vivo. The last possibility, and the one favored in our laboratory at this time, is that the steroid hormone directly interacts in some way with the histone acetokinase enzyme to activate this enzyme. The mechanism by which this takes place is totally unknown. Because we are working in crude systems with an ill-defined enzyme and an ill-defined substrate, I feel that such questions will remain unanswered until studies can be carried out with purified enzyme and substrate.

Acknowledgments

This investigation was supported in part by grant G-65-RP-9 from the United Health Fund and grant CA-04632-11 from the National Cancer Institute, National Institutes of Health.

References

1. Mueller, G. C.; Herranen, A. M.; and Jervell, D. F. 1958. Studies on the mechanism of action of estrogens. *Rec. Prog. Hormone Res.* 14: 95.
2. Gorski, J.; Notides, A.; Toft, D.; and Smith, D. E. 1967. Mechanism of sex steroid action. *Clin. Obstet. Gynecol.* 10: 17.
3. Hamilton, T. H. 1968. Control by estrogen of genetic transcription and translation. *Science* 161: 649.
4. Jensen, E. V.; Suzuki, T.; Kawashima, T.; Stumpf, W. E.; Jungblut, P. W.; and DeSombre, E. R. 1968. *Proc. Nat. Acad. Sci. USA.* 59: 632.
5. Toft, D., and Gorski, J. 1966. A receptor molecule for estrogens: Isolation from the rat uterus and preliminary characterization. *Proc. Nat. Acad. Sci. USA* 55: 1574.
6. Pogo, B. G. T.; Allfrey, V. G.; and Mirsky, A. E. 1966. RNA synthesis and histone acetylation during the course of gene activation in lymphocytes. *Proc. Nat. Acad. Sci. USA* 55: 805.
7. Means, A. R., and Hamilton, T. H. 1966. Early estrogen action: Concomitant stimulations within two minutes of nuclear RNA synthesis and uptake of RNA precursor by the uterus. *Proc. Nat. Acad. Sci. USA* 56: 1595.
8. Barker, K. L., and Warren, J. C. 1966. Template capacity of uterine chromatin: Control by estradiol. *Proc. Nat. Acad. Sci. USA.* 56: 1298.
9. O'Malley, B. W.; McGuire, W. J.; Kohler, P. O.; and Korenman, S. G. 1969. Studies on the mechanism of steroid hormone regulation of synthesis of specific proteins. *Rec. Proc. Hormone Res.* 25: 105.
10. Dahmas, M. E., and Bonner, J. 1965. Increased template activity of

liver chromatin, a result of hydrocortisone administration. *Proc. Nat. Acad. Sci. USA* 56: 1370.
11. Libby, P. R. Unpublished observations.
12. Libby, P. R. 1968. Histone acetylation by cell-free preparations from rat uterus: *In vitro* stimulation by estradiol-17β. *Biochem. Biophys. Res. Commun.* 31: 59.
13. Duncan, G. W.; Lyster, S. G.; Clark, J. J.; and Lednicer, D. 1963. Antifertility activities of two diphenyl-dihydro-naphthalene derivatives. *Proc. Soc. Exp. Biol. Med.* 112: 439.
14. Jensen, E. V.; Jacobson, H. I.; Flesher, J. W.; Saha, N. N.; Grupta, G. N.; Smith, S.; Colucci, V.; Shiplacoff, D.; Neumann, H. G.; DeSombre, E. R.; and Jungblut, P. W. 1966. Estrogen receptors in target tissues. In *Steroid dynamics,* ed. G. Pincus, T. Nakao, and J. F. Tait, p. 133. New York: Academic Press.
15. Libby, P. R. Unpublished observations.
16. Edelman, I. S., and Fimognari, G. M. 1968. On the biochemical mechanism of action of aldosterone. *Rec. Prog. Hormone Res.* 24: 1.
17. Libby, P. R. 1969. *In vitro* acetylation of histones by rat kidney: Stimulation by mineralocorticoids. Abst. #B86, 158th Meeting Amer. Chem. Soc., New York.
18. Sharp, G. W. G., and Leaf, A. 1966. Studies on the mode of action of aldosterone. *Rec. Prog. Hormone Res.* 22: 431.
19. Fanestil, D. D. 1968. Mode of spirolactone action: Competitive inhibition of aldosterone binding to kidney mineralocorticoid receptors. *Biochem. Pharmacol.* 17: 2240.
20. Robison, G. A.; Butcher, R. W.; and Sutherland, E. W. 1968. Cyclic AMP. *Ann. Rev. Biochem.* 37: 149.
21. Walsh, D. A.; Perkins, J. P.; and Krebs, E. A. 1968. An adenosine 3′,5′-monophosphate-dependent protein kinase from rabbit skeletal muscle. *J. Biol. Chem.* 243: 3763.
22. Miyamoto, E., Kuo, J. F.; and Greengard, P. 1969. Cyclic nucleotide-dependent protein kinases. II. Purification and properties of adenosine 3′,5′-monophosphate-dependent protein kinase from bovine brain. *J. Biol. Chem.* 244: 6395.
23. Langan, T. A. 1968. Histone phosphorylation: Stimulation by adenosine 3′,5′-monophosphate. *Science* 162: 579.
24. ———. 1968. Phosphorylation of liver histone following the administration of glucagon and insulin. *Fed. Proc.* 28: 1899.
25. Ogawa, Y.; Quagliarotti, G.; Jordan, J.; Taylor, C. W.; Starbuck, W. C.; and Busch, H. 1969. Structural analysis of the glycine-rich arginine-rich histone. III. Sequence of the amino-terminal half of the molecule containing the modified lysine residues and the total sequence. *J. Biol. Chem.* 244: 4387.
26. Stedman, E., and Stedman, E. 1950. Cell specificity of histones. *Nature (Lond.)* 166: 780.
27. DeLange, R. J.; Fanbrough, D. M.; Smith, E. L.; and Bonner, J. 1968.

Calf and pea histone. IV. Amino acid composition and the identical COOH-terminal 19-residue sequence. *J. Biol. Chem.* 243: 5906.

28. Pogo, B. G. T.; Pogo, A. O.; and Allfrey, V. G. 1969. Histone acetylation and RNA synthesis in rat liver regeneration, *Genet. Suppl.* 61: 373.

29. Takaku, F.; Nakao, K.; Ono T.; and Terayama, H. 1969. Changes in histone acetylation and RNA synthesis in the spleen of polycythemic mouse after erythroporetin injection. *Biochim. Biophys. Acta* 195: 396.

30. Paul, J., and Gilmour, S. 1968. Organ-specific restriction of transcription in mammalian chromatin. *J. Molec. Biol.* 34: 305.

31. Wang, T. Y. 1968. Restoration of histone-inhibited DNA-dependent RNA synthesis by acidic chromatin proteins. *Exp. Cell Res.* 53: 288.

32. Spelsberg, T. C., and Hnilica, L. S. 1969. Effects of acidic proteins and RNA on histone inhibition of DNA-dependent RNA synthesis *in vitro. Biochim. Biophys. Acta* 195: 63.

33. Bekhor, I.; Kung, G. M.; and Bonner, J. 1969. Sequence-specific interaction of DNA and chromosomal protein. *J. Molec. Biol.* 39: 351.

34. Huang, R. C., and Huang, P. C. 1969. Effect of protein-bound RNA associated with chick embryo chromatin on template specificity of the chromatin. *J. Molec. Biol.* 39: 365.

35. Lewin, S. 1970. Possible selective genetic controls in synthesis of messenger RNA by means of "paired" histones along the wide groove of the double helix of DNA. *Biochem. J.* 117: 19P.

36. Libby, P. R. 1970. Activity of histone deacetylase in rat liver and Novikoff hepatoma. *Biochim. Biophys. Acta* 213: 234.

Guy Williams–Ashman, *Chairman*

Discussion: Part I — 6

DR. WILLIAMS-ASHMAN: We have heard a wide range of approaches to the problem of how estrogens act on normal and neoplastic tissues. A general question emerges about the functional significance, from the standpoint of estrogen action, of those proteins present in estrogen-responsive tissues which bind estrogens very tightly and with high stereospecificity. The binding of estrogens can clearly be impeded by various so-called estrogen antagonists. Also, there is much evidence, particularly discussed by Dr. Jensen, that cytoplasmic estrogen binding proteins may be involved in two-step mechanisms for the entry of estrogens into cell nuclei and for their retention in these organelles in combination with specific intranuclear forms of the binding proteins. We can easily imagine three possibilities of what this might mean physiologically. First, the cytoplasmic estrogen binding proteins may simply be a device to allow capture of the hormone by responsive cells and to transport the estrogen into the cell nucleus. The second possibility, alluded to in a number of the presentations, is that the estradiol-"receptor" protein complexes (and particularly the nuclear forms thereof) are the true "active forms" of the hormones. If this is indeed so it has immediate bearing on the large number of experimental failures to influence various intranuclear biochemical processes involved in gene expression (RNA biosynthesis, etc.) by direct addition of estrogens. Another imaginable function for these hormone binding proteins involves turning a previous hypothesis around 180 degrees, so to speak. We can postulate that it is not the function of the binding proteins to get the hormone into the nucleus, but rather that the hormone (by combining with

The chairman is affiliated with the Ben May Laboratory for Cancer Research and the Department of Biochemistry at the University of Chicago.

specific groups and perhaps changing the conformation or other features of the macromolecule) gets the protein into the nucleus; once the protein is inside the nucleus it can serve a regulatory function which no longer requires the hormone. According to this hypothesis, the action of the hormone would be essentially "permissive." I am sure that over the next few years experiments will be carried out all over the world to test these and perhaps other hypotheses regarding the function of specific intracellular sex hormone-binding proteins.

I would also like to bring up the assumption made in most of the presentations that the presence of estrogen binding proteins in large amounts may be used as some sort of definition of an estrogen "target organ." I agree with Dr. Korenman that we have to be wary of circular reasoning here. It is important, in my opinion, not to disregard experiments which point to apparent exceptions to this hypothesis. I think this is especially true for the "hormone dependence" of various mammary cancers. This term was introduced by Huggins in a strictly operational sense, that is, to indicate that the growth of certain tumors is altered by removing or administering what might in the natural course of the tumor's history be regarded as sustaining hormones. I mention this because it is by no means clear whether changes in growth of a neoplasm after levels of circulating estrogens are altered in an animal with a mammary tumor, for example, necessarily imply that the tumor as such is responding to circulating estrogens. Some of the effects on the tumor of administering or removing estrogens could conceivably relate to other factors, such as regulation by estrogen levels of the output of prolactin or other hormones by the pituitary.

DR. MEITES: I have some questions for Dr. Jensen. The first, already alluded to by Dr. Williams-Ashman, is What is the meaning of the term "hormone-independent" rat mammary tumor which you mentioned in your talk? The second question is What is known about the nature of the estrogen binding proteins?

DR. JENSEN: I gave the definition of the "hormone-independent" rat mammary tumor as that small percentage of the total, about 12%, which continues to grow when the ovaries are removed. It is strictly an operational definition; what it is that the ovaries are supplying, we don't know. It is a completely empirical observation that tumors which continue to grow in the ovariectomized rat have less of the estradiol binding protein than do those which regress. As for the nature of the protein, the 8S protein in the cytosol apparently is an aggregate of 4S units, with either themselves or possibly some other nonbinding unit present in the cytosol. The cytosol receptor is a rather difficult substance to work with, because it both decomposes and aggregates on storage or manipulation. If you partially purify it on a small scale by sucrose gradient density centrifugation it is considerably more stable, indicating that there are instability factors in the cytosol. The purified material shows a molecular weight by elution from Sephadex of about 200,000, has an isoelectric point by isoelectric focusing of 5.8, and apparently contains sulfhydryl groups, because the complex is decomposed by treatment with p-hydroxymercuribenzoate. When estradiol is attached to this protein, it acquires the ability to bind to many things, including the nucleus. It also associates with basic proteins such as RNase, protamine, and polylysine. If one first treats the 8S protein with KCl to deaggregate it into 4S subunits, and then adds calcium (1mM concentration), one can stabilize the 4S subunit so that it will not go back to 8S form when the salt is removed and does not aggregate on precipitation with ammonium sulfate or on purification on Sephadex G-200. This calcium-stabilized 4S unit is what we've purified about five thousand-fold. The 5S complex, which we extract from the nucleus, appears to be derived from the 4S subunit of the cytosol protein. We think it also has a sulfhydryl group, but it is much less reactive. In the transformation of 4S to 5S, the sulfhydryl group may have become masked, or buried in some way. This 5S unit apparently has an isoelectric point of about 5.8, whereas the calcium-stabilized 4S unit has an isoelectric point of 6.4 and a molecular weight of 75,000. Both the cytosol and the nuclear receptors appear to be primarily protein in nature. As Gorski first showed for cytosol protein, and we for the nuclear one, they are decomposed by trypsin or pronase, but not by DNase or RNase, although the 8S protein forms a complex with RNase. We have preliminary evidence that the 8S protein may contain phosphorus.

DR. MC GUIRE: I've been examining estradiol receptors in the DMBA-induced tumors. The tumors can be classified into three groups: they either grow continuously, are actively growing, or do not regress after ovariectomy. Figure 1 shows data on the hormone-dependent tumor cytosol. This animal was given radioactive estradiol in vivo; the cytosol was applied to a G-100 column, and you can see in the early fractions the bulk of the radioactivity, or at least a large amount of it, came right through in the void volume with the macromolecular fraction. Albumin on this column is partially retarded.

Figure 2 shows data on tumor cytosol from hormone-independent tumor by the criteria I just mentioned. The radioactivity is insignificant in the macromolecular fraction, and it is found almost entirely again with the OD 260 material that is retained on the column. The R 3230 AC transplantable mammary carcinoma in Fisher rat which apparently responds to estradiol with certain enzyme changes does not respond to ovariectomy. There is no change in tumor growth and there is no macromolecular binding of estradiol with this tumor. If you take the macromolec-

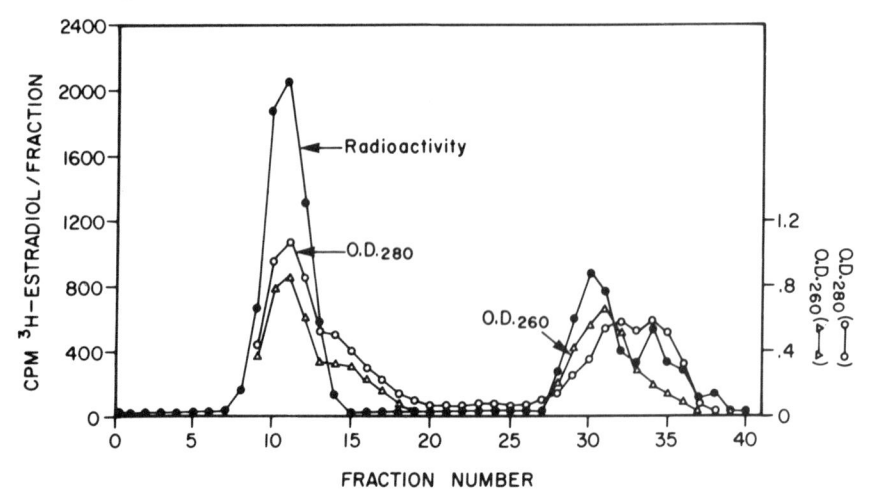

Fig. 1. G-100 Sephadex chromatography of a 105,000 g supernatant from a hormone-sensitive DMBA mammary tumor injected in vivo with radioactive estradiol.

ular fraction off the G-100 column of a DMBA hormone-sensitive tumor and put it on a DEAE cellulose column, you find two peaks of radioactivity with sodium chloride gradient elution as shown in figure 3. If you decrease the slope of this gradient, or use a stepwise elution, these peaks will separate even better. So I think the DMBA tumor has attractive features, in terms of hormone dependence, but I agree with previous comments that the criteria of the dependence and independence must be fairly rigid.

DR. LIPSETT: Dr. Jensen, to determine the presence or absence of receptor you have to separate the bound estrogen from the free estrogen, and you are doing this by sucrose gradient analysis. Have you tried comparing your method with the Korenman method of using charcoal to separate bound from free steroid, which seems to offer some degree of simplicity?

DR. JENSEN: Whether we use the Korenman (charcoal) method to remove the free hormone from the bound or the Sephadex G-25

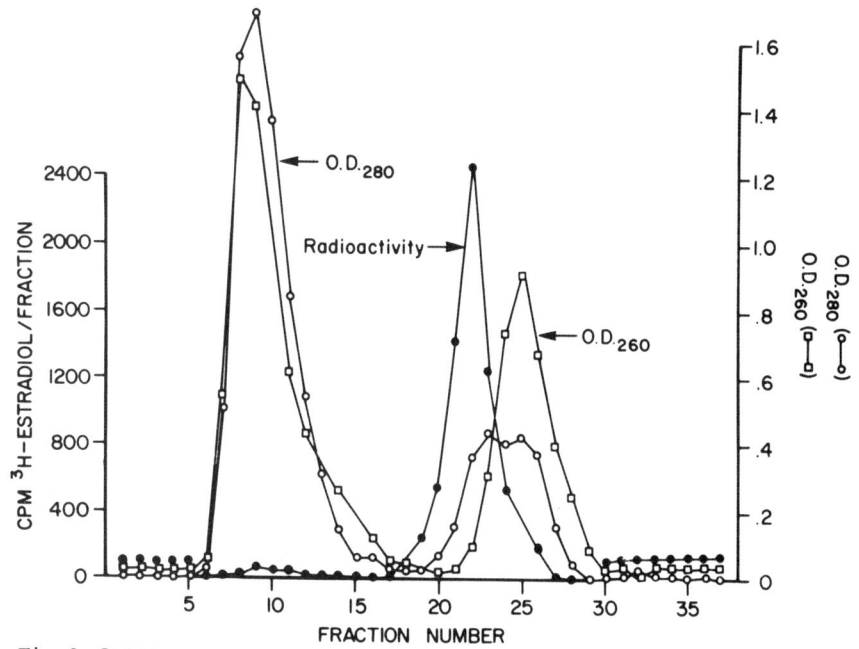

Fig. 2. G-100 Sephadex chromatography of a 105,000 g supernatant from a hormone-insensitive DMBA mammary tumor injected in vivo with radioactive estradiol.

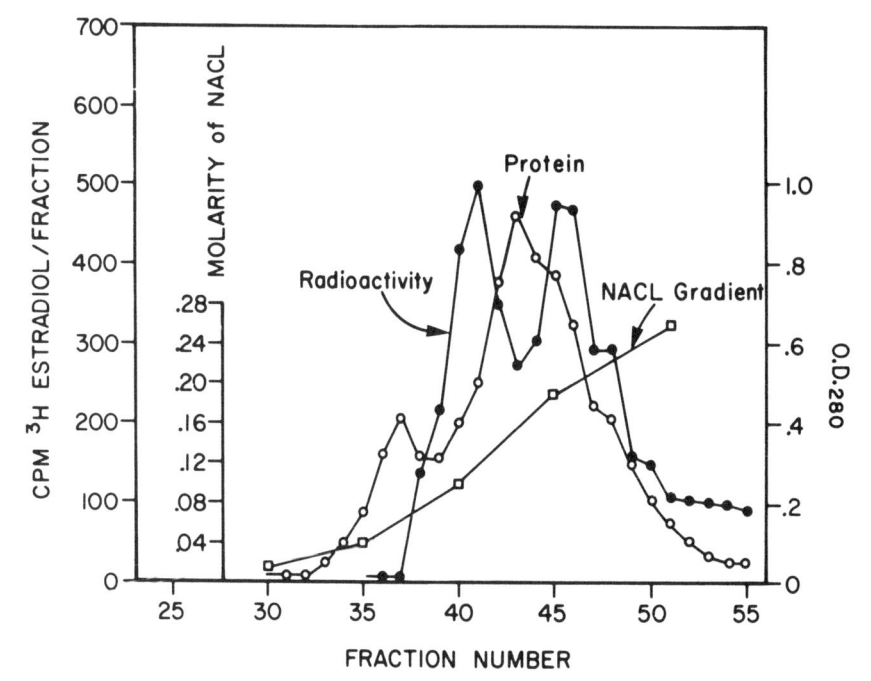

Fig. 3. DEAE cellulose chromatography of the macromolecular fraction from G-100 Sephadex chromatography of the 105,000 g supernatant of a hormone-sensitive DMBA mammary tumor.

method that I illustrated, we get a similar general pattern. Perhaps we aren't as careful as Dr. Korenman in using charcoal, because we observe considerably less total binding capacity than we find with the sucrose gradient method. In our experience, the Sephadex column method of removing the excess hormone gives values closer to the density gradient procedures than does the charcoal method, but they both give essentially the same qualitative pattern.

DR. KORENMAN: I have actually compared samples treated with charcoal and not treated with charcoal on a sucrose density gradient. We get very similar answers. The system is sufficiently sensitive that we can use 100 mg of tissue to determine whether there is binding or not, although we cannot do all the specificity experiments. If there is a gram or so of active tissue, it is possible to determine the association constant as well as the total number of binding sites. One technician can work up a breast cancer in an afternoon; an ultracentrifuge is required, however, to make cytosol.

Another point I might make is the role of Sephadex. Sephadex is not simply a molecular sieve. Sephadex retains estrogen beyond sodium chloride. In fact Sephadex is a very efficient means of separating the three principal estrogens, if you use a mixture of G-15 and G-25. However, Sephadex preparations above G-25 are less effective than the more highly cross-linked gels. I would recommend, if one is using a simple protein separation procedure, that at least G-50 should be employed, because then there will be less removal of bound hormone from the protein by the action of Sephadex itself.

DR. JENSEN: I agree with Dr. Korenman about the problems of Sephadex removing the bound hormone; we feel that all these other binding methods probably do this simply because of the dissociation constants obtained by these methods. Investigators report values which vary from 10^{-10} to 10^{-9}, whereas the dissociation constant as measured by our procedure lies between 10^{-11} and 10^{-12}. Since we feel that the actual binding is much tighter than is indicated by these procedures, it makes us somewhat apprehensive of values obtained by either Sephadex or charcoal.

DR. TORGERSON: I would like to ask Dr. Jensen to comment on the possibility of getting these receptor substances to such purity that they might act as specific antigens in the fluorescent antibody technique. As a pathologist, I am very much interested in this possibility.

DR. JENSEN: One of our high priority endeavors is isolating substantial amounts of both the 4S binding unit from cytosol and the 5S protein from nucleus in purified form. When we do, we certainly

Discussion

want to use these proteins to make antibodies. From older work that we have done with inactivated but still purified receptor proteins, we know already that these proteins are fairly active antigens, so I am optimistic about obtaining antibodies to them.

DR. GRIFFITHS: It seems that in these breast cancer studies, the homogenization of tissue must be done very carefully. It is normally a very difficult process; Dr. Jensen, would you care to comment on how you do this?

DR. JENSEN: We have found that the best way is to freeze the tumor specimen in liquid nitrogen, pulverize the frozen tissue with a stainless steel device called the Thermovac Autopulverizer, and then homogenize the powder in a glass homogenizer. Here one must be very careful not to destroy the receptor by local heating. One homogenizes in the cold for no more than 10 sec at a time with an intermittent 50-sec cooling period.

DR. O'MALLEY: Do any of you have an idea of the physical shape of estrogen receptor? The progesterone receptor has shown remarkable similarity to the estrogen receptor. But when we try to calculate molecular weight or size, there is absolutely no agreement between sucrose gradient and column methods. This seems to be because the receptors are not globular proteins. Using the gel electrophoresis method of Rodbard and Chrambach, and working only with molecular radius, we are able to get a straight line mass/charge relationship between the monomer and multimer binding protein forms. The progesterone receptor now looks like a monomer of 90,000 molecular weight and a tetramer of 360,000. There are the 4S and 8S, and I would guess that estrogen may be similar to this and the monomer form can aggregate into multimer depending on the experimental conditions.

I would also like to mention that some of us agree with Dr. Williams-Ashman's comment that the hormone may be acting to simply get the receptor inside the nucleus. I say this because DNA and chromatin appear to have a limited number of binding sites for the hormone-receptor complex. More interesting, these sites can be saturated by receptor alone. These data could be interpreted so that the active molecule may be the receptor protein and the hormone simply the mechanism responsible for transfer to the nucleus.

I have two additional questions. One is directed to those working on histone. Do you think that histones have the specificity required to play a major role in regulation? The following evidence seems to mitigate against this hypothesis. (1) When one does column chromatography or electrophoresis, the numbers of different histone proteins in different organs or even species seem to be all the same.

(2) Recently sequenced histone fractions from different species seem to have the same sequence. If one takes two chromatins (e.g., liver and thymus), removes the histones but leaves the acidic proteins on the DNA, switches the histones from one chromatin to the other by reconstituting by methods of Bonner, and then transcribes them, the transcription rates for the chromatin are the same as the DNA of origin. Furthermore, if one looks at hybridization competition of the newly transcribed RNAs, it seems that the histones also do not qualitatively change the type of RNA made. If one alters the acidic proteins, however, transcription is quantitatively and qualitatively altered.

My other question is for Dr. Turkington. I don't quite understand the last figure showing your theory that you need an activator DNA that doesn't amplify response. You mentioned that this molecule is needed to translate the "language" into the "genetic code" so that it can interact better with DNA; but we already know that repressors and inducers interact with operones; these molecules are proteins. Therefore, why would you need an intermediate RNA unless you need an amplification mechanism?

DR. TURKINGTON: It is clear that the histones of various species are very similar. As you point out, they don't contain in their amino acid sequences the specificity for recognizing specific nucleotide sequences in DNA. What seems to be very important, and perhaps the reason this highly specific structure has persisted in the histones throughout phylogeny, is that the basic residues of the histones bind very tightly to the negatively charged phosphate groups on the DNA. The data from Harris Busch's lab on the complete amino acid sequence of the GAR histone provides a three-dimensional model in which basic residues on the histone pair vary specifically with the constellations of phosphate groups in the three-dimensional DNA helix. Perhaps this is why histone amino acid sequences have been very constant to meet the steric requirements to preserve this tight binding in the major groove of DNA. So in that sense, the histones would not seem to carry information which could specifically recognize nucleotide sequences. The studies of Hans Ris on the electron microscopic structure of chromatin suggest that what we are really dealing with is a problem in molecular engineering or modeling. If one of these genes so tightly bound to the histone is to be activated, how is the histone to be removed so the RNA polymerase can copy it? It could be that some of the structural modifications of histones which occur at the same time that genes are activated may relate to the fact that some of these sites for phosphorylation are exposed and just become phosphorylated or that the phosphorylation step or acetylation step is a prerequisite for altering the interaction of DNA with histones.

DR. LIBBY: In general, I agree with Dr. Turkington. We must accept the fact that these changes we observe are crude modifications of the structure. We cannot expect to find a specific histone for, say, liver tyrosine amino transferase or oviduct avidin. However, we must remember that after hormone treatment, we often find observable differences in chromatin, as is evidenced by template capability. Also, the report of Lewin (*Biochem. J.* 117:19, 1970) suggests that the sequences of nucleotides along the helix of DNA will control the exposure of various side groups of the histone amino acids, allowing for much more selective control of potential acetylation (or phosphorylation) sites.

DR. DE OME: I would like to raise a question concerning the relative proportions of the epithelial and the stromal elements in these experiments. Both tumors and the normal mammary gland may contain an enormous amount of stromal tissues. Normally, the virgin mammary gland contains about 95% of stroma and only about 5% epithelial elements. One is constantly faced with this problem; however, in these experiments we are talking about receptor proteins and receptor systems in the epithelial elements.

DR. JENSEN: In regard to the uterus, where you have well-defined epithelium, lamina propria, and myometrium, the difference between these regions is only quantitative and not very great even at that. Myometrium seems to behave just like endometrium in regard to all the phenomena I mentioned. With the immature rat we work with the whole uterus, but with the calf we have worked with endometrium and myometrium separated and we see no striking difference in vitro. The uptake of estradiol is somewhat higher in the endometrium than in the myometrium, but except for that the picture is very similar. I don't know whether this is true with the mammary gland.

DR. WILLIAMS-ASHMAN: One point that seems to be almost universally ignored in considering sex-hormone action on both normal and malignant tissues is whether the blood vessels in these tissues are under the control of the hormones. When mammary gland or uterus grows in response to ovarian hormones, for example, blood vessels in these organs proliferate, and of course tumor growth is utterly dependent on an adequate blood supply. The ingrowth and elaboration of new blood vessels is often assumed to be a rather passive process, but perhaps, endothelial cells in appropriate biological regions are themselves very hormone dependent.

DR. PEARSON: I would like to ask Dr. Jensen whether there is any evidence that the endocrine status of the animal affects the concentration of estrogen binding protein. For example, if you had a hormone-responsive DMBA tumor and took out the pituitary, you'd have that tumor, say, halfway shrunken. Would the concentration of estrogen binding protein be any different?

DR. JENSEN: I can't answer that specific question, but it appears from the little work we've done and the considerable work other people have done that the concentration of the 8S receptor in the uterine tissue does depend somewhat on the endocrine status of the animal. The concentration is highest in the immature rat and is lower in the mature rat. After ovariectomy of the mature rat there is first an apparent increase in receptor concentration, probably reflecting

TABLE 1: EFFECT OF OVARIECTOMY ON ESTROGEN RECEPTOR IN HORMONE-DEPENDENT MAMMARY TUMORS AND NORMAL MAMMARY TISSUE

DPM 17β-Estradiol Added/10 mg Tissue	DPM 17β-Estradiol Bound/10 mg Tissue			
	Normal Mammary Gland		Mammary Tumor	
	+Ovaries	−Ovaries	+Ovaries	−Ovaries
0.22×10^5	—	—	620	101
0.77×10^5	31	85	1,645	261
2.3×10^5	98	215	2,470	488
3.9×10^5	165	360	2,825	828
8.0×10^5	287	665	3,700	1,197
12.1×10^5	495	900	4,080	1,675

depletion of endogenous hormone which is tying up some receptor; but within a week after ovariectomy there is a progressive decline in receptor content, suggesting that something from the ovary is necessary to maintain the level of estrogen receptor in the mature animal.

Other studies have shown a significant fluctuation during the ovarian cycle from estrus to diestrus, reaching a peak when estrogen has been there. These studies are unpublished and I don't know the specific details.

DR. BROOKS: We have obtained data which may give some indication about the fate of estrogen receptor in hormone-dependent mammary tumors after ovariectomy (table 1).

The analyses of the receptor in these experiments was carried out exactly as Dr. Jensen described earlier, utilizing Sephadex G-25

Discussion

columns to separate the unbound tritiated 17β-estradiol from that bound to the receptor. Increasing concentrations of 17β-estradiol were incubated with a constant level of protein from the cytosol. In this way it was possible to show the saturation of the receptor. The cytosol from the normal rat mammary gland displayed only nonspecific binding (straight line extrapolating to zero). A small amount of estrophile protein was apparent in the absence of the ovaries. In the intact animal endogenous estrogen is presumed to have saturated the receptor.

In the cytosol from a biopsy of a DMBA-induced mammary tumor, there is a steep initial slope to the 17β-estradiol binding curve. In the intact animal this continues until the receptor molecules are saturated with the steroid. Twelve days after ovariectomy, the initial slope of the binding curve decreases sharply, indicating a greatly decreased concentration of receptor molecule in the remaining mammary tumor. During the 12-day period following ovariectomy the mammary tumor had regressed to approximately 10% of its original size.

DR. KORENMAN: The degree of saturation is very relevant here, and particularly in our series, in which we did not find one premenopausal woman whose tumor had a significant amount of binding. We were very concerned about this. But the negative statement that when there was binding the binding sites were not saturated doesn't really answer the question. It has another order of complexity which I would like to bring up to this group. If, as Dr. Jensen and others suggest, in the presence of estrogen 80% or so of the cytosol receptor is found in the nucleus (we are studying the cytosol receptor), we have eliminated four-fifths of the material we can possibly find if there is estrogen circulating. Therefore it is quite conceivable that in all our studies of cytosol alone we may be subject to a self-induced error in the premenopausal woman, and this technique may be principally useful in those patients in whom endogenous estrogen is at a low concentration. We don't know this. We are studying the concentration of hormone both in the nucleus and in the cytoplasm to try to determine this.

DR. TURKINGTON: Many of the data from the study of different tumors suggest that one of the defects the tumor cell exhibits is a marked alteration in the regulation of gene expression, so that the tumor cell itself is not like the normal cell. It may very well be different from any cell the body has ever had. In that sense, one might expect to find a multiplicity of responses to the hormone or the hormone-receptor complex among various tumors. Even if the hormone receptor is present, it might still not be possible to predict the response of the cell, since it may now have an unpredictable combination of expressed genes which might confer a wider and more variable range of responses. We tend to see, in general, two populations of cancers with growth rates hormonally responsive or not hormonally responsive, but I wonder if among these two populations we may be seeing a wide spectrum of responses to hormones, and whether these may be conditioned largely by the modes of gene expression made possible by the neoplastic transformation.

DR. BRENNAN: If the estrogen receptor is induced by estrogen, would studies of the male mammary gland help determine the inducibility of the receptor? The male mammary gland is not responding to small amounts of testicular and adrenal estrogen. But under the influence of chorionic gonadotrophin, for example, or after direct administration of large amounts of estrogen, the mammary gland grows.

DR. JENSEN: I cannot comment on this interesting suggestion, but I can say that the only male tissue with a substantial amount of the receptor substance is the anterior pituitary. In both male and female rats, the anterior pituitary seems very similar in receptor content. If you need estrogen to induce or stimulate it, then there is the question of what does this for the male.

DR. SARFATY: If estrogen is responsible for inducing the receptor protein and hence for the continuation of tumor growth, how is it that pharmacological doses of estrogen on certain occasions will cause regression of the tumor?

DR. MEITES: I can give you one possible answer. I believe that large doses of estrogen as well as small doses increase prolactin secretion, but large doses prevent prolactin from having any direct effect on mammary carcinogenesis. Similarly, large doses of estrogen increase prolactin secretion but also prevent prolactin from stimulating lactation, and hence inhibit lactation. How this is done from the biochemical and molecular point of view, I don't know.

DR. LIPSETT: With respect to the question raised to Dr. Meites about the large dose of estrogen ameliorating breast cancer, of course we don't even understand how estrogen can accelerate breast cancer, either in the ovariectomized rat with the DMBA tumor or in the ovariectomized woman with breast cancer, but at least there is some biological specificity to this phenomenon. However, there is little biologic specificity to the inhibition of tumor growth in women where large doses of androgen, estrogen, progestational agents, or glucocorticoids may be effective. We have taken too simplistic a view of tumor growth; a tumor is not just a collection of cells, all of which are growing and going through phases G1, S, G2, and M.

Most of the cells, in fact, are not growing at all; they are so-called G0. Now it seems probable from ancillary evidence that the length of the cell cycle is not affected. We also know that not all the cells that go through the cycle and divide become tumor cells; there is a very appreciable rate of cell loss. To explain the nonspecific effects of these many different steroids in large doses, one might propose that they affect the rate of cell loss rather than decelerate the rate at which cells pass from G0 to G1.

I think there is biological specificity in the response of DMBA-induced mammary tumors to either removal or administration of estrogen. This mechanism is unknown. But the regression induced in man by many steroids has little specificity, and, practically, any steroid agents we know will induce remissions.

DR. BRENNAN: I think it is important to realize that although massive doses of several hormonal steroids, estrogens, androgens, corticoids, and progestins will produce regressions, some patients will respond to one agent and not to others. In other words, the various hormonal steroids are not really equivalent, even though response rates are similar. Some women respond to large doses of estrogen and don't respond at all to large doses of testosterone or progesterone or corticosteroids. So there is some level of specificity, even at the pharmacological dosage level, and this suggests that the mechanism of inducing regression may be multiple.

DR. PEARSON: I would like to ask Dr. Turkington about his schema of the action of estrogen and prolactin in normal mammary explants. As I recall, you had estrogen stimulating growth of mouse mammary epithelial cells.

DR. TURKINGTON: Over a wide range of prolactin concentrations in the medium, we have never seen any effect of prolactin on the growth of the explants in terms of the incorporation of tritiated thymidine in DNA or of mitotic indexes, except with very high concentrations of prolactin. We now use the NIH ovine preparations, and with such high concentrations as 100 μg/ml or more we do begin to see very small increases in cell proliferation. But these increases seem to follow the same sort of dose-response relationship we observed with very low concentrations ("physiologic" concentrations) of growth hormone. It is really the old question whether this represents prolactin activity or growth hormone-like activity. We tentatively regard this as representing more the growth hormone-like activity of the prolactin preparation and we feel that at least at "physiologic" concentrations the growth hormone preparation stimulates cell proliferation and the prolactin preparation only induces milk proteins.

DR. DAO: Dr. Korenman mentioned that binding sites in tumor in premenopausal women may be saturated because of the presence of endogenous hormone. Do you have any evidence that the binding sites of estriol and estradiol are not the same?

DR. KORENMAN: Two things: (1) All the evidence we have from measuring cytosol estrogen concentration indicates that the binding sites are never saturated. (2) Estriol does compete for the estradiol receptor. That does not mean that there is not a different receptor somewhere else, which estradiol does not compete with, but estriol does compete for estradiol receptor when there is a specific receptor present.

DR. NANDI: Insulin does not either promote thymidine uptake or increase mitosis in rat mammary gland, whereas prolactin significantly increases both mitosis and thymidine uptake. If you also have aldosterone, aldosterone and prolactin seem to act in synergism in rat mammary gland, whereas in mouse the situation is quite different. Has anybody ever looked at the effect of progesterone, aldosterone, or any other kind of steroid on estrogen binding in mammary gland or mammary tumor system?

DR. KORENMAN: I did show the progesterone data, and so far we haven't found any high affinity receptor for progesterone at all in about seven cases. I've tried aldosterone as a competitor for estradiol, and it does not compete. The most interesting observation is that dihydrotestosterone not only binds well but also competes to a small extent for the estrophile both in the uterus and in the mammary gland.

DR. SINGH: I would like to ask Dr. Turkington a question. What percentage of mammary gland epithelial cells are able to synthesize casein in the presence of insulin, hydrocortisone, and prolactin? A recent publication (Mills and Topper, *J. Cell Biol.* 44:310–28, 1970) has shown that in the presence of insulin and hydrocortisone some cells are able to produce rough endoplasmic reticulum which is acted on by prolactin to produce casein. However, some do not. Therefore, it seems to me that not all of the epithelial cells present in the mammary gland are able to produce casein.

DR. TURKINGTON: It is quite clear that the organ culture system is very unphysiological, in the sense that one does not have continuous proliferation as one has in vivo. In vitro, and in chemically defined medium containing insulin, cell proliferation occurs as a single synchronized wave of division confined to a period of 48–60 hr and involving a majority of the epithelial cell population. One cannot regard this as the kind of population which is functional in the same sense in the animal. We find that by immunofluorescence staining with anticasein and antilactalbumin all of the secretory cells seem to make both of these milk proteins and the ductal cells do not. It may be that in the organ culture system some of the cells are not given the opportunity to develop to the point where they generate the endoplasmic reticulum. I don't know. It is very difficult to quantitate, that is to compare in a quantitative sense, the in vitro and in vivo systems. I would like to respond to Dr. Nandi's question, which no one has answered very well. We have never found any response to DNA synthesis in the organ culture system in response to either prolactin or the steroids in either the rat or the mouse. Again, there may be factors in the animal which would permit these hormones to have these effects. The effect of insulin in the organ culture is artificial in the sense that physiological concentrations of insulin in vitro do not elicit the effect, and injections of insulin and so forth in the intact animal, as was pointed out, really do not mediate growth responses as the other hormones do. And so this may really be an effect which is specific for the organ culture system and which replaces something that is provided in the animal.

Certainly the effect of insulin can be supplemented or replaced by other factors, like epithelial growth factor, which seem to have the same effect at levels which might be considered physiologic, although those levels are not really known. Some other factors extractable from the plasma also have this effect of stimulating DNA synthesis in vitro. Possibly the other hormones which are also present in the animal are the primary regulators of growth in vivo, but insulin does provide the means for analyzing regulatory events in the cell cycle in vitro.

DR. MEITES: Later we are going to discuss tumorigenesis, but not from the biochemical point of view. The biochemists spoke about the relationship of the biochemical events that occur after estrogen is administered in the uterus and mammary gland. What is the relationship of estrogen to mammary tumorigenesis from the biochemical point of view?

DR. JENSEN: I will give you my opinion, which may or may not be valid; that is estrogens are not tumorigenic or carcinogenic themselves, but they put the tissue in a state of active metabolism so that it can be subject to the influences of carcinogenic agents or factors, whether they be hereditary, viral, or chemical. I think it is difficult to have neoplastic transformation in atrophic tissue.

DR. NANDI: I would like to make precisely an opposite comment. I think there are systems like the mouse mammary tumor systems where the tumor is virally induced, but I do not think that the virus itself could cause cancer. The virus perhaps alters the surface of the cells somehow, so that they become more responsive to estrogen and other hormones. At least, I think that the virus itself may not be the causative agent.

DR. MEITES: Whatever it is, viruses are not necessarily involved in mammary tumorigenesis in the rat.

DR. NANDI: There is absolutely no evidence that viruses are involved in rat mammary tumorigenesis. However, if one doesn't find a virus in a tumor, it does not mean that a virus cannot be involved in its genesis. In the case of DNA tumor viruses, once the virus causes the transformation it can no longer be detected in tumors unless one uses some special technique such as rescue of virus by fusing transformed cells with permissive cells.

DR. ADAMS: I'd like to direct a question to Dr. Turkington. A paper appeared in *Science* (W. G. Dilley and S. Nandi, *Science* 161:59, 1961), dealing with the maintenence of explants of mammary glands from immature rats in culture and studying the differentiation of lobular tissue. Differentiation occurred in the presence of insulin, corticosteroid, and prolactin. In one of the control experiments, they left out the steroid hormone and found that it made little difference to the subsequent differentiation of lobular tissue. Now does this mean that there is no need for steroid hormone, or, if there is, what is the source of the steroid hormone in this case? What I'm driving at is, Does the breast possibly have the ability to produce steroid hormone for differentiation and changing structural requirements?

DR. TURKINGTON: It may be that the tissue cultured in those experiments did in fact have a very low requirement for hydrocortisone such as might persist in the tissue after explantation. I believe that the tissue was from the rat rather than from the mouse system that we have primarily studied, but the end point for hormone action was really morphological rather than one of the biochemical parameters we have studied. Perhaps Dr. Nandi would like to comment on that.

DR. NANDI: I think Dr. Turkington may be right. There is a possibility that endogenous steroid hormone like corticosteroid might have been present in the mammary gland at the time of explantation. However, if you keep the explants of mammary glands from immature rats in a medium containing only insulin for 3 or 4 days, so that you can dilute out some endogenous corticosteroid, and then add prolactin to this particular explant, it will also differentiate to show signs of secretion, and lobuloalveolar stimulation. I think it is most likely that there are differences between the rat system and the mouse system. The mouse system appears to

Discussion

be much more dependent on corticosteroids than rat mammary gland. I think Dr. Meites did some experiments on this; he might like to comment.

DR. MEITES: What we did—and I believe it has been substantiated by other methods—was to show that in hypophysectomized-ovariectomized-adrenalectomized rats, in which presumably all the steroid hormones and anterior pituitary hormones have been removed, administering large doses of prolactin and growth hormone alone can sitmulate lobuloalveolar growth. Of course, one may argue that estrogen may still be present somewhere, perhaps in the mammary gland; I think Dr. Dao and we have shown that if one transplants a rat pituitary directly over the mammary tissue, one of the mammary glands of adrenalectomized-ovariectomized rats, one sees localized lobuloalveolar growth. This raises the possibility that mammary gland differentiation and growth and perhaps mammary tumor growth can occur in the absence of steroid hormones.

DR. FORREST: May I ask if Dr. Jensen has done any work on the estrogen receptor proteins in the normal human breast? I note also that he has pooled his results on hypophysectomy and adrenalectomy, and I wonder if he has observed any difference in pattern between them. The number is small, but I wonder if one is justified in putting them together when looking for this responsiveness. Third, what other tumors have been looked at for estrogen receptor activity?

DR. JENSEN: I will start with the last question. The only other studies I know of have been carried out with endometrial cancer. Some endometrial tumors appear to contain the receptor substance. As far as the hyphophysectomy goes, we have had only three such patients; one was positive and the other two were negative. We haven't tried to break these down as yet; when we get more cases, I think we shall. We haven't been very successful in studying normal breast tissue, either in vivo or in vitro. In vivo there is very little uptake, probably because there is much adipose tissue, and we are not skillful enough to study only the duct cells. In vitro, as Dr. Korenman mentioned, we find no evidence of any significant uptake. However, Bresciani and Puca in Italy have looked at normal breast tissue and have reported that the situation is quite similar to that in uterus except that the number of receptor-bearing cells is rather low and so the concentration of the receptor is lower in breast than in uterus.

Guy Williams–Ashman, *Chairman*

Summary: Part I   7

I feel that this meeting has been most valuable, especially because it has brought into the open certain issues which everyone in the field must contend with. I am not going to rehash or summarize what the speakers have already said; rather, I shall make a few general comments on the preceding session, which dealt with the mode of action of estrogens on target tissues. We heard presentations dealing with both of the major approaches to the problem of steroid hormone action which investigators have taken in recent years. The first approach, which we might label the "forward approach," rests on the assumption that a hormone must first recognize and combine with specific receptor molecules, and that this receptor-hormone combination can, so to speak, "do something." For obvious reasons, receptor substances for all hormones must presumably be macromolecules of one form or another, and proteins seem the most likely candidates for such receptor functions, although it is conceivable that polynucleotides or even polysaccharides or complex lipids could function in this regard. So the strategy is to try to find out the chemical nature of these "receptors" by examining the fate of labeled steroid hormones in tissues. The second approach, which can be called the "backward approach," is to determine the nature and time sequence of biochemical events set in motion by the hormonal stimulus in vivo, usually putting great stress on the earliest detectable biochemical changes, in the hope that this might enable one to "work back" to the primary sites of action of the hormones. After the explosive developments in molecular biology in the early 1960s, which provided a chemical basis for the intermediate steps in the transfer of genetic information from the DNA

The chairman is affiliated with the Ben May Laboratory for Cancer Research and the Department of Biochemistry at the University of Chicago.

genome to the amino acid sequences of specific proteins, and with the gradual acceptance of the view that the action of growth-promoting hormones such as sex hormones may be regarded as a facet of the general problem of the biochemistry of true or functional differentiation, it is only natural that in recent times much effort has been directed toward mapping alterations in RNA and protein biosynthesis and turnover induced by sex hormones in responsive cells and tissues. But to my knowledge there is still no evidence that any sex hormone directly influences any well-defined enzymatic process involved in RNA transcription or translation, even though large changes in RNA and protein synthesis occur in many tissues soon after administration of appropriate sex hormones, and in some instances, changes in transcriptive events occur before detectable alterations in protein synthesis by polyribosomal systems. In this connection, I believe that the chick oviduct system Dr. O'Malley discussed is especially useful, because it has the signal advantage that the synthesis of the specific proteins ovalbumin (induced by estrogens) and avidin (induced by progesterone) can be measured. However, we sometimes forget that in many experiments involving stimulation of secondary sexual tissues by various sex hormones, details of the biochemical changes so induced are essentially a property of the tissue under examination rather than of the particular hormone used as a trigger.

We have heard an excellent account from Dr. Jensen of his pioneering studies on the uptake and retention of labeled estrogens by various female reproductive organs, and Dr. Korenman discussed some new developments in this field. This leads me to consider a rather general issue. For many years, a number of investigators have cautioned against assuming any unitary hypothesis for the molecular basis of steroid hormone action. There is no doubt that the estrogen receptor proteins ("estrophilic proteins," in Dr. Jensen's terminology) in various target tissues are responsible for the selective uptake and retention of estrogenic hormones, mainly in cell nuclei. But how far these proteins are involved in the early hormone-induced alteration of biochemical happenings in estrogen-target tissues is still far from clear. So I think we must be careful in assuming that various specific estrogen binding proteins are necessarily involved in more than the intracellular uptake and translocation of these hormones. Moreover, although in the case of 17β-estradiol most of the hormone in uterus is found in nuclei in firm combination with a 5S-receptor protein, this does not necessarily mean that the cytoplasmic 8S-receptor protein may not exert regulatory functions in extranuclear regions of the cell. I would like, moreover, to make a plea for more comparative studies on proteins in responsive cells that bind sex hormones or their metabolites with a high degree of affinity and stereospecificity. For if an examination is made of other than the rather few organs studied up to now (mainly rat and calf uterus), we may well find variants in the nature and intracellular location of such macromolecules which would throw an entirely new light on their possible functions.

I would like to comment on a matter arising out of the lectures by Dr. O'Malley and Dr. Turkington—the possible participation of intracellular "second messengers" in the action of mammalian sex hormones. Since Sutherland's pioneer work, there is now a large body of experimental evidence that many of the actions of peptide hormones like glucagon and vasopressin, and also of the catecholamine hormones, can be accounted for by their ability to enhance adenylcyclase reactions, so as to increase the intracellular levels of cyclic adenosine 3'-5'monophosphate (cyclic AMP), which in turn influences a host of biochemical processes. But although there are some claims to the contrary, I think it is fair to state that there is little compelling evidence to suggest that cyclic AMP serves a major intermediary role in the actions of either estrogens or androgens. Dr. Turkington did describe some effects of hormones on the enzymatic phosphorylation of certain histones in his mammary gland organ culture system. It is interesting that recently a class of cyclic AMP-activated protein phosphokinases have been discovered which utilize some histones as substrates, and this has led T. A. Langan and others to speculate that such reactions could be involved in certain cells, particularly at the transcriptive level.

Both Dr. Turkington in his discussion of histone phosphorylation and Dr. Libby in his consideration of enzymatic acetylation of histones considered reactions in which proteins (histones) of well-defined amino acid sequences can be modified by adding or subtracting adventitious phosphoryl or acetyl groups. This could conceivably alter the conformational and charge properties of histones so that their interaction with DNA might be perturbed. Experiments from a number of other laboratories (notably these of T. A. Langan and V. Allfrey) have suggested that histones in living cells may be subject to such modifications. But in these instances I am not sure whether it has been rigorously proved that the histone phosphorylation or acetylation estimated in vivo really reflected addition of such groupings to histones in living cell nuclei. There is strong evidence that histones are synthesized not in cell nuclei but in the cytoplasm, and it is not impossible that phosphorylation, acetylation, and so on of histones is functionally related to other processes besides histone-DNA interactions, such as intracellular transport of newly formed histones from the cytoplasm into the nucleus.

Dr. O'Malley showed us some interesting new findings concerning rapid hormonal stimulation or ornithine decarboxylase in chick oviduct. Large and swift increases in ornithine decarboxylase activity are now known to accompany the growth of a number of tissues. This brings up the possibility that putrescine formation by this enzyme is related to a rapid increase in the polyamines spermidine and spermine during growth, since putrescine is a precursor of both of these substances. Since spermidine and spermine can influence the enzymatic synthesis of RNA and proteins, and can stabilize polynucleotides and also membranous structures in mammalian cells, there have been recent suggestions that these polyamines might serve a second-messenger function in the action of some growth-promoting hormones. Recent studies from my laboratory (A. E. Pegg, D. H. Lockwood, and H. G. Williams-Ashman, *Biochem. J.* 117:17, 1970) suggest, however, that at least in androgen-induced prostatic growth, there is no evidence for any cause-and-effect relationship between increases in polyamine levels and early enhancement of nuclear RNA synthesis, even though androgens induced rapid increases in this organ. Rather, it appears that in many rapidly growing tissues, a coupling occurs between polyamine formation and the synthesis of ribonucleic acids, especially of ribosomal RNA. This may help to neutralize excessive negative electrical charges due to accumulation of new RNA molecules.

Metabolism of Steroids by Mammary Cancer   II

John B. Adams and Michael Wong

Paraendocrine Behavior of Human Breast Cancer 8

INTRODUCTION

The vast majority of completed scientific projects are by necessity reported in an overwhelmingly logical manner. The reader gains the impression that each planned experiment led on to the next until the final answer was obtained. Actually, as most of us realize, these results were sifted from a conglomeration of abortive experiments, false leads, time-wasting artifacts, and some chance observations. On rarer occasions, one hears or reads accounts of research presented in a true chronological order. It is the latter type of presentation that I have always found more interesting and to a degree I will use this approach.

Some years ago I was working on a study of the possible implication of the amorphous ground substance on the spread and invasion of neoplastic cells. Early histochemical reports had described changes, usually metachromatic, which took place in the ground substance in the vicinity of tumor spread. For these reasons we initiated a study on the biosynthesis of the sulfated mucopolysaccharide components of the ground substance, and possible changes therein, in the presence of invading tumors (1). Radioactive ^{35}S sulfate of high specific activity was employed, and when it was incubated with tissue extracts, a large number of ^{35}S ester sulfates were formed. Since some of these labeled metabolites may have represented intermediates involved in overall biosynthesis of mucopolysaccharide, we attempted to identify them. Some possessed unusual chromatographic properties on paper, since, despite having a highly polar sulfate ester moiety,

The authors are affiliated with the School of Biochemistry at the University of New South Wales.

they still exhibited high R_F values in most solvent systems employed. A bulky hydrophobic molecule was indicated, and one possibility was a sterol, or steroid sulfate. Hence steroids were added to the incubation mixtures. When we examined human adrenal tissue containing extensive deposits of metastatic breast cancer, we found powerful steroid sulfotransferase enzymes. We examined some properties of the crude enzyme system of adrenals removed from breast cancer patients and found that steroids, possessing a wide variety of functional hydroxyl groups, could be sulfated (2). Normal ovarian tissue was then examined, and in surprising contrast, contained virtually no steroid sulfotransferase activity (3). We did not determine whether any functional corpora lutea were present in the specimens examined, but metastatic breast carcinoma, which had grossly replaced normal ovarian tissue, did possess sulfotransferase activity for dehydroepiandrosterone (DHEA) and estrone. Fifteen primary breast tumors were next examined and all were found to possess steroid sulfotransferase activity. Normal tissue, obtained from the radical mastectomy specimens, did possess very weak activity in a few cases (3). This contrast between normal and cancerous tissues may have been due to the great difference in their cellularity. Since DHEA sulfate could be formed by adrenal gland, and evidence had been obtained that this was the form in which the steroid was secreted (4), then obviously the accepted concept at the time, that steroid sulfates represented detoxication products, was untenable. Steroid sulfates were shown shortly after to be capable of undergoing reactions in which the sulfate moiety remained intact (5). In the breast tumors, the steroid sulfokinase may have been involved in similar reactions in which changes of physiological significance occurred in the steroid moiety. Accordingly, we undertook experiments to test this hypothesis.

OUTLINE OF METHODS OF INVESTIGATING
STEROID TRANSFORMATIONS IN VITRO

Usually the tumor obtained at radical mastectomy was dissected free of fat and normal tissue and incubated as a slice or mince with labeled steroid in Krebs-Ringer phosphate buffer, with or without added cofactors (6). After carrier steroids were added, the lipid-soluble extract was partitioned between pentane and 90% methanol, and the methanol layer was further fractionated into estrone, estradiol, estriol, and neutral fractions by the method of Ryan and Smith (7).

Radioactive metabolites were separated by paper and thin-layer chromatography.

In later experiments, we examined the possible cleavage of 4-^{14}C cholesterol to pregnenolone, but dilution of isotope with endogenous cholesterol made it necessary to isolate mitochondrial fractions (8). It proved extremely difficult to obtain these from the comparatively plentiful primary breast tumors, and we resorted to isolating them from involved lymph nodes, usually obtained from the axilla. However, the shortage of such secondary tumors has greatly hampered progress in studies on the cholesterol-cleavage reaction, used as a criterion of endocrinelike behavior. We examined cleavage of C_{21} steroids to C_{19} steroids by using homogenates of tissues, since dilution of isotope by endogenous steroid did not occur in these cases (8).

Steroid Analyses in Urine of Cancer Patients and Controls

One characteristic feature of breast tumor tissue revealed by the above in vitro studies was the presence of a powerful steroid 16α-hydroxylase (6). Accordingly, we analyzed 16-oxygenated-Δ^5-C_{19} steroids in urine of cancer patients and controls, using the selective cleavage of sulfate esters of Δ^5-steroids when the urine was boiled (9). Fractionation into ketonic, neutral, and polar metabolites was made, separation was achieved on silica gel thin-layer chromatography plates, and quantitation was carried out by the method of Shackleton and Mitchell (10) The separated steroids were characterized by comparing the following properties with authentic specimens: chromatography of the free steroids and their acetates, sulfuric acid spectra, spectra in the Eik-Nes reagent, and retention times of trimethylsilyl derivatives on gas chromatography.

Results and Discussion

Using DHEA and pregnenolone as substrates, we established the presence of an isomerase-dehydrogenase system as shown by conversion to Δ^4-androstenedione and progesterone respectively (table 1). The "estriol" fraction of the procedure of working up the incubation mixture, as described by Ryan and Smith (7), contained considerable radioactivity when 4-^{14}C DHEA was used as substrate. The major component of this fraction behaved exactly like estriol on thin-layer chromatography, but was shown not to be identical to this estrogen when the radioactivity remained in the mother liquors on

TABLE 1: CRYSTALLIZATION OF RADIOACTIVE METABOLITES TO CONSTANT SPECIFIC ABILITY

Precursor	Metabolite	Solvent	Original Pool	Specific Activity (counts/min/mg)						
				Crystals			Mother Liquors		
				1	2	3	1	2	3
4-^{14}C DHEA	Androstenedione	Acetone-ligroin	300	290	313	—	273	283	—
4-^{14}C Pregnenolone	Progesterone	Hexane	1,000	936	725	751	1,457	975	731
4-^{14}C Androstenedione		Acetone-ligroin	999	833	785	763	1,154	822	733
4-^{14}C Testosterone	Estriol	Aqueous methanol	1,462	996	900	1,045	1,883	1,074	809

cocrystallization with estriol (6). Identical behavior occurred on cocrystallization with 16-epiestriol. This radioactive metabolite was finally identified as androst-5-ene-3β-16α-17β-triol (α-triol) (6); 16α-hydroxy-DHEA was also identified among the metabolites formed from 4-^{14}C DHEA. The percentage conversion of isotope to labeled metabolites is shown in table 2.

We could not demonstrate conversion of DHEA to estrogen even with microsomal preparations, which are known to transform DHEA to estrogen in the placenta (11). Only 16α-hydroxy-DHEA and α-triol were obtained in this experiment. One factor which might possibly influence the course of transformation to estrogen is the rapid hydroxylation at position 16. Possession of a 16α-hydroxyl group has been reported to inhibit the isomerase-dehydrogenase system (12).

That some of these transformations may occur by the involvement of sulfate esters was of course the original premise on which these experiments were based. It has been suggested that conversion of Δ^5-steroid sulfates, synthesized in the fetus, to estrogens in the placenta involves the preliminary removal of the sulfate ester group (13). We found that a sulfatase capable of hydrolyzing DHEA sulfate was present in homogenates of breast carcinoma tissue (6). This is also demonstrated in table 3, where the metabolism of DHEA and DHEA sulfate is compared in homogenates of primary breast carcinoma and normal tissue from radical mastectomy specimens. Extensive hydrolysis occurs in both cases, but not in the control, using boiled homogenate. A comparison of the relative proportions of metabolites from DHEA and its sulfate ester is also shown. In this experiment the identity of the metabolites is only tentative, since it is based only on the position of radioactive zones on thin-layer chromatograms and is included only for comparison. Some other evidence for the possible involvement of sulfate esters of steroids in biosynthesis arose out of the finding that human breast tumor extracts, when incubated with ^{35}S adenosine-3'-phosphate-5'-phosphosulfate of high specific activity and then chromatographed on paper in two dimensions, yielded a labeled metabolite in the steroid sulfate area of the chromatogram. Upon elution this was identified as cholesteryl ^{35}S sulfate (3, 14). Cholesteryl sulfate occurs in small quantities in bovine adrenals (15) and has been shown to undergo transformation to DHEA ^{35}S sulfate when administered to a patient with an adrenal adenoma (5).

TABLE 2: SUMMARY OF RESULTS CONCERNING TISSUE SPECIMENS AND YIELDS OF METABOLITES

Precursor	Tumor No.	Patient	Pre- or Postmenopausal	Tissue	Metabolite	Conversion (%)
4-¹⁴C DHEA	1	R. McW.	Pre-	Adenocarcinoma (secondary)	Androstenedione α-Triol[a]	0.9 1.2
	2	E. B.	Post-	Adenocarcinoma (secondary)	Androstenedione α-Triol[a]	0.7 6.8
	3	P. C.	Post-	Adenocarcinoma (primary)	Androstenedione α-Triol[a]	0.7 4.1
	4	M. M.	Post-	Schirrous (secondary)	Androstenedione α-Triol[a]	1.3 2.2
	5	L. S.	Post-	Poorly differentiated	16α-Hydroxy DHEA α-Triol	5.4[b] 4.3[b]
4-¹⁴C Pregnenolone		M. C.	Post-	Adenocarcinoma (secondary)	Progesterone 3 neutral polar steroids	1.3 8.0
4-¹⁴C Testosterone		J. M.	Post-	Mucus-secreting adenocarcinoma	Androstenedione 16α-Hydroxytestosterone Estriol	0.6 0.2 0.2

[a] An additional component tentatively identified as the 16α-hydroxy DHEA was present in the neutral fraction in about half the concentration of the α-Triol.
[b] Microsome preparation used.

TABLE 3: COMPARISON OF THE METABOLISM OF $(7\alpha$-^{3}H$)$ DHEA SULFATE AND $(7\alpha$-^{3}H$)$ DHEA

Patient	Diagnosis	Substrate Used	% Radioactivity Recovered in Fractions "Conjugated"	% Radioactivity Recovered in Fractions "Free"	DHEA Sulfate	DHEA	16α-Hydroxy-DHEA Sulfate	16α-Hydroxy-DHEA	α-Triol Sulfate	α-Triol	Androstenediol Sulfate	Androstenediol
F.S.	Breast carcinoma	$(7\alpha$-^{3}H$)$ DHEA sulfate	29	52	++++	+++++	0	++	0	0	++	++
F.S.	Breast carcinoma	$(7\alpha$-^{3}H$)$ DHEA	4	81	++	++++++	0	0	0	++	++	+
Control		$(7\alpha$-^{3}H$)$ DHEA sulfate	80	1	++++++	+	0	0	0	0	0	0
K. K.	Normal breast	$(7\alpha$-^{3}H$)$ DHEA sulfate	47	28	+++++	++++	0	0	0	0	+	0
O. T.	Normal breast	$(7\alpha$-^{3}H$)$ DHEA sulfate	52	40	+++++	++++	0	++	0	0	+	0

NOTE: Minced preparations were used in Krebs-Ringer bicarbonate glucose medium (10 ml to 2 g tissue). Flasks contained 30 mµmole of $(7\alpha$-^{3}H$)$ DHEA or $(7\alpha$-^{3}H$)$ DHEA sulfate (s.a. 0.48 µc/µmole for both steroids). Incubation time was 3 hr with shaking in carbogen. In a control experiment $(7\alpha$-^{3}H$)$ DHEA sulfate was incubated with 10 ml of tissue preparation, previously heated at 100° for 5 min. After addition of carrier steroids, separation into neutral and conjugated steroid fractions was as described by Fahmy et al. (48).

Aromatase System

On incubation in air with 4-^{14}C testosterone in the presence of NADPH, breast tumor microsomes yielded Δ4-androstenedione, identified by its chromatographic behavior and by cocrystallization with authentic material (table 1). Another metabolite was identified as 16α-hydroxytestosterone. Its identification was based on comparison of chromatographic properties of the free steroid and its acetate with authentic material, and by the constancy of specific activity determinations on mixing with reference material, followed by chromatography in three systems. Sufficient reference compound was not available for cocrystallization studies. The radioactive metabolite in the "estriol" fraction behaved exactly like estriol on prolonged paper chromatography (72 hr) in propylene glycol/ligroin, and again after elution and thin-layer chromatography. It was identified as estriol by cocrystallization (table 1). Although the isomerase-dehydrogenase for conversion of Δ^5-C_{19} steroids to Δ^4-C_{19} steroids is reversible (16), and therefore the "estriol" fraction could theoretically contain some α-triol, it was shown previously that radioactive α-triol did not cocrystallize with estriol; virtually all the counts remained in the mother liquors in the first crystallization. Jones et al. (17) recently described how a breast tumor slice preparation, when incubated with labeled testosterone without added cofactors, failed to form estriol. They suggested that the estriol formed in the experiment shown in table 1 could have been α-triol. However, in view of the above remarks, this suggestion would be untenable. It is of considerable interest that these authors described the conversion of DHEA to 16α-hydroxytestosterone, and they also obtained some evidence for estrone formation. Conversion in vitro of C_{19} to C_{18} steroids by breast cancer tissue is described in this volume by Dao, Varela, and Morreal (chap 10).

Desmolase Activity

Ability to convert cholesterol to pregnenolone, and thence to physiologically active steroid hormones, is confined to the endocrine organs, adrenal, ovary, and testes, and to the placenta (18). This cleavage reaction is catalyzed by a C_{27} desmolase. We examined human breast carcinoma tissue for the presence of this enzyme system in order to further explore its "endocrinelike" properties (8). Early experiments using 4-^{14}C cholesterol and breast tumor homogenates were not very rewarding, but in one case We obtained a labeled metabolite with chromatographic properties resembling pregnenolone. As was previously mentioned, dilution of labeled cholesterol by endogenous cholesterol may have been responsible for failure to demonstrate this reaction. Mitochrondrial preparations, which contain the enzyme system in steroid-producing endocrine tissue, were then isolated and examined. Tables 4 and 5 demonstrate the formation of pregnenolone from secondary breast carcinoma obtained from axillary lymph nodes. In the first instance a mitochondrial fraction was used, and the pregnenolone peak was eluted from the chromatogram (propylene glycol/ligroin), rechromatographed in a different system, and finally cocrystallized with pregnenolone. In the second instance, slices of secondary tumor were employed and the pregnenolone peak was eluted, acetylated, rerun in the same system, and then chromatographed twice in the Bush A system. The radioactive zone corresponding to pregnenolone acetate was eluted and cocrystallized with carrier. Percentage conversion of labeled cholesterol to pregnenolone in these two cases was about 0.5 and 0.2, respectively. Some evidence for estriol formation was also obtained in this experiment, as judged by persistency of radioactivity during cocrystallization of the eluate of a radioactive peak, which corresponded to estriol on thin-layer chromatography of the polar fraction, obtained from the incubation. Because of the predominately fibrous nature of normal breast tissue (obtained from radical mastectomy specimens), particulate fractions which contained significant proportions of mitochondria could not be obtained. Since the C_{27}-desmolase which occurs in adrenal mitochondria can be solubilized by acetone treatment (19), such treatment would also serve to remove endogenous cholesterol which could reduce the sensitivity of detection of the desmolase. A preparation derived by acetone treatment of a homogenate of normal breast tissue yielded a radioactive metabolite which was similar to pregnenolone chromatographically, both as free steroid and as acetate, but which could not be satisfactorily characterized by cocrystallization data (8). Although it was claimed at the time that pregnenolone had been formed, and thus that the C_{27}-desmolase was not confined to the tumor, we feel that this interpretation was premature and that the question whether normal breast tissue is similar to breast tumor in endocrinelike properties is still unresolved. Some further evidence for the presence of the C_{27}-desmolase was obtained using 26-^{14}C cholesterol and mitochondria derived from secondary breast

TABLE 4: DESMOLASE ACTIVITY OF BREAST CANCER TISSUE: ISOLATION OF METABOLITES BY PAPER CHROMATOGRAPHY

				Specific Activity (dpm/mg)							
			Original Pool	Crystals					Mother Liquors		
Precursor	Tissue	Metabolite		1	2	3	4	5	1	2	3	4
4-^{14}C Cholesterol	Secondary breast cancer particulate fraction	Pregnenolone	2,300	701	797	760	748	—	3,700	903	1,100	767
4-^{14}C Cholesterol	Secondary breast cancer slices	Pregnenolone (as acetate)	—	1,345	1,265	1,405	1,470	—	8,270	1,460	1,285	1,180
7α-^{3}H 17α-Hydroxy-progesterone	Secondary breast cancer homogenate	Androstene-dione	28,400	21,000	17,900	14,300	15,000	15,300	31,500	33,400	22,600	15,500

tumor. Experimental procedures for preparing mitochondria, etc., and conditions of incubation were as described by Ichii, Forchielli, and Dorfman (20). Steam distillation and fractionation of volatile metabolites were as described by Menon et al. (21). Results are shown in table 5. Although isocaproic acid is normally the main volatile product from the side-chain cleavage of cholesterol, it has been shown that the immediate product in, for example, the adrenal gland, is the aldehyde (22). Results suggest that the aldehyde is formed with

TABLE 5: DESMOLASE ACTIVITY OF BREAST CANCER TISSUE: RADIOACTIVITY IN STEAM VOLATILE FRACTIONS USING 26-^{14}C CHOLESTEROL

			Radioactivity (dpm)	
Precursor	Tissue	HCG[a]	Alkali-Soluble	Alkali-Insoluble
26-^{14}C Cholesterol	Secondary breast cancer mitochondria	— +	1,800 700	3,500 11,100
26-^{14}C Cholesterol	Primary breast cancer acetone powder	— +	70 20	4,500 5,400

[a] Human chorionic gonadotrophin (Sigma, 100 IU) in 2 ml of incubation mixture.

the breast tumor mitochondria and there is only limited conversion to the acid. Adding human chorionic gonadotrophin appears to be effective in stimulating side-chain cleavage of cholesterol. It should be emphasized, however, that lack of suitable secondary tumor specimens has prevented confirmation of this effect of chorionic gonadotrophin and chemical verification of whether the aldehyde is formed. We have included results of this particular experiment in the hope that someone with access to a better supply of human secondary breast tumors will be interested enough to seek confirmation.

Cleavage of 7α-^{3}H 17α-hydroxyprogesterone to Δ^4-androstenedione by a C$_{21}$-desmolase was also demonstrated in homogenates of secondary breast carcinoma (table 4). This metabolite was accompanied by 17α, 20α-dihydroxypregn-4-en-3-one and its 17α, 20β-epimer. Unlike C$_{27}$-desmolase, which is confined to steroid-producing endocrine organs, the C$_{21}$-desmolase, although present in these organs, also occurs in the liver (18).

CONVERSION OF ACETATE TO CHOLESTEROL

We examined the ability of breast tumor tissue to incorporate labeled acetate and mevalonate into steroids by using slices of primary and secondary tumors in Krebs-Ringer phosphate buffer, without added cofactors. After incubation, carrier steroids were added and subsequent partitioning into various fractions was carried out as described previously (6). There was low incorporation of radioactivity into these fractions with labeled mevalonate. This parallels results obtained with endocrine tissues (23). Unidentified polar metabolites were present in the "neutral" fraction from incubations with labeled acetate. The "pentane" fraction contained radioactive material with the chromatographic mobility, on paper, of cholesterol in the system propylene glycol/ligroin, although this area was sometimes compounded of more than one peak on scanning. Results of specific activity determinations, obtained after elution, chromatography on alumina, bromination and debromination, and cocrystallization with cholesterol, are shown for one case in table 6. In all but one of the primary tumors incubated with labeled acetate, the alkali-soluble fraction contained an unidentified metabolite with an R_F value of 0.35 (estradiol 0.70; estrone 0.85) upon thin-layer chromatography in cyclohexane: ethylacetate (1:1).

Figure 1 summarizes the steroid conversions discussed above. Results of experiments on the metabolism of 4-^{14}C estradiol by breast tumor mince preparations (carried out under conditions similar to those used for 4-^{14}C DHEA[6]) are also shown. Characterization of these metabolites is only tentative and was confined to comparison with authentic substances in a number of chromatographic systems.

STUDIES ON 16-HYDROXYLATED-Δ^5-C_{19} STEROIDS IN URINE

A significant increase in urinary estriol occurs in postmenopausal women with breast cancer (24, 25, 26, 27, 28). Marmorston et al. (28) suggested that this specific elevation in estriol could reflect a process in which estriol is formed directly, that is, is not in direct equilibrium with estrone and estradiol. One such pathway is known: the formation of estriol from 16α-hydroxylated-Δ^5-C_{19} steroids in the fetal/placental unit. Because of the marked ability of breast cancer tissue to form 16α-hydroxylated products from DHEA, the determination of such compounds was made in the urine of breast cancer patients and controls (9). It was indeed found that α-triol, which was formed

TABLE 6: CONVERSION OF U-^{14}C ACETATE TO CHOLESTEROL IN BREAST CANCER IN VITRO

			Specific Activity (dpm/mg)							
		Original Pool	Crystals				Mother Liquors			
Precursor	Tissue	Metabolite		1	2	3	4	1	2	3	4
U-^{14}C Acetate	Primary breast cancer slices	Cholesterol	484	486	466	446	425	470	495	530	—

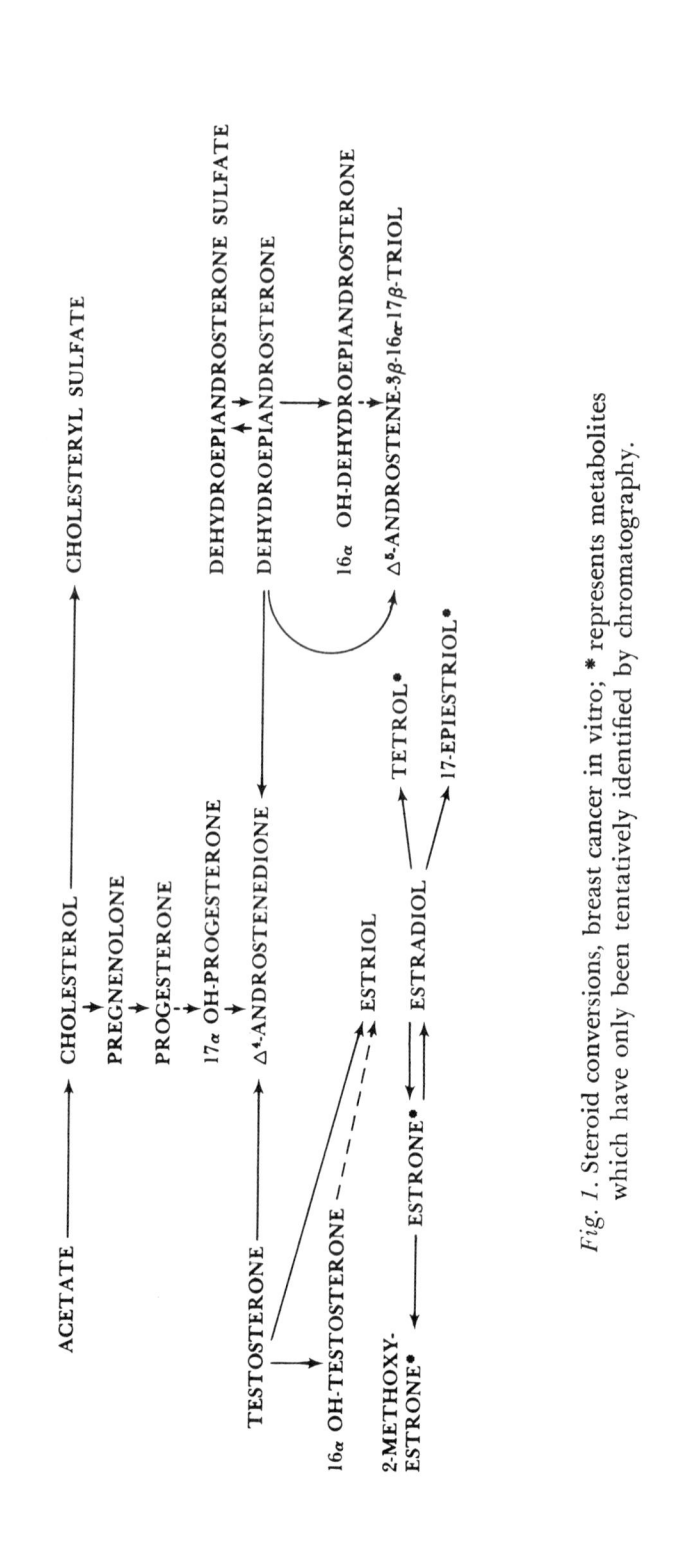

ACETATE → CHOLESTEROL → CHOLESTERYL SULFATE

PREGNENOLONE

PROGESTERONE

17α OH-PROGESTERONE

DEHYDROEPIANDROSTERONE SULFATE

DEHYDROEPIANDROSTERONE

TESTOSTERONE → Δ⁴-ANDROSTENEDIONE

16α OH-DEHYDROEPIANDROSTERONE

Δ⁵-ANDROSTENE-3β-16α-17β-TRIOL

ESTRIOL

TETROL*

17-EPIESTRIOL*

ESTRADIOL

16α OH-TESTOSTERONE

ESTRONE*

2-METHOXY-ESTRONE*

Fig. 1. Steroid conversions, breast cancer in vitro; * represents metabolites which have only been tentatively identified by chromatography.

Paraendocrine Behavior of Human Breast Cancer

in greatest yield among the metabolites of ^{14}C DHEA in vitro, was significantly increased in the urine of premenopausal breast cancer patients and subjects with benign breast disease (Figs. 2, 4a). When this was expressed as a ratio of α-triol to the sum of DHEA, 16α-hydroxy-DHEA, and 16-oxoandrostenediol, controls had values less than 1 and the cancer and benign group had values, with one exception, greater than 1 (Fig. 4b). In postmenopausal women the

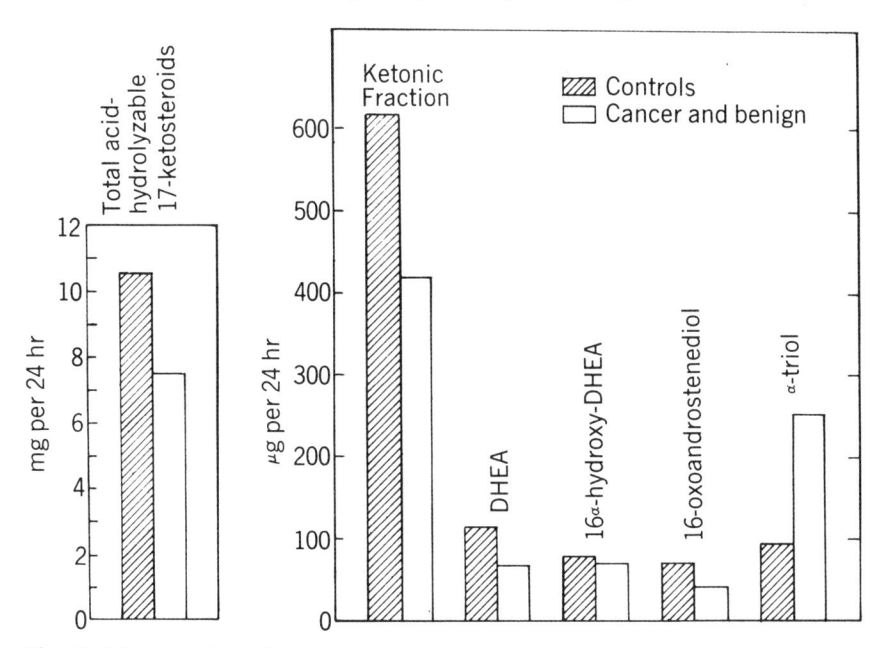

Fig. 2. Mean values in premenopausal women of urinary acid-hydrolyzable 17-ketosteroids (*left*) and 3β-hydroxy-Δ⁵-steroids formed from ester sulfates by boiling the urine samples (*right*).

α-triol levels, and the above ratios, were not significantly different from those of controls (Figs. 3, 5). However, there was a trend in the same direction as the premenopausal group. Thus a correlation was established between the in vitro studies and the situation in vivo, but of course did not establish that breast cancer tissue was responsible for the increased urinary levels of α-triol or estriol. When DHEA sulfate was given by infusion to an oophorectomized, adrenalectomized breast cancer subject, then α-triol, which was not detectable in the urine before infusion, appeared in substantial amount (table 7). In a similar experiment conducted later on the same patient, the level of estriol in the urine also increased after infusion. This will be discussed later. The formation of α-triol in the above experiment thus eliminated the ovaries and adrenals as unique sites of synthesis—the liver or peripheral sites or both, including breast tumor and normal breast, could then be implicated. One very interesting finding was the presence of DHEA, 16α-hydroxy-DHEA, and 16-oxoandrostenediol in the urine of this patient before

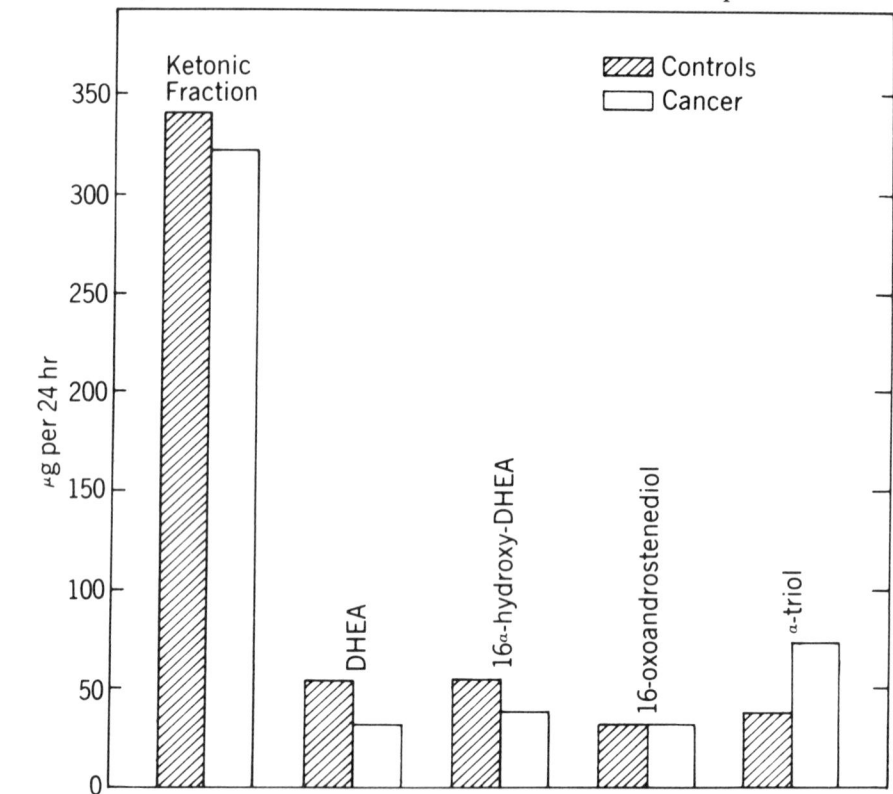

Fig. 3. Mean values of urinary 3β-hydroxy-Δ⁵-steroids in postmenopausal women.

infusion (table 7). The source of these steroids is unknown. Cortisone was used to maintain the patient, but the above compounds are not among the known metabolites of cortisone.

The effect of radical mastectomy on the urinary levels of DHEA and its 16-oxygenated derivatives was examined next. In three patients studied, there was an increase in the sum of Δ^5-C_{19} steroids analyzed 1 wk postoperatively, and this increase was reflected in the 16-oxygenated derivatives, DHEA remaining near preoperative levels. One subject was studied for 16 wk postoperatively and results

Paraendocrine Behavior of Human Breast Cancer

are shown in figure 6. It can be observed that the total Δ^5-C_{19} steroids remained high for a considerable time postoperatively and did not return to preoperative levels until sometime after the 10th wk. This result is complicated by the possible effects of radiotherapy, which continued for 4 wk, commencing 1 wk postoperatively. Nevertheless,

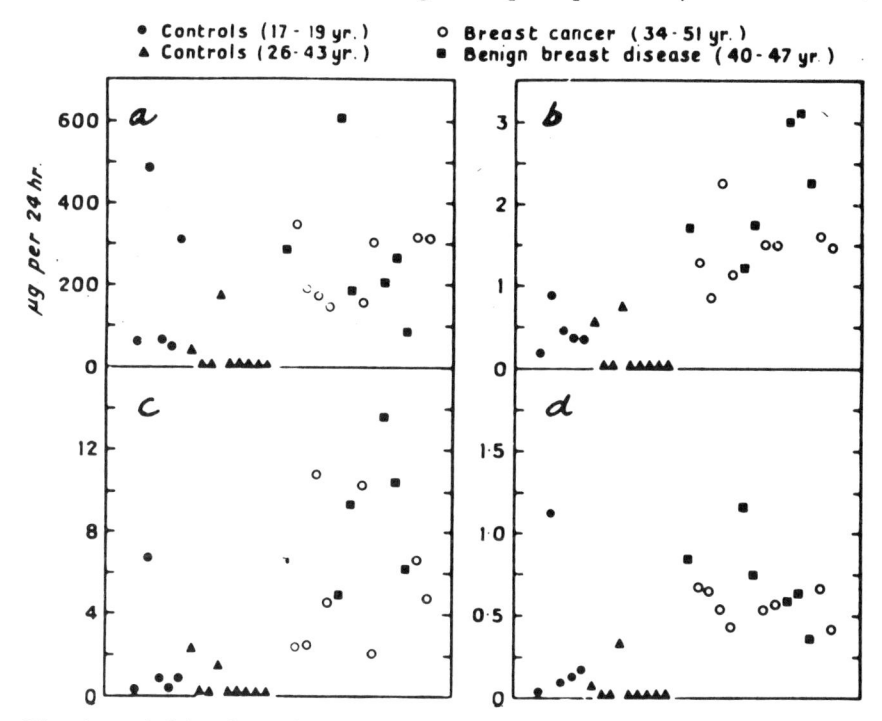

Fig. 4. α-triol levels and ratios in premenopausal women; (*a*) individual values for urinary α-triol; (*b*) α-triol expressed as ratios to the sum of DHEA, 16α-hydroxy-DHEA, and 16-oxoandrostenediol; (*c*) α-triol as ratio to DHEA; (*d*) α-triol as ratio to the ketonic fraction determined colorimetrically. Individual values have been plotted in the same sequence along the abscissa for comparison.

it appears that stress can cause increased adrenal secretion of DHEA, which is metabolized, probably to the greatest degree in the liver, to 16-oxygenated derivatives. Thus we might reason that increased urinary levels of α-triol, and the high ratios of α-triol to DHEA, as shown in figures 2–5, could reflect a stress phenomenon already present in the cancer patients and subjects with benign breast disease. An increased miscible pool of cortisol in advanced breast cancer was demonstrated by Jensen et al. (29), and was shown to be due to a higher production rate. These authors concluded that such patients were being subjected to considerable stress, or, alternatively, that ectopic production of corticotrophin by tumor tissue was involved. Bulbrook (30) noted that mastectomy had a persistent effect, lasting many months, on urinary 11-deoxy-17-oxosteroids and 17-hydroxycorticosteroids and also on the discriminant function, based on the ratio of the former to the latter. This varied from a persistent depression of the discriminant for 17 mo after mastectomy to a rebound at 18 and 31 mo, after a prolonged period of depression of the discriminant. If the lowered levels of 11-deoxy-17-oxosteroids relative to 17-hydroxycorticosteroids in breast cancer is due to altered activity of adrenal C_{21}-desmolase (31), then changes in the discriminant after mastectomy suggest that there is some interplay

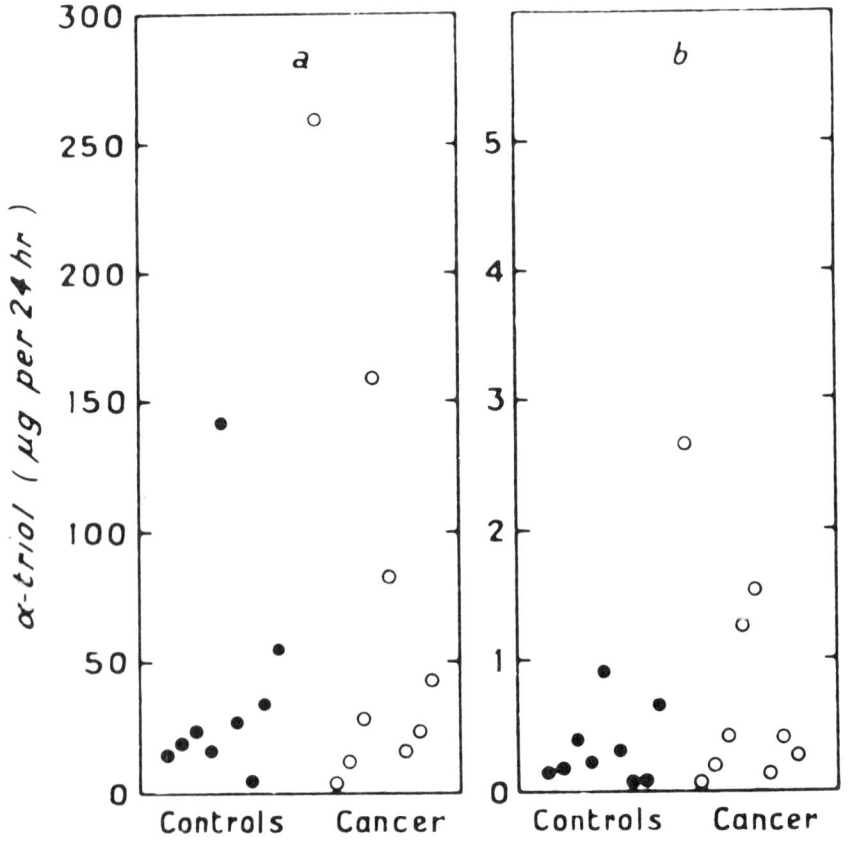

Fig. 5. Individual values in postmenopausal controls and breast cancer patients (see fig. 4): (*a*) urinary α-triol; (*b*) ratio of α-triol to DHEA plus 16α-hydroxy-DHEA plus 16-oxoandrostenediol.

TABLE 7: URINARY ANALYSIS OF 3β-HYDROXY-Δ^5-STEROIDS IN AN ADRENAL-ECTOMIZED AND CASTRATED WOMAN BEFORE AND AFTER INFUSION OF DHEA SULPHATE

Treatment	Urinary Steroids (μg/ 24 hr)					
	Ketonic Fraction	DHEA	16α-Hydroxy-DHEA	16-Oxo-DHEA	α-Triol	β-Triol[a]
Before infusion	120	30	24	17	0	0
After infusion of 110 mg DHEA sulphate/ 24 hr:						
Day 1	1,200	630	470	90	960	166
Day 2	1,000	540	320	85	920	196

[a] Androst-5-ene-3β-16β-17β-triol tentatively identified by chromatographic comparison with authentic material.

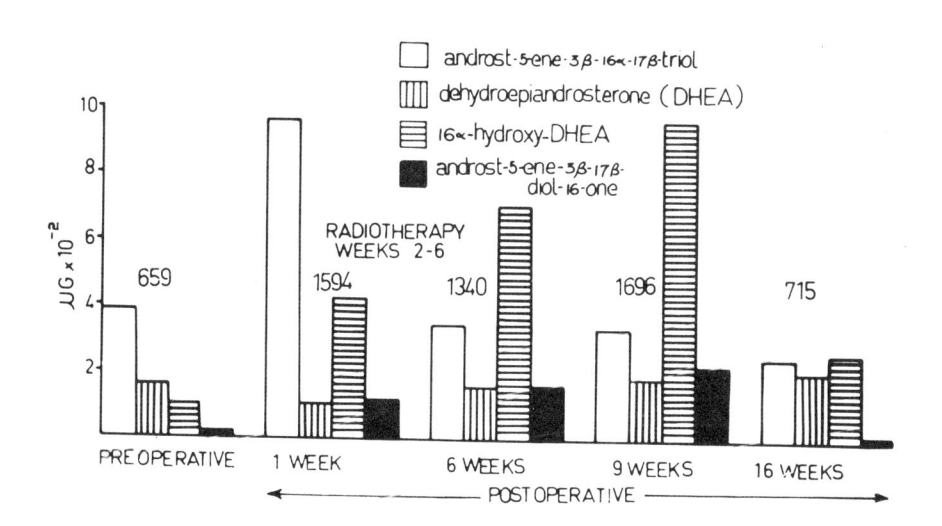

Fig. 6. Effect of mastectomy on urinary Δ^5-C_{19} steroids. Steroids were estimated as in fig. 2. The patient was 41 years old and had not received treatment before radical mastectomy. Numbers represent the sum total of the steroids indicated.

between breast tumor and adrenal cortex, or between the breast and adrenal cortex. If so, this could be by way of production of steroid, or some trophic factor, perhaps influencing adrenal synthesis of DHEA sulfate.

Estrogens are known to persist in the urine of breast cancer patients after oophorectomy and adrenalectomy. Conversion of

TABLE 8: URINARY ESTROGENS BEFORE AND AFTER INFUSION OF DEHYDROEPIANDROSTERONE SULFATE TO OOPHORECTOMIZED, ADRENALECTOMIZED SUBJECTS WITH BREAST CANCER

| | μg/24 hr ||||
Condition	Estrone	Estradiol	Estriol	Total
Before infusion	0.23	0.17	0.14	0.54
After infusion...	1.96	0.42	1.22	3.60
20 Postmenopausal women[a]				
Mean	1.0	0.3	3.6	4.9
Range	0.4–2.0	0.1–0.6	1.0–6.2	1.7–8.5
20 Postmenopausal or oophorectomized women after adrenalectomy[a]				
Mean	0.075	0.046	0.24	0.36
Range	0.02–0.20	0.01–0.12	0.06–0.43	0.12–0.75

[a] Unpublished data, J. B. Brown, F. I. R. Martin, and W. J. Moon, from 20 normal post-menopausal women and 20 women with breast cancer after adrenalectomy.
Infusion of DHEA sulfate (55 mg/day) was carried out for 14 days and estrogen measured on a 24-hr urine collected on days 13 to 14. Adams and Brown (49).

administered testosterone to estrogen has been shown to occur in such subjects (32, 33), and Chang and Dao (34) demonstrated conversion of ^{14}C cortisone to 11β-hydroxyestrone and 11β-hydroxyestradiol. Table 8 shows results on estrogens in the urine of an oophorectomized, adrenalectomized breast cancer patient before and after infusion of DHEA sulfate. After infusion the levels are increased, predominately into estrone and estriol, and fall into the range determined on twenty normal postmenopausal women. The increase in estrogen excretion is equivalent to a yield of approximately 0.006%.

Results reported here show that dehydroepiandrosterone sulfate can be converted to estrogen by peripheral tissue. Breast cancer tissue contains both 3β-hydroxy-Δ^5 steroid isomerase-dehydrogenase and aromatase systems and could contribute to this transformation. The liver is distinctly possible as a site for aromatization, but although human fetal liver is able to convert androgen to estrogen (35) this property is apparently not shared by adult human liver (36). However, it is doubtful that conversions as low as those reported here would have been detected by the methods employed. The presence of an undefined peripheral aromatase system is also implicated by the finding that the estrogenic activity of dehydroepiandrosterone sulfate in rats, as measured by uterotrophic response, is not affected by oophorectomy and adrenalectomy (37). Skin tissue has been shown to transform dehydroepiandrosterone to testosterone (38, 39). Oertel and Treiber (40) claimed that skin tissue may be able to metabolize C_{19} steroids, such as dehydroepiandrosterone, to estrogens. This was based on the observation that, after a male subject was perfused with 7α-^{3}H-dehydroepiandrosterone ^{35}S sulfate, double-labeled C_{19} and C_{18} steroids were present in skin extracts which differed from the usual pattern found in peripheral plasma.

CONCLUSIONS

Paraendocrine behavior of human tumors is a well-recognized phenomenon, but apart from the carcinoid syndrome it appears to be associated with clinical manifestations suggestive of polypeptide hormone or chorionic gonadotrophin secretion (41, 42, 43, 44). Evidence for the direct production of a hormone identical to ACTH by bronchogenic carcinoma is substantial (43). The paraendocrine behavior of human breast carcinoma is the first instance of a tumor associated with steroid hormone production. However, a corticosteroidlike substance was produced by transplanted prostatic squamous-cell carcinoma after ACTH stimulation in the rat (45). It seems quite possible that steroidogenesis in breast cancer could explain the development of hormone independence. The question is immediately raised, however, whether we are dealing with dedifferentiation by the tumor cell or, alternatively, with a manifestation of an activity which may perhaps normally occur at some stage in the life span of the gland, for example, in pregnancy or lactation, since the biosynthetic directive seems to be toward steroid hormones associated with this state. Again, the changes in structure which take place in the mammary gland during the normal menstrual cycle could conceivably be partially controlled by localized steroid hormone production, or utilization of circulating prehormones as defined by Baird et al. (46). While speculating on the possibility that the normal breast may on occasion possess endocrinelike properties, could the onset of the menopause, for example, result in a "triggering" mechanism effective on mammary tissue as a result of the altered hormonal milieu and increased gonadotrophin levels? Luteinizing hormone has recently been shown to be markedly increased in the premenopausal state (47). Could response to this stimulation be a contributing factor toward the onset of malignancy? We know that menopausal status has a dramatic effect on response to oophorectomy, adrenalectomy, or hypophysectomy in breast cancer patients with negative discriminants. In premenopausal subjects, as in subjects 6 or more yr postmenopausal with negative discriminants, a 20% regression rate was observed, whereas the regression rate was nil in subjects 1–6 yr after menopause (30).

It is important that this question whether normal mammary tissue has potential endocrine properties be settled, since an answer would help to define more clearly the factors involved in neoplastic change in the human mammary gland and perhaps would open up new approaches for control and treatment.

ADDENDUM

The extent of hydrolysis of sulfate esters of 3β-hydroxy-C_{19}–Δ^5 steroids on boiling urine samples and the recovery of the liberated free steroids have been determined under the controlled conditions used in the analysis of these compounds. The urinary levels of 16α-hydroxy-C_{19}-Δ^5 steroids as presented in figs. 2, 3, 4, 5, and 6 in table 7 should be multiplied by a factor of approximately 3.4 to adjust them to absolute values.

References

1. Adams, J. B. 1954. *The role of the stroma in tumor spread and invasion.* New State Cancer Council Special Unit for Investigation and Treatment, publication no. 10, p. 18. Sydney: Australasian Medical Publishing Co.
2. ———. 1964. Enzymic synthesis of steroid sulphates. I. Sulphation of steroids by human adrenal extracts. *Biochim. Biophys. Acta* 82: 572.

3. ———. 1964. Enzymic synthesis of steroid sulphates. II. Presence of steroid sulfokinase in human mammary carcinoma extracts. *J. Clin. Endocr.* 24: 988.
4. Baulieu, E. E. 1962. Studies of conjugated 17-ketosteroids in a case of adrenal tumor. *J. Clin. Endocr.* 22: 501.
5. Roberts, K. D.; Bandy, L.; Calvin, H. I., Drucker, W. D.; and Lieberman, S. 1964. Evidence that steroid sulphates serve as biosynthetic intermediates. IV. Conversion of cholesterol sulphate *in vivo* to urinary C_{19} to C_{21} steroidal sulphates. *Biochemistry* 3: 1983.
6. Adams, J. B., and Wong, M. S. F. 1968. Paraendocrine behavior of human breast carcinoma: *In vitro* transformation of steroids to physiologically active hormones. *J. Endocr.* 41: 41.
7. Ryan, K. J., and Smith, O. W. 1961. Biogenesis of estrogens by human ovary. I. Conversion of acetate-1-^{14}C to estrone and estradiol. *J. Biol. Chem.* 236: 705.
8. Adams, J. B., and Wong, M. S. F. Desmolase activity of normal and malignant human breast tissue. *J. Endocr.* 44: 69.
9. ———. 1968. Correlation between urinary steroid metabolites and pathways of steroidogenesis in human breast tumor tissue. *Lancet* 2: 1163.
10. Shackleton, C. H. L., and Mitchell, F. L. 1967. The measurement of 3β-hydroxy-Δ^5 steroids in human fetal blood, amniotic fluid, infant urine, and adult urine. *Steroids* 10: 359.
11. Ryan, K. J. 1959. Biological aromatization of steroids. *J. Biol. Chem.* 234: 268.
12. Younglai, E., and Solomon, S. 1966. The *in vivo* metabolism of 16α-hydroxydehydroisoandrosterone. *Fed. Proc.* 25: 281.
13. Pulkkinen, M. O. 1961. Arylsulphatase and the hydrolysis of some steroid sulphates in developing organism and placenta. *Acta Physiol. Scand.* 52, suppl. 180.
14. Adams, J. B., and Wong M. S. F. 1968. Enzymic synthesis of steroid sulfates. VI. Formation of cholesteryl-3 ^{35}S-sulfate in incubation of human breast carcinoma extracts with adenosine-3′-phosphate-5′-phospho-^{35}S-sulfate. *Steroids* 11: 313.
15. Drayer, N. M.; Roberts, K. D.; Bandy, L.; and Leiberman, S. 1964. Isolation of cholesterol sulfate from bovine adrenals. *J. Biol. Chem.* 239: 3112.
16. Ward, M. G., and Engel, L. L. 1964. Reversal of the 3β-hyroxysteroid dehydrogenase-isomerase reactions: Conversion of androst-4-ene-3,17-dione-4-C^{14} to 3β-hydroxyandrost-4-en-17-one-^{14}C and 3β-hydroxyandrost-5-en-17-one-^{14}C. *J. Biol. Chem.* 239: 3604.
17. Jones, D.; Cameron, E. H. D.; Griffiths, K.; Gleave, E. N.; and Forrest, A. P. M. 1970. Steroid metabolism by human breast tumors. *Biochem. J.* 116: 919.
18. Dorfman, R. I., and Ungar, F. 1965. *Metabolism of steroid hormones.* New York and London: Academic Press.

19. Halkerston, I. D. K.; Eichhorn, T.; and Hechter, O. 1961. A requirement for reduced triphosphopyridine nucleotide for cholesterol side-chain cleavage by mitochondrial fractions of bovine adrenal cortex. *J. Biol. Chem.* 236: 374.
20. Ichii, S.; Forchielli, E.; and Dorfman, R. I. 1963. In vivo effect of gonadotrophins on the soluble cholesterol side-chain cleaving enzyme system of bovine corpus luteum. *Steroids* 2: 631.
21. Menon, K. M. J.; Drosdowsky, M.; Dorfman, R. I.; and Forchielli, E. 1965. Side-chain cleavage of cholesterol-26-^{14}C and 20α-hydroxycholesterol-22-^{14}C by rat testis mitochondrial preparations and the effects of gonadotrophin administration and hypophysectomy. *Steroids*, suppl. 1: 95.
22. Constantopoulos, G.; and Tchen, T. T. 1961. Cleavage of cholesterol side-chain by adrenal cortex. I. Cofactor requirement and product of cleavage. *J. Biol. Chem.* 236: 65.
23. Bryson, M. J., and Sweat, M. L. 1962. Is mevalonic acid a precursor of the corticosteroids? *Arch. Biochem. Biophys.* 96: 1.
24. Brown, J. B. 1958. Urinary oestrogen excretion in the study of mammary cancer. In *Endocrine aspects of breast cancer*, ed. A. R. Currie, p. 197. London: E. and S. Livingstone.
25. Nissen-Meyer, R., and Sanner, T. 1963. The excretion of oestrone pregnanediol and pregnanetriol in breast cancer patients. *Acta Endocr. (Kbh.)* 44: 334.
26. Persson, B. H., and Risholm, L. 1964. Oophorectomy and cortisone treatment as a method of eliminating oestrogen production in patients with breast cancer. *Acta Endocr. (Kbh.)* 47: 15.
27. Stern, E.; Hopkins, C. E.; Weiner, J. M.; and Marmorston, J. 1964. Hormone excretion patterns in breast and prostate cancer are abnormal. *Science* 145: 716.
28. Marmorston, J.; Crowley, L. G.; Myers, S. M.; Stern, E.; and Hopkins, C. E. 1965. Urinary excretion of estrone, estradiol and estriol by patients with breast cancer and benign breast disease. *Amer. J. Obstet. Gynec.* 92: 460.
29. Jensen, V.; Deshpande, N.; Bulbrook, R. D.; and Doouss, T. W. 1968. Adrenal function in breast cancer: Production and metabolic clearance rate of cortisol in patients with early or advanced breast cancer and in normal women. *J. Endocr.* 42: 425.
30. Bulbrook, R. D. 1967. Endocrine studies in patients with advanced breast cancer. In *Current concepts in breast cancer.* ed. A. Segaloff, K. K. Meyer, and S. DeBakey, p. 139. Baltimore: Williams and Wilkins.
31. Doouss, T. W., and Desphande, N. 1968. *In vivo* perfusion of the human adrenal gland and ovary in patients with mammary cancer. *Brit. J. Surg.* 55: 673.
32. West, C. D.; Damast, B. L.; Sarro, S. D.; and Pearson, O. H. 1956.

Conversion of testosterone to estrogens in castrated, adrenalectomized human females. *J. Biol. Chem.* 218: 409.
33. Dao, T., and Morreal, C. E. 1968. Isolation and identification of estriol in urine of castrated and adrenalectomized women receiving 4-C^{14} testosterone. *Steroids* 12: 651.
34. Chang, E., and Dao, T. 1961. Adrenal estrogens. I. Conversion of 4-C^{14} cortisone acetate to 11-oxygenated estrogens in women. *J. Clin. Endocr.* 21: 624.
35. Slaunwhite, W. R.; Karsay, M. A.; Hollmer, A; Sandberg, A. A; and Niswander, K. 1956. Fetal liver as an endocrine tissue. *Steroids,* suppl. 11: 211.
36. Slaunwhite, W. R.; Karsay, M.A.; and Sandberg, A. A. 1966. *In vivo* biosynthetic reaction of human adult liver. In *Second International Congress on hormonal steroids,* International Congress Series no. 111, ed. E. B. Romanoff and L. Martin. *Excerpta Med. Foundation,* abst. no. 285.
37. Harper, M. J. K. 1969. Estrogenic effects of dehydroepiandrosterone and its sulfate in cats. *Endocrinology* 84: 229.
38. Cameron, E. H. D.; Baillie, A. H.; and Grant, J. F. 1966. Transformation *in vitro* of [7 —^{3}H] DHEA to [^{3}H] testosterone by skin from men. *J. Endocr.* 35: xix.
39. Gallegos, A. J., and Berliner, D. L. 1967. Transformation and conjugation of dehydroepiandrosterone by human skin. *J. Clin. Endocr.* 27: 1214.
40. Oertel, G. W., and Treiber, L. 1969. Metabolism and excretion of C_{19} and C_{18} steroids by human skin. *Europ. J. Biochem.* 7: 234.
41. McArthur, J. 1963. Para-endocrine phenomena in obstetrics and gynecology. In *Progress in gynaecology,* ed. J. V. Meigs and S. H. Sturgis, p. 146. New York: Grune and Stratton.
42. Lipsett, M. B.; Odell, W. D.; Rosenberg, L. E.; and Waldmann, T. A. 1964. Humoral syndromes associated with nonendocrine tumors. *Ann. Intern. Med.* 61: 733.
43. Bower, B. F., and Gordan, G. S. 1965. Hormonal effects of nonendocrine tumors. *Ann. Rev. Med.* 16: 83.
44. Hobbs, C. G., and Miller, A. C. 1966. Review of endocrine syndromes associated with tumors of non-endocrine origin. *J. Clin. Path.* 19: 119.
45. Sediyama, S.; Hirai, M.; and Pincus, G. 1966. Release of corticosterone-like substance from a transplanted prostatic squamous cell carcinoma after exogenous ACTH stimulation. In *Second International Congress on hormonal steroids,* International Congress Series no. 111, ed. E. B. Romanoff and L. Martin. *Excerpta Med. Foundation,* abst. no. 603.
46. Baird, D.; Horton, R.; Longcope, C.; and Tait, J. F. 1968. Steroid prehormones. *Perspect. Biol. Med.* 11: 384.
47. Dove, G. A.; Papanicolaou, A. D.; Adamopoulos, D.; Loraine, J. A.;

Mackay Mairi, A.; and Lunn, S. F. 1969. Further studies on endocrine function in perimenopausal women with special reference to the excretion of follicle-stimulating hormone (FSH) and luteinising hormone (LH). *Acta Endocr. (Kbh.)*, suppl. 138: 225.

48. Fahmy, D.; Griffiths, K.; Turnbull, A. C.; and Symington, T. 1968. A comparison of the metabolism in vitro of [7α—^{3}H] DHEA sulfate and [4—^{14}C] pregnenolone by tissue from a hilus cell tumor of the ovary. *J. Endocr.* 41: 61.

49. Adams, J. B., and Brown, J. B. 1971. Increase in urinary excretion of estrogen on administration of dehydroepiandrosterone sulfate to an adrenalectomized, oophorectomized patient with breast cancer. *Steroidologica* 2: 1.

Keith Griffiths, D. Jones, E. H. D. Cameron,
E. N. Gleave, and A. P. M. Forrest

Transformation of Steroids by Mammary Cancer Tissue   9

The extensive studies of Bulbrook and his colleagues (1, 2, 3) relating 11-deoxy-17-oxosteroids and prognosis in patients with cancer of the breast directed attention to the major source of these urinary C_{19} steroids, dehydroepiandrosterone sulfate (DHEA sulfate), which is secreted by the adrenal gland and is normally present in high concentrations in plasma (4). It seemed that abnormalities in the secretion or metabolism of DHEA sulfate could in some way be concerned with the etiology of breast cancer and so, concurrently with Dr. Adams and his colleagues, we in Cardiff commenced a series of experiments designed to assess the capacity of human breast tumor tissue to metabolize various C_{19} steroids.

Tumor tissue, which was maintained at 0° C after removal from the patient until it was incubated, usually 30 min later, was thinly sliced with a razor blade and chopped into smaller segments. Tissue was then incubated with radioactive steroids in Krebs-Ringer bicarbonate glucose medium (12.5 ml/g tissue) shaking at 37° C, in an atmosphere of $O_2:CO_2$ (95:5) for 2 hr. No cofactors were added to the incubation. The arbitrary nature of such in vitro studies makes it difficult to decide the nature and amount of cofactors which could be added, and in their absence we routinely incubate whole cell preparation of endocrine tissues. Purity of the incubated radioactive steroid precursors was checked by isotope-dilution analysis.

Figure 1 shows the metabolites formed and their yields from the incubation in vitro of labeled DHEA sulfate, DHEA, androstene-

K. Griffiths, D. Jones, and E. Cameron are affiliated with the Tenovus Institute for Cancer Research and E. Gleave and A. Forrest with the Surgical Unit of the Welsh National School of Medicine, in Cardiff, Wales.

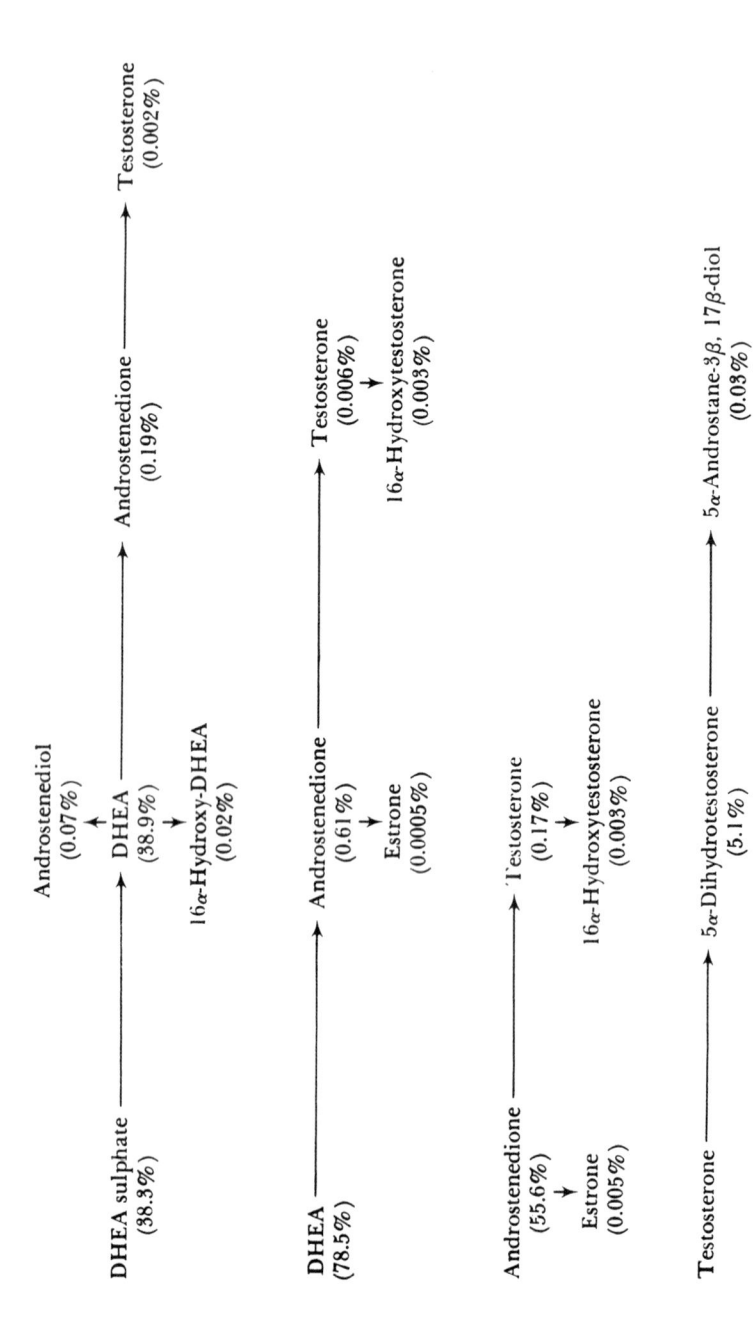

DHEA sulphate ⟶ Androstenediol
(38.3%)   (0.07%)
               DHEA ⟶ Androstenedione ⟶ Testosterone
               (38.9%)   (0.19%)   (0.002%)
               ↓
               16α-Hydroxy-DHEA
               (0.02%)

DHEA ⟶ Androstenedione ⟶ Testosterone
(78.5%)   (0.61%)   (0.006%)
          ↓   ↓
          Estrone   16α-Hydroxytestosterone
          (0.0005%)   (0.003%)

Androstenedione ⟶ Testosterone
(55.6%)   (0.17%)
↓   ↓
Estrone   16α-Hydroxytestosterone
(0.005%)   (0.003%)

Testosterone ⟶ 5α-Dihydrotestosterone ⟶ 5α-Androstane-3β, 17β-diol
                (5.1%)   (0.03%)

Fig. 1. Incubation of labeled steroids with breast tumor tissue.

dione, and testosterone with the breast tumor preparations. A preliminary account of these experiments has already been communicated (5).

An observation which Dr. Adams has described (see chap. 8), the deconjugation of DHEA sulfate and its transformation to other steroids including androstenedione and testosterone, was shown with these tissue preparations. Since we obtained no evidence for the synthesis of 16α-hydroxy-DHEA sulfate or androst-5-ene-3β,17β-diol sulfate, we must assume at present that 16α-hydroxy-DHEA is formed from DHEA.

Estrone was synthesized in small yields from both DHEA and androstenedione, although, contrary to the observation of Dr. Adams, no estriol could be detected despite repeated attempts to demonstrate its formation. A radioactive material with a chromatographic mobility identical to that of estriol was formed, but also separated completely from authentic carrier after methyl ether or acetate formation. Dr. Dao (6) has suggested that this "contaminant" may well be the androst-5-ene-3β,16α,17β-triol which is difficult to separate from estriol, and this possibility has now been verified (7). Noteworthy was the demonstrated 16α-hydroxylation of testosterone, also described by Adams and Wong (8).

Of particular interest however, was the formation of 5α-dihydrotestosterone (17β-hydroxy-5α-androstan-3-one) from testosterone, a compound which was shown by Huggins and Mainzer (9) to inhibit growth of 17β-estradiol-dependent rat mammary fibroadenoma and is currently considered to be the principal androgen within the cells of the prostate gland. The basis for this concept has been the finding that 5α-dihydrotestosterone was preferentially retained by rat prostatic nuclei after the tissue was incubated with labeled testosterone (10) or after testosterone was administered in vivo (11). Baulieu, Lasnitzki, and Robel (12, 13) have further shown that this compound will stimulate cell division and induce epithelial hyperplasia of the prostate tissue maintained in culture media. King (14) has also demonstrated the transformation of testosterone to 5α-dihydrotestosterone in rat mammary fibroadenoma and adenocarcinoma.

Results from investigations in which labeled steroids were perfused through human breast tumor tissue have tended to confirm these in vitro biosynthetic patterns. Perfusion studies were performed on tumors localized in the medial half of the breast, supplied predominantly by the internal mammary artery, which was exposed during exploration of the second or third intercostal space for lymph-node biopsy. A ligature was tied proximal to the point of injection and either (7α-³H) DHEA sulfate (ca. 33 nmole, specific activity 0.36 μCi/nmole) or (7α-³H) androstenedione (ca. 2 nmole, specific activity 5 μCi/nmole) administered as a single injection within 30 sec (fig. 2).

After the breast was removed, the tumor was dissected from surrounding tissues and maintained at 0° C until it was transferred to the laboratory, and then the radioactive steroids were analyzed

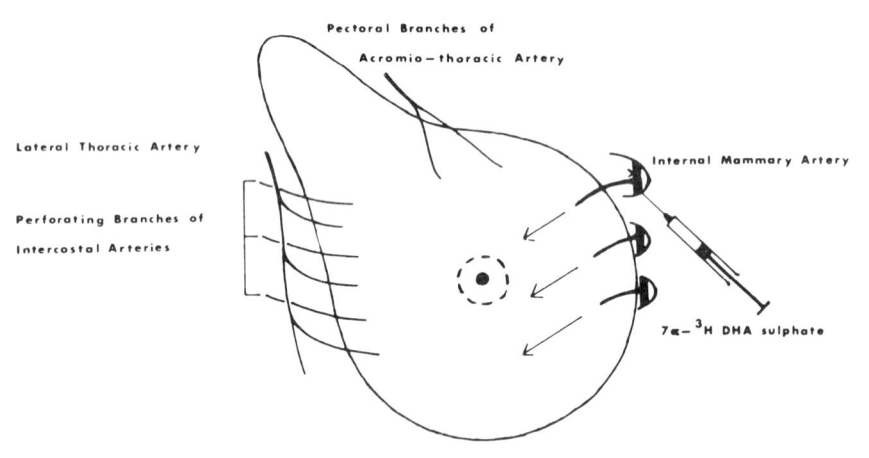

Fig. 2. Schematic diagram of the mammary gland illustrating the point of injection of (7α-³H) DHEA sulfate into the internal mammary artery.

(5). In one experiment, venous blood was collected from the side of the tumor opposite the point of substrate infusion and the radioactive steroids were measured. Results are shown in tables 1 and 2. Total radioactivity extracted from each tumor is listed together with the identity of the metabolites, and the radioactivity associated with each is listed as a percentage of the total.

DHEA sulfate was transformed to DHEA and androstenedione, and carrier testosterone was also labeled, although there was insufficient radioactivity for good identification. Testosterone and 5α-dihydrotestosterone were formed from the (7α-³H) androstenedione in reasonable yields. In the one experiment—and it must be regarded as a preliminary finding—it was interesting that no 5α-dihydrotestosterone was isolated in the venous blood which was collected. This could mean that 5α-dihydrotestosterone is retained by the tumor cell and is subsequently metabolized to the various saturated C_{19} steroids.

The close relationship between the metabolism of testosterone by the breast tumor tissue and by the prostate is interesting. Some of the metabolites formed from testosterone by human breast tissue in vitro are shown in table 3. Table 4 shows the metabolic products from the incubation of testosterone with canine prostatic tissue (16). Similar metabolic activity has been described for human prostatic

TABLE 1: PERFUSIONS OF HUMAN BREAST TUMORS WITH (7α-^{3}H) DHEA SULFATE

Total Radioactivity Isolated (dpm)	Steroid Isolated	Radioactivity Associated with Steroid (as % of total dpm isolated)
1. 260,000 (tissue)	DHEA	3.27
	Δ^4-Androstenedione	0.11
2. 49,600 (tissue)	DHEA	16.25
	Δ^4-Androstenedione	0.51
3. 96,000 (tissue)	DHEA	8.88
	Δ^4-Androstenedione	0.31
4. 14,000 (tissue)	DHEA	1.89
	Δ^4-Androstenedione	0

TABLE 2: PERFUSION OF HUMAN BREAST TUMORS WITH (7α-^{3}H) Δ^4-ANDROSTENEDIONE

Total Radioactivity Isolated (dpm)	Steroid Isolated	Radioactivity Associated with Steroid (as % of total dpm isolated)
1. 29,600 (tissue)	Δ^4-Androstenedione	23.0
	Testosterone	43.0
	5α-Dihydrotestosterone	4.3
	Epitestosterone	0
2. 47,700 (tissue)	Δ^4-Androstenedione	63.0
	Testosterone	7.0
	5α-Dihydrotestosterone	0.43
3. 19,800 (blood)	Δ^4-Androstenedione	50.4
	Testosterone	5.9
	5α-Dihydrotestosterone	0

TABLE 3: INCUBATIONS OF MINCED HUMAN BREAST TISSUE WITH RADIOACTIVE STEROID SUBSTRATES

Substrate	Steroid Isolated	% Radioactivity Associated with Steroid Isolated
(4-^{14}C) Testosterone	Testosterone	80.70
	5α-Dihydrotestosterone	5.10
	5α-Androstane-3β, 17β-diol	0.03
	5α-Androstane-3α, 17β-diol	0.0
	5α-Androstane-3β, 17α-diol	0.0
	5α-Androstane-3α, 17β-diol	Trace
	Epitestosterone	Trace
(4-^{14}C) Testosterone	Testosterone	86.60
	5α-Dihydrotestosterone	0.21
	Androstenedione	1.15
	5α-Androstanediols	0.0
	Epitestosterone	0.56

SOURCE: Jones et al. (5).

TABLE 4: NORMAL DOG PROSTATE MINCE INCUBATED WITH 50 μCi (7α-^{3}H) TESTOSTERONE FOR 1 HR

Steroid Investigated	% Radioactivity Found in Carrier Steroid of Total Radioactivity Taken up by Mince	
	Whole Tissue	Nuclear Fraction
Testosterone	51.36	1.25
Epitestosterone	0.62	0.59
5α-Dihydrotestosterone	19.96	1.30
5α-Androstane-3α, 17α-diol	0.06	0.06
5α-Androstane-3α, 17β-diol	0.86	0.03
5α-Androstane-3β, 17α-diol	0.06	0.01
5α-Androstane-3β-17β-diol	0.30	0.02

SOURCE: Harper et al. (15).

tissue (16, 17). Although 5α-androstanediols were formed by the prostatic tissue, no 5β-epimers were found in these studies; 5α-dihydrotestosterone, epitestosterone, and androstenedione were all synthesized from testosterone. Further, a similar pattern of metabolism was obtained (table 5) by incubating testosterone with nuclei isolated from human breast tumor tissue by procedures described by King, Cowan, and Inman (18). The presence of the 5α-reductase

TABLE 5: INCUBATION OF HUMAN BREAST TISSUE NUCLEI WITH RADIOACTIVE STEROID SUBSTRATES

Substrate	Steroid Isolated	% Radioactivity Associated with Steroid Isolated
(7α-³H) Testosterone	Testosterone	88.94
	Epitestosterone	0.83
	5α-Dihydrotestosterone	1.97
	5α-Androstane-3α,17β-diol	0.05
	5α-Androstane-3β,17β-diol	0.03
	5α-Androstane-3α,17α-diol	0
	5α-Androstane-3β,17α-diol	0
(7α-³H) Testosterone	Testosterone	95.64
	Epitestosterone	0.86
	5α-Dihydrotestosterone	0.20
	5α-Androstane-3α,17β-diol	0
	5α-Androstane-3β,17β-diol	0
	5α-Androstane-3α,17α-diol	0
	5α-Androstane-3β,17α-diol	0

in the breast tumor nuclear preparation is of considerable interest in relation to the observations of Bruchovsky and Wilson (19) that this enzyme is normally found in the nuclei of androgen-responsive tissues. The possibility that 5α-dihydrotestosterone may be concerned in some regulatory mechanism within the breast tumor cell is thus worthy of serious consideration, and the identification of a 5α-dihydrotestosterone-protein receptor in human breast tumor tissue would open up new fields in the endocrinology of breast cancer. The 5α-androstanediols which have been shown to have biological activity in the prostate (12, 13) may also have some role in the breast tissue cell.

Two observations may therefore be made from the studies described. First, in vitro and in vivo studies have proved conclusively that breast tumor tissue can synthesize steroid hormones from C_{19} steroid precursors present in the plasma. That such hormones can be synthesized from endogenous cholesterol, as suggested by Dr. Adams, is also a possibility, but it may be that the pathway from cholesterol → DHEA, excluding pregnenolone and recently shown to be present in endocrine tissues (20), is of more importance. This biosynthetic capacity of the breast tumor tissue could provide a particular intracellular hormone environment on which the growth and metabolism of the tissue depended. The relatively low conversions shown to occur also suggest that the abnormal urinary steroid excretion pattern described by Bulbrook and his colleagues (2, 3) is not the result of extensive steroid metabolism by the tumor tissue. Some of our clinical studies on patients with breast disease in South Wales appear to add further support to this contention.

Estimation of urinary steroids have been made on 177 women with breast disease; 63 patients had benign disease of the breast, proved by excision biopsy of a palpable lump, 30 had primary cancer, and 63 had advanced cancer of the breast subsequently treated by hormone administration or ablation of endocrine glands. Twenty-one patients in the advanced group had disease limited to the breasts, chest wall, regional lymph nodes, or pleural cavity (localized disease), and 42 had osseous or visceral metastases (generalized disease), with or without local disease. Steroid analysis was also performed on 21 patients without known breast disease or malignant disease of any kind who had been admitted to the hospital for elective general surgery. Procedures involved in the analysis of 17-hydroxycorticosteroids and 11-deoxy-17-ketosteroids were described by Gleave (21) in the first Tenovus Workshop on Breast Cancer and have been described elsewhere (22). Comparison of the logarithmic values of etiocholanolone showed that, although there was no difference between the mean values of the normal, benign, and primary groups, there was a difference when the advanced group as a whole was compared with each of the other groups. Regression lines were drawn confirming that patients with advanced disease were different from others and had significantly lower logarithmic levels of etiocholanolone regardless of age (fig. 3). Further examination of this difference indicated that patients with advanced *localized* disease were distinct from all others and that these patients had significantly lower levels

Transformation of Steroids by Mammary Cancer Tissue

of etiocholanolone when adjusted for age (fig. 4) (22). Thus, it would seem that these abnormal levels of urinary steroids are confined to patients with advanced cancer, and primarily to those with *localized* disease. Of further interest are the results from the analysis of DHEA sulfate in the plasma from patients in these various groups. Again, the plasma DHEA sulfate was lower in the advanced group than in the others (fig. 5).

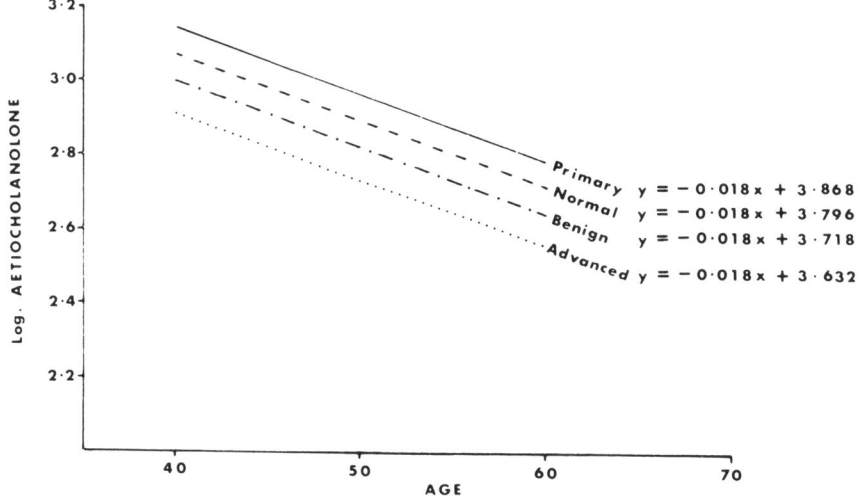

Fig. 3. All groups of patients over thirty-eight years of age; pooled regression of log. etiocholanolone on age.

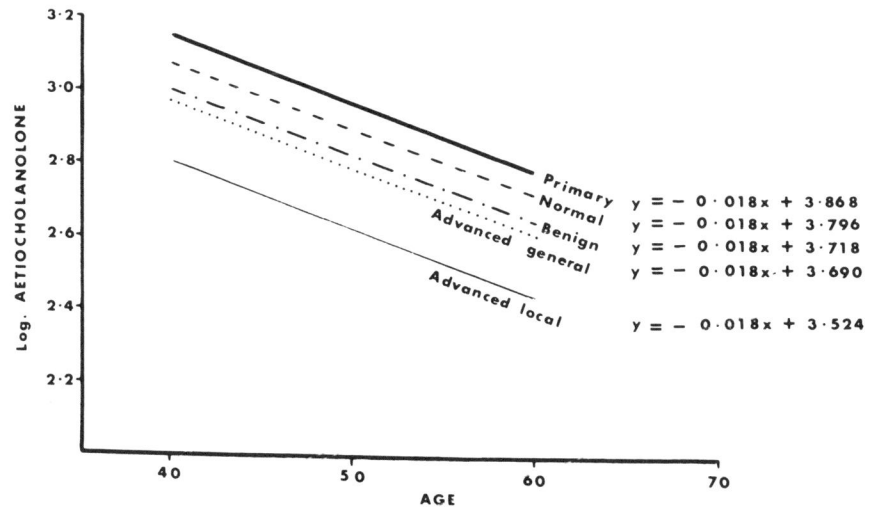

Primary $y = -0.018x + 3.868$
Normal $y = -0.018x + 3.796$
Benign $y = -0.018x + 3.718$
Advanced $y = -0.018x + 3.632$

Fig. 4. All groups of patients over thirty-eight years of age; pooled regression of log. etiocholanolone on age (including subgroups).

Primary $y = -0.018x + 3.868$
Normal $y = -0.018x + 3.796$
Benign $y = -0.018x + 3.718$
Advanced general $y = -0.018x + 3.690$
Advanced local $y = -0.018x + 3.524$

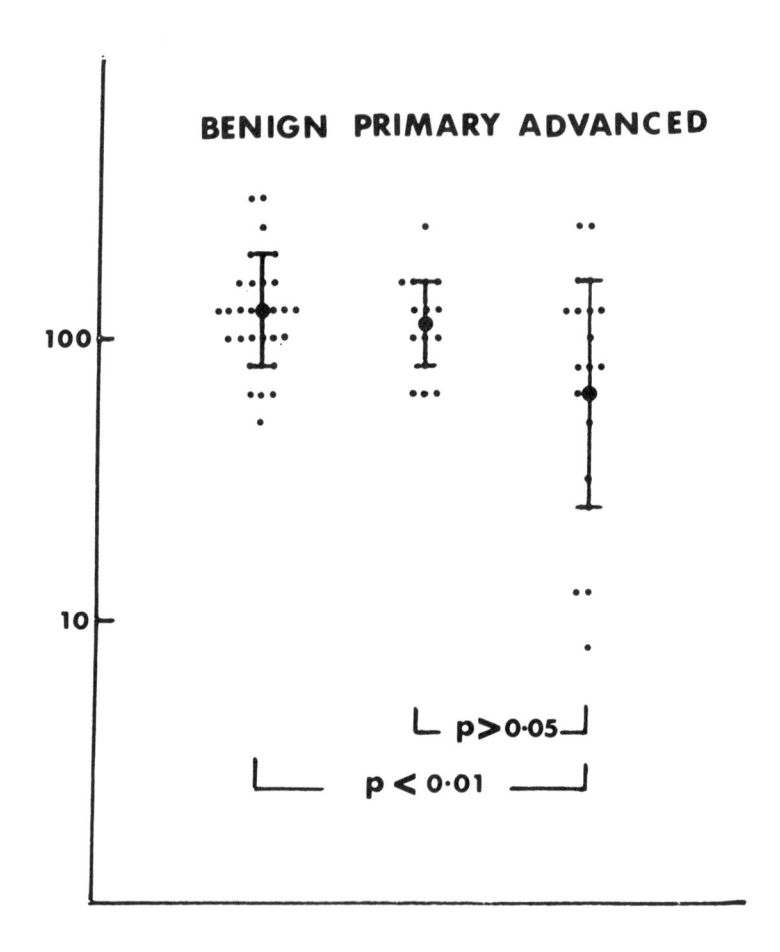

Fig. 5. Log plasma DHEA-S

Acknowledgments

The authors wish to acknowledge the generous financial support of the Tenovus Organization and also wish to thank Mr. Ralph Marshal, Department of Medical Illustrations, Royal Infirmary, Cardiff, for his help in preparing the illustrations.

References

1. Bulbrook, R. D.; Greenwood, F. C.; and Hayward, J. L. 1960. Selection of breast cancer patients for adrenalectomy or hypophysectomy by determination of urinary 17-hydroxycorticosteroids and aetiocholanolone. *Lancet* 1: 1154.

2. Bulbrook, R. D. 1965. Hormone assays in human breast cancer. *Vitamins Hormones* 23: 329.
3. Hayward, J. L., and Bulbrook, R. D. 1968. Urinary steroids and prognosis in breast cancer. In *Prognostic factors in breast cancer,* ed. A. P. M. Forrest and P. B. Kunkler. Edinburgh: E. and S. Livingstone.
4. Yamaji, T., and Ibayashi, J. 1969. Plasma dehydroepiandrosterone sulfate in normal and pathological conditions. *J. Clin. Endocr.* 29: 273.
5. Jones, D.; Cameron, E. H. D.; Griffiths, K.; Gleave, E. N.; and Forrest, A. P. M. 1970. Steroid metabolism by human breast tissue. *Biochem. J.* 116: 919.
6. Dao, T. L. 1969. Studies on the mechanism of regression of mammary cancer after adrenalectomy. *The human adrenal gland and its relation to breast cancer,* ed. K. Griffiths and E. H. D. Cameron, p. 99. Caerphilly: Alpha Omega Alpha Publishing Co.
7. Morreal, C. E.; Dao, T. L.; and Lonergan, P. 1970. A method for the separation of polar androgens from estrogens. *Anal. Biochem.* 34: 352.
8. Adams, J. B., and Wong, M. S. F. 1968. Paraendocrine behaviour of human breast carcinoma: *In vitro* transformation of steroids to physiologically active hormones. *J. Endocr.* 41: 41.
9. Huggins, C. B., and Mainzer, K. 1957. Hormonal influences on mammary tumors of the rat. II. Retardation of growth of a transplanted fibroadenoma in intact female rats by steroids in the androstane series. *J. Exp. Med.* 105: 485.
10. Anderson, K. M., and Liao, S. 1968. Selective retention of dihydrotestosterone by prostatic nuclei. *Nature (Lond.)* 219: 277.
11. Bruchovsky, N., and Wilson, J. D. 1968. The intranuclear binding of testosterone and 5α-androstan-17β-ol-3-one by rat prostate. *J. Biol. Chem.* 243: 5953.
12. Baulieu, E. E.; Lasnitzki, I.; and Robel, P. 1968. Testosterone, prostate gland and hormone action. *Biochem. Biophys. Res. Commun.* 32: 575.
13. ———. 1968. Metabolism of testosterone and action of metabolites on prostate glands grown in organ culture. *Nature (Lond.)* 219: 1155.
14. King, R. J. B.; Gordon, J.; and Helfenstein, J. E. 1964. The metabolism of testosterone by tissues from normal and neoplastic rat breast. *J. Endocr.* 29: 103.
15. Harper, M. E.; Pierrepoint, C. G.; Fahmy, A. R.; and Griffiths, K. 1971. The metabolism of steroids in the dog prostate and testis. *J. Endocr.* 49: 213.
16. Farnsworth, W. E. 1970. The normal prostate and its endocrine control. *Some aspects of the etiology and biochemistry of prostatic cancer,* ed. K. Griffiths and C. G. Pierrepoint. Caerphilly: Alpha Omega Alpha Publishing Co.

17. Ofner, P. 1969. Metabolism of hormones in normal and neoplastic prostate tissue. *Vitamins Hormones* 26: 237.
18. King, R. J. B.; Cowan, D. M.; and Inman, D. R. 1965. The uptake of (6,7-^{3}H) oestradiol by dimethylbenzanthracene-induced rat mammary tumors. *J. Endocr.* 32: 83.
19. Bruchovsky, N.; and Wilson, J. D. 1968. The conversion of testosterone to 5α-androstan-17β-ol-3-one by rat prostate *in vivo* and *in vitro*. *J. Biol. Chem.* 243: 2012.
20. Jungmann, R. A. 1968. Androgen biosynthesis. I. Enzymatic cleavage of the cholesterol side chain to dehydroepiandrosterone and 2-methylheptan-6-one. *Biochim. Biophys. Acta* 164: 110.
21. Gleave, E. N. 1969. Primary and advanced breast cancer in South Wales: A study of urinary steroids. *The human adrenal gland and its relation to breast cancer,* ed. K. Griffiths and E. H. D. Cameron, p. 86. Caerphilly: Alpha Omega Alpha Publishing Co.
22. Cameron, E. H. D.; Griffiths, K.; Gleave, E. N.; Stewart, H. J.; Forrest, A. P. M.; and Campbell, H. 1970. Benign and malignant breast disease in South Wales: A study of urinary steroids. *Brit. Med. J.* 4: 768–71.

Thomas L. Dao, R. Varela, and Charles Morreal

Metabolic Transformation of Steroids by Human Breast Cancer   10

The mechanism by which the removal of adrenal glands induces regression of breast cancer is not understood. Although it is generally believed that adrenalectomy removes the extragonadal site of estrogen production, conclusive evidence is lacking to support such a hypothesis, since we do not know whether human adrenals secrete estrogens. On the other hand, studies of urinary estrogen excretion before and after adrenalectomy disclosed that estrogenic substances in the urine were either greatly decreased or nonmeasurable after adrenalectomy in women with metastatic cancer of the breast (1). This observation raises an interesting question: What is the role of the adrenal glands in estrogen synthesis?

Conversion of administered testosterone to estrogens has been shown to occur in patients without ovaries and adrenals: estrone and estradiol were found by West et al. (2), and estriol and estrone by Dao and Morreal (3). A similar study reported evidence for conversion of 4-^{14}C-cortisone to 11β-hydroxyestrone and 11β-hydroxyestradiol (4). These studies led to a search for one or more sites for such metabolic transformations.

Although transformation of 4-^{14}C-cortisone to 11β-hydroxyestrone has been reported in human breast tumor slices (5), the data await confirmation. The present study examined conversion of cholesterol and of C_{19} steroid precursors, including testosterone and dehydroepiandrosterone (DHEA), to estrogens by mammary tumor and liver microsomal preparations. This chapter reports that human breast

The authors are affiliated with the Department of Breast Surgery and Endocrine Research Laboratory at the Roswell Park Memorial Institute of the New York State Department of Health at Buffalo.

cancer tissue contains aromatizing, hydroxylating, and dehydrogenase enzyme systems to transform C_{19} precursor steroids into estrogens. Desmolase activity in the tumors is demonstrated by the isolation of several C_{19} steroids as metabolites of cholesterol. In contrast, the liver does not have the aromatase enzyme system to perform a similar metabolic transformation.

METHODS OF STUDY AND RESULTS

Breast tumors obtained at surgery were carefully dissected free of fat and adjacent connective tissues, and a section of each tumor was prepared for histological study. The remaining tissue of the tumor, approximately 1.5 to 2.5 g, was homogenized in 10 ml of 0.25 M sucrose in a Virtis "23" homogenizer. The nuclei and mitochondria were removed by centrifuging at 10,000 g for 10 min. The supernatant fluid was centrifuged for 1 hr at 50,000 rpm, using rotor 65 in a Beckman L265B ultracentrifuge. The precipitate was resuspended in 5 ml of 0.25 M sucrose.

To the microsomal suspension were added 2 mg of DPN, 2 mg of TPN, 10 μmole of ATP, 50 μmole of glucose-6-phosphate, 2 units of glucose-6-phosphate dehydrogenase, 1 ml of tris buffer (pH 7.6), and 10 μCi of ^{14}C-labeled or 25μCi of ^{3}H-labeled steroids. The incubations were carried out at 37° C for 3 hr in an oxygen atmosphere.

The incubation media was purified according to methods previously described by Ryan and Smith (6). The steroid pool was next separated into a neutral fraction and a crude phenolic fraction as described by Engel (7). The phenols were then partially separated and freed of contaminating neutral polar compounds by multiple partition between diethyl ether and 1 N NaOH (n = 8) according to the method of Morreal, Dao, and Lonergan (8). Three pools were collected: tube 0, containing estriol and other polyoxy phenols; tubes 1–4, containing estrone and estradiol; and tubes 5–8, containing neutral compounds.

The contents of tube 0 and tubes 5–8 were subjected to thin-layer chromatography on silica gel plates in 0.5% ethanol in ethyl acetate (system A), and the contents of tubes 1–4 were chromatographed in 8% ethylene glycol monomethyl ether in benzene (system B).

The objective of our experiments was to compare the efficiencies of the possible metabolic conversion of testosterone and DHEA and their sulfates to estrogens by mammary tumor tissue and normal liver tissue.

Conversion of Steroids in Vitro by Tumor Tissue

The tumor from patient C. S., who underwent radical mastectomy for cancer of the breast, was studied with testosterone, testosterone sulfate, DHEA, and DHEA sulfate by the method just outlined. The purified phenolic fractions were analyzed as follows.

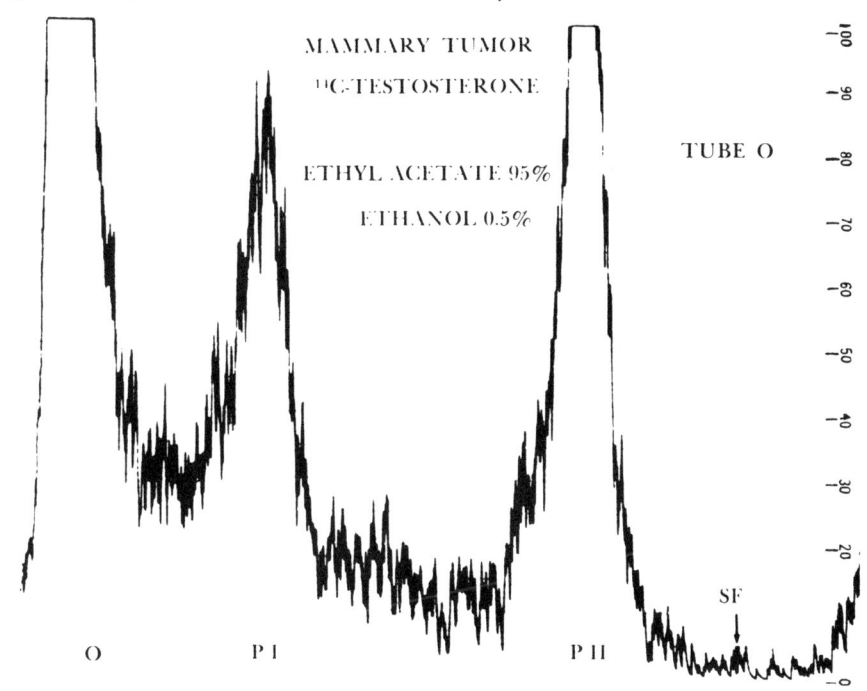

Fig. 1. Thin-layer chromatography in system A of contents in tube 0 gives three radioactive peaks; peak at origin, peak I, and peak II, which corresponds to standard 16α-hydroxyestrone run in parallel with the radiochromatogram.

Conversion of Testosterone (Case C. S.)

The microsomal preparation of tumor tissue was incubated with 10 μCi of 4-^{14}C-testosterone and the purified phenolic fraction of the incubation mixture was analyzed. Thin-layer chromatography of the contents of tube 0 in system A gave three distinct peaks of radioactivity: one more polar than estriol (PI), a radioactive zone at the origin, and a less polar peak (PII) near the solvent front (fig. 1). On rechromatography in system B, Peak I gave a metabolite with mobility identical to that of standard 2-hydroxyestriol. The less polar material (PII), on rechromatography in system B, showed radioactivity in the zone of 16α-hydroxyestrone. There was considerable degradation of this nonpolar material, as evidenced by the persistent appearance of radioactivity at the origins of the chromatograms. Countercurrent distribution of this metabolite with pure 16α-hydroxyestrone in 70% methanol/40% chloroform in carbon tetrachloride (n = 50) gave coincident peaks of radioactivity and gravimetric assay (fig. 2).

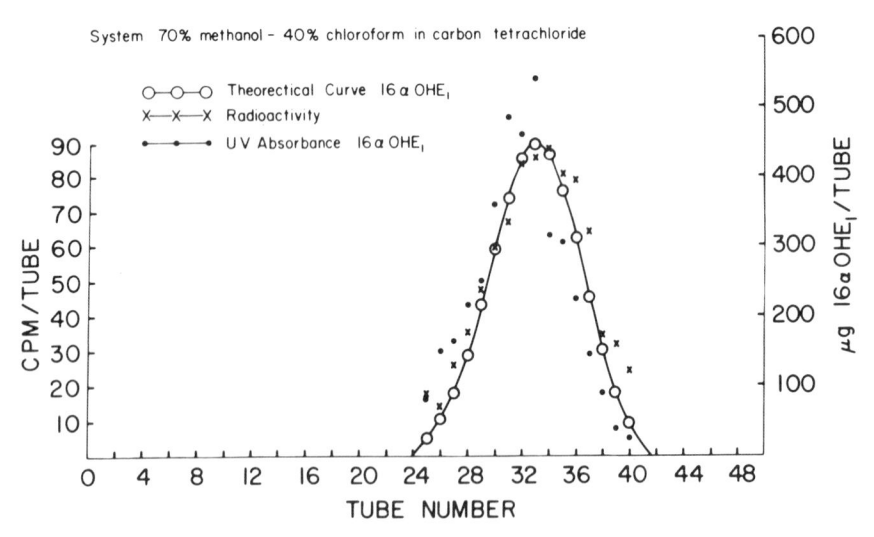

Fig. 2. Rechromatography of PII in system B showed radioactivity in the zone of 16α-hydroxyestrone. Countercurrent distribution of this metabolite with pure 16α-hydroxyestrone gave coincident peaks of radioactivity and gravimetric assay.

Chromatography of the contents of tubes 1–4 in system B showed a radioactive peak corresponding to estrone, with a shoulder similar in mobility to estradiol. Rechromatography of this area in 2% methanol in methylene chloride gave a peak identical in mobility to estrone, but carrier recrystallization with added standard estrone was negative. Similarly, the presence of estradiol could not be verified. Also appearing in tubes 1–4 was a metabolite more polar than estrone, with a mobility similar to that of epiestriol. This substance has not been characterized further.

In tubes 5–8 we found a large amount of unreacted testosterone. On elution and rechromatography in 10% ethanol in chloroform, the zone corresponding to 16α-hydroxytestosterone gave a peak identical in mobility to this compound. Coincident peaks of radioactivity and gravimetric assay were obtained on countercurrent distribution of this metabolite with authentic 16α-hydroxytestosterone in 50% ethyl acetate in hexane/33% ethanol (n = 50) (fig. 3).

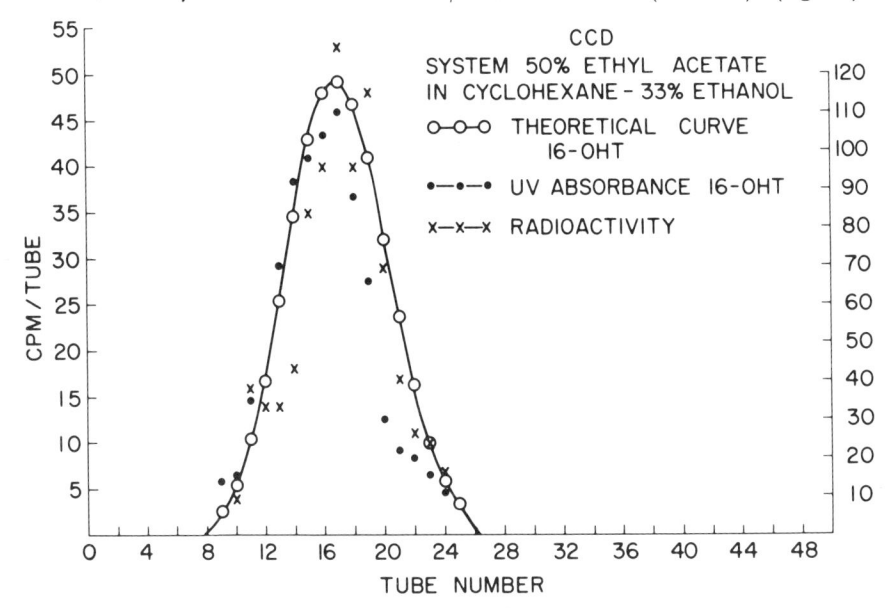

Fig. 3. Countercurrent distribution of the metabolite with pure 16α-hydroxytestosterone gave coincident peaks of radioactivity and gravimetric assay.

Conversion of Testosterone Sulfate

Incubating the same tumor (C. S.) with 25 μCi of ³H-testosterone sulfate gave, in tube 0, a peak following thin-layer chromatography in system A at the origin, which is attributable to the uncleaved conjugated precursor. Conspicuous by its absence was any radioactive zone in the area that contained 16α-hydroxyestrone in the comparable analysis with free testosterone. The contents of tubes 1–4 were chromatographed in system B but showed no radioactivity in the estrone and estradiol areas. Thin-layer chromatography of the contents of tubes 5–8 in system A revealed a small peak in the area corresponding to testosterone.

Conversion of DHEA

The same tumor was incubated with 25 μCi ³H-DHEA. Thin-layer chromatography of the contents of tube 0 in system A showed all the radioactivity concentrated in a zone more polar than estriol. These polar metabolites are probably tetroxy phenols, but have not yet been identified. The contents of tubes 1–4 showed a large peak with a mobility similar to that of estriol, and probably represent an overlap of the neutral contaminants from tubes 5–8, since estriol can be present only in tube 0. Metabolites corresponding in mobility to estrone or estradiol were not present.

A polar peak in the zone attributable to either androst-5-ene-3β, 16α,17β-triol (the α-triol) or 16α-hydroxytestosterone was found in tubes 5–8 after thin-layer chromatography in system A. Rechromatography of this peak material in 10% ethanol in chloroform gave two peaks. The smaller peak had the same mobility as the α-triol on further purification in the same system. Carrier recrystallization of both peaks with the α-triol, and a 50-tube CCD of the larger peak with 16α-hydroxytestosterone, were all negative. A portion of the larger peak was reduced with NaBH₄, giving a product that now had the same mobility as the α-triol in 10% ethanol-chloroform. Nevertheless, a carrier recrystallization of the reduced product with the α-triol was negative. This eliminates the possibility that the original peak was 16α-hydroxy-DHEA or its isomer androst-5-ene-3β, 17β-diol-16-one. It is possible that this peak represents a different hydroxy-DHEA isomer, such as 2-, 6-, 7-, 11-, or 15-hydroxy-DHEA, which, on reduction with NaBH₄, gave the corresponding triol.

Conversion of DHEA Sulfate

In this experiment the same tumor was incubated with 25 μCi of ³H-DHEA sulfate. The contents of tube 0, on thin-layer chromatography in system A, showed no radioactivity beyond the origin. A sharp peak occurring in tubes 1–4 on thin-layer chromatography in system A is probably an overlap of the abundant polar material found in tubes 5–8, which on thin-layer chromatography in system B gave a radioactive peak with a mobility identical to that of the α-triol. Rechromatography in ethanol and CHCl₃ revealed that the radioactive peak coincided with the authentic α-triol running concurrently. Carrier recrystallization with authentic α-triol, however, was negative. This metabolite appears to be the same as the one found in incubation with DHEA. They probably are dihydroxy-ketone compounds, and have yet to be identified.

Conversion of Cholesterol (Case O. U.)

The microsomal preparation from the tumor specimen was incubated with 10 μCi 4-^{14}C-cholesterol and was chromatographed on paper by the method of Feher (9), using propylene glycol as the stationary phase and heptane-benzene-methanol (130:60:10) as the mobile phase. Radioactive zones with mobilities identical to testosterone, androsterone, androst-4-ene-3,17-dione, 5α-androstane-3,

TABLE 1: IDENTIFICATION OF ANDROST-4-ENE-3-17-DIONE BY CARRIER RECRYSTALLIZATION (CASE O. U.)

Recrystallization (Number)	Specific Activity (dpm/mg)	
	Crystals	Filtrate
Start	2,340	
1	2,330	2,215
2	2,380	2,160
3	2,290	2,500
4	2,320	2,510
5	2,480	2,360

17-dione, and 5α-androstane-3α,17β-diol were found. Thin-layer chromatography of these metabolites in 50% ethyl acetate in heptane showed mobilities identical to authentic standards run concurrently. Final confirmation was evidenced by positive carrier recrystallizations of these five metabolites in ethyl acetate and heptane with standard material. Two representative examples, androst-4-ene-3,17-dione and androsterone, are shown in tables 1 and 2.

Conversion of Steroids in Vitro by Liver Tissue

Liver biopsy was perfomed in patients D. B. and D. F., who underwent bilateral oophorectomies for metastatic cancer of the breast. The liver tissue from patient D. B. was incubated with 4-^{14}C-testosterone, and that from patient D. F. with 4-^{14}C-DHEA. Incubation, extraction, separation, and purification of the phenolic fraction were carried out as already described. The analyses of the purified phenolic fractions were performed as follows.

Conversion of Testosterone in Vitro (Case D. B.)

Thin-layer chromatography of the contents of tube 0 in System A did not give a pattern identical to that obtained in the tumor

TABLE 2: IDENTIFICATION OF ANDROSTERONE BY CARRIER RECRYSTALLIZATION (CASE O. U.)

Recrystallization (Number)	Specific Activity (dpm/mg)	
	Crystals	Filtrate
Start	1,460	
1	1,310	1,540
2	1,380	1,510
3	1,390	1,350
4	1,260	1,380
5	1,310	1,400

incubation. The radioactivity in the nonpolar area of the chromatogram was so low as to preclude further identification.

The unidentified nonpolar peak in the chromatogram of the contents of tubes 1–4 from the tumor sample was absent from the metabolites isolated from the liver preparation. As in the tumor sample, though, the polar zone in the vicinity of estriol was probably due to an overlap of neutral contaminants from tubes 5–8.

A greater conversion to polar neutral metabolites was noticeable in the contents of tubes 5–8 from the liver incubation compared with those of the tumor analysis with testosterone as a precursor (fig. 4). The zone attributable to 16α-hydroxytestosterone, on rechromatography in system B and in 10% ethanol in chloroform, gave peaks of radioactivity identical to concurrently run authentic material (fig. 5). Carrier recrystallization of this metabolite with added

16α-hydroxytestosterone confirmed its identity as 16α-hydroxytestosterone.

Conversion of DHEA (Case D. F.)

Like the contents of tube 0 of the tumor incubation with DHEA, the liver tissue provided a polar peak followed by a band of radioactivity corresponding to estriol in system A. Carrier recrystallization

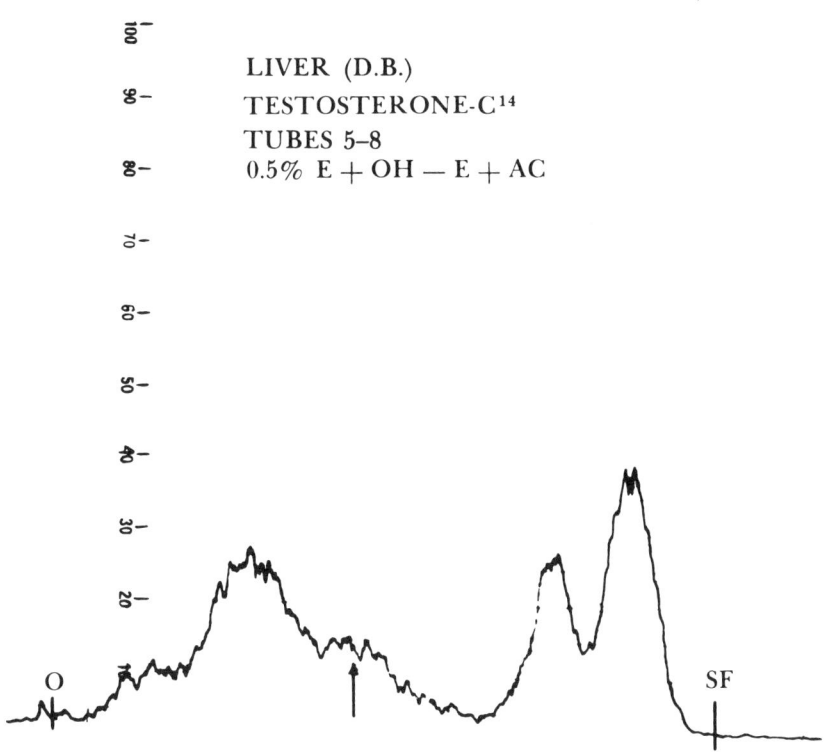

Fig. 4. Thin-layer chromatography of contents of tubes 5–8 from liver incubation. The arrow indicates the radioactive zone corresponding to standard 16α-hydroxytestosterone run concurrently. Radiochromatogram run on strip counter at 10 K.

of the area corresponding to estriol proved negative. The polar metabolite remained in the aqueous layer on ether extraction, indicating that the material was probably conjugated. Thin-layer chromatography in system A of the contents of tubes 1–4 showed peaks identical in mobility to estrone and estradiol, but subsequent purification and carrier recrystallization proved negative for these estrogens. A prominent peak intermediate in mobility between estriol and epiestriol remains unidentified. There was a polar peak close to the origin, identical in mobility to a similar metabolite obtained in the tumor incubation with DHEA. As in the tumor analysis, the liver tissue showed a peak, after thin-layer chromatography, in system A of the contents in tubes 5–8, with a mobility identical to

LIVER (D.B.)

TESTOSTERONE-C^{14} TUBES 5–8

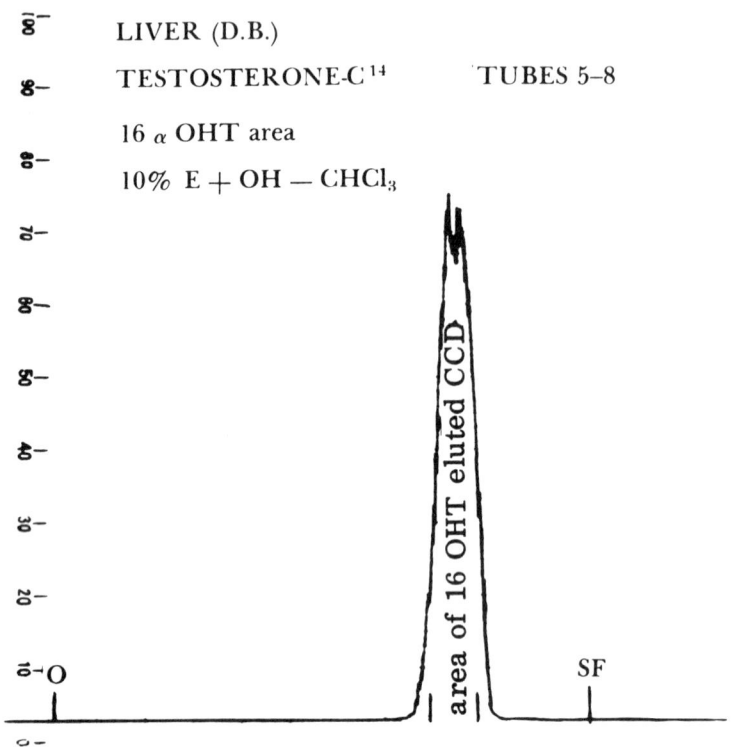

16 α OHT area

10% E + OH — CHCl$_3$

Fig. 5. Thin-layer chromatography of the radioactive zone corresponding to 16α-hydroxytestosterone in 10% ethanol in CHCl$_3$ again gives radioactive peaks identical to concurrently run standard 16α-hydroxytestosterone. Radiochromatogram run on strip counter at 3 K.

that of the α-triol. On rechromatography in 10% ethanol in CHCl$_3$ this material did not have the same mobility as the authentic α-triol.

CONVERSION OF ESTRONE IN VITRO BY MAMMARY TUMOR TISSUE

16α-Hydroxyestrone is susceptible to isomerization and degradation in alkaline solution. The method used in the present study can easily cause degradation of this metabolite, and hence it is not surprising that tumor specimens gave only a small radioactive peak corresponding to 16α-hydroxyestrone. To ascertain the presence of 16α-hydroxylase in the mammary tumors, we have carried out experiments to study the metabolism of estrone by breast cancer tissue. Tumors from two patients were incubated with ^{14}C-estrone. The total steroid pool from the incubation extracts (case M. Z.) was directly chromatographed on paper in the Bush B1 system without prior partition between diethyl ether and 1 N NaOH. Most of the radioactive peaks were reserved for future analysis, but a polar zone in the area of 16α-hydroxyestrone was eluted, and, on further chromatography in

TABLE 3: IDENTIFICATION OF 16α-HYDROXYESTRONE BY CARRIER RECRYSTALLIZATION (CASE M. Z.)

Recrystallization (Number)	Specific Activity (dpm/mg) Crystals	Filtrate
Start	842	
1	499	6,620
2	333	2,310
3	299	337
4	252	200
5	266	225
6	285	264

system B and 50% ethyl acetate in heptane, gave sharp peaks coincident with authentic standard run concurrently. Carrier recrystallization of this metabolite with pure standard material verified its identity as 16α-hydroxyestrone (table 3).

A metabolite with the same R_F value as estradiol in the Bush B1 system was rechromatographed on thin-layer chromatography in system B (fig. 6). The peak still ran the same as estradiol, and carrier recrystallization of the radioactivity verified the metabolite as estradiol (table 4).

A radioactive shoulder less polar than estrone was apparent in the thin-layer chromatogram of the steroid extract. Rechromatography gave what appeared to be a homogeneous peak, but it was rounded at the top rather than sharp (fig. 7). Nevertheless, carrier recrystallization was conducted with authentic 2-methoxyestrone; and although there was a gradual decline in specific activity, there were still significant counts in the crystals after seven recrystallizations (table 5). Thus we believe that this metabolite may indeed be 2-methoxyestrone, although impure.

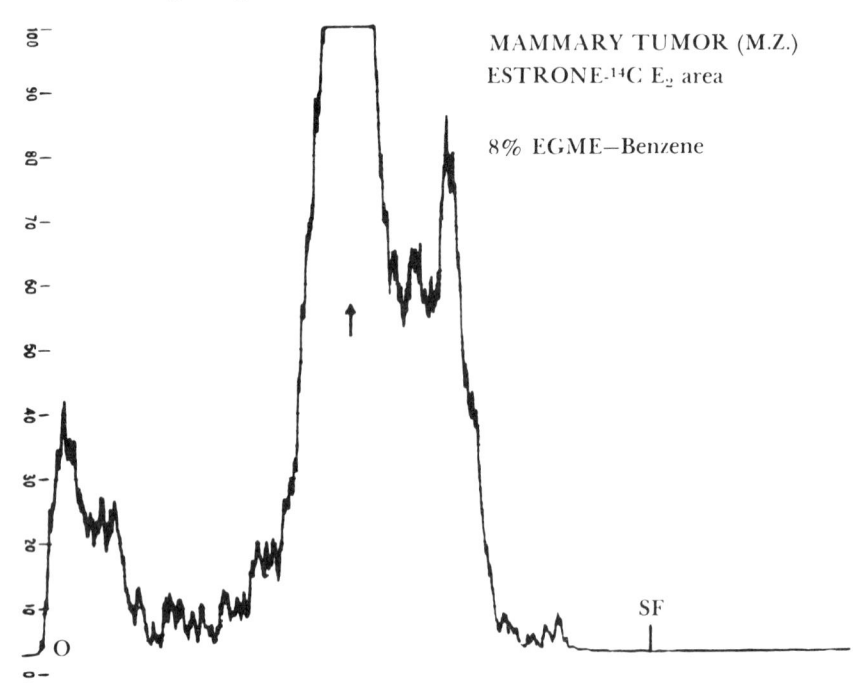

Fig. 6. Thin-layer chromatography in system B of a metabolite with the same mobility as estradiol in Bush B1 system again gave the same R_F value as standard estradiol. Radiochromatogram run on strip counter at 3 K.

Discussion

Several human tumors of nonendocrine origin have been shown to induce humoral syndromes as a result of the production by the neoplastic tissues of substances with hormonal activity (10). For example, Cushing's syndrome has been observed in patients with bronchogenic carcinoma of the lungs. In these patients, the cancer tissues were found to secrete a substance that was biologically, physiologically, and chemically indistinguishable from human ACTH (11). It is thus not surprising that tumors of endocrine target tissues may have the ability to synthesize hormones. Such a possibility, if proved to occur, say, in

TABLE 4: IDENTIFICATION OF ESTRADIOL BY
CARRIER RECRYSTALLIZATION (CASE M. Z.)

Recrystallization (Number)	Specific Activity (dpm/mg) Crystals	Filtrate
Start	1,910	
1	1,530	2,340
2	1,360	2,083
3	1,380	2,320
4	1,700	1,407
5	1,560	1,395
6	1,680	1,584

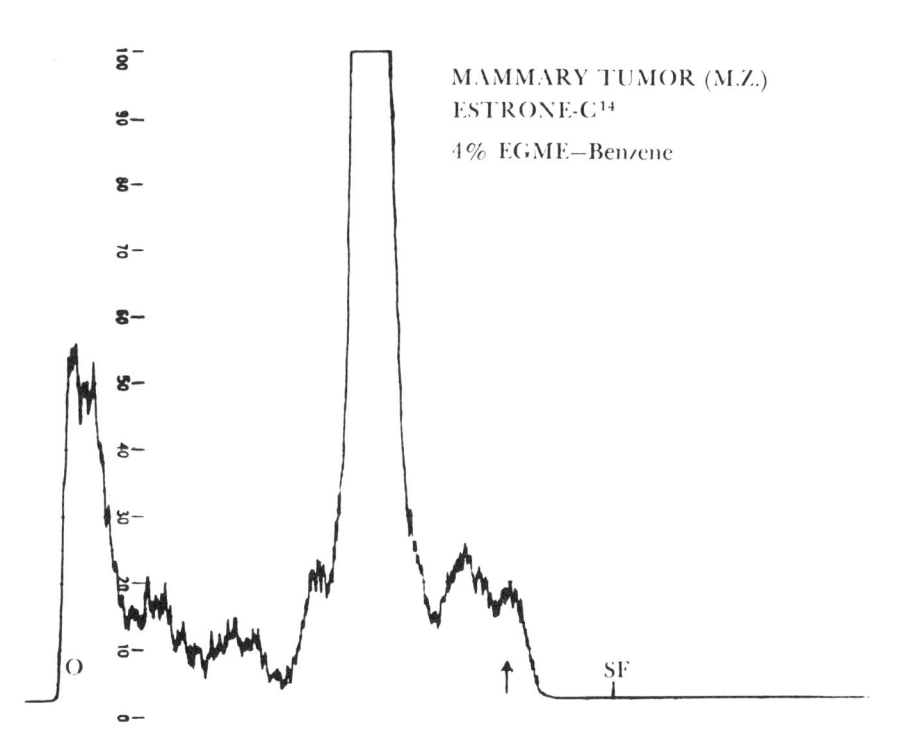

MAMMARY TUMOR (M.Z.)
ESTRONE-C[14]
4% EGME—Benzene

Fig. 7. Thin-layer chromatography in system B of a metabolite with same mobility as 2-methoxyestrone in Bush B1 system. The arrow indicates the radioactive peak that has the same R_F value as standard 2-methoxyestrone run concurrently. Radiochromatogram run on strip counter at 10 K. The more polar larger peak has the same mobility as estrone. It is probably the unmetabolized estrone.

human breast cancer tissue, may have far-reaching implications in our understanding of the pathogenesis of breast cancer.

Table 6, summarizing the results of this study, shows at least one underlying factor presenting a clue that facilitates an understanding of the possible metabolic pathways leading to phenolic steroids in breast cancer patients. All three of the androgenic precursors that were used in incubation with tumor tissue (testosterone, DHEA, and DHEA sulfate) gave 16α-hydroxy derivatives of the parent compounds.

TABLE 5: IDENTIFICATION OF METHOXYESTRONE BY CARRIER RECRYSTALLIZATION (CASE M. Z.)

Recrystallization (Number)	Specific Activity (dpm/mg) Crystals	Filtrate
Start	2,090	
1	836	11,090
2	556	2,330
3	312	1,310
4	225	645
5	190	875
6	147	288
7	108	155

In addition, when mammary tissue was incubated in the presence of estrone, 16α-hydroxyestrone and 17 β-estradiol were identified as conversion products. These results demonstrate conclusively that mammary cancer tissues possess both 16α-hydroxylating and 17β-estradiol dehydrogenase enzyme systems. The persistent presence of estriol as the major phenolic metabolite of testosterone in adrenalectomized and ovariectomized women with breast cancer can be viewed as the final excretory product of the 16α-hydroxyestrone formed in mammary tumor tissue (3), since it is well known that liver homogenates possess the 17 β-estradiol dehydrogenase enzyme system (12).

Baulieu (13) has implicated DHEA sulfate as an important estrogen precursor and Shubert (14) has shown a greater rise in estrogen excretion after infusion of DHEA sulfate than after infusion of either testosterone or androstenedione in normal women. Our experiments

TABLE 6: METABOLIC PRODUCTS OF SOME STEROIDS INCUBATED WITH BREAST TUMOR AND LIVER TISSUE

Precursor Steroid	Metabolic Conversion Product (%) Tumor	Liver
4-^{14}C-Testosterone	16α-Hydroxyestrone 0.01% 16α-Hydroxytestosterone 0.015% 2 Hydroxyestriol (?) 0.013%	16α-Hydroxytestosterone 0.08%
4-^{14}C-Estrone	Estradiol-17β 0.3% 16α-Hydroxyestrone 0.03% 2-Methoxyestrone 0.34%	Not done
^{3}H-Testosterone sulfate	Tetroxyestrogens[a]	Not done
^{3}H-DHEA	Tetroxyestrogens[a] Dihydroxyketone compounds[a] 4.7%	Dihydroxyketone compounds (0.1%)
^{3}H-DHEA sulfate	Dihydroxyketone compounds[a] 1.5%	Not done
4-^{14}C-Cholesterol	Testosterone 1.50% Androsterone 10.0% Androst-4-ene-3,17-dione 4.1% 5α-Androstane-3,17-dione 0.10% 5α-Androstane-3α,17β-diol 0.61%	Not done

[a] Nature of these compounds is to be identified.

of tumor incubation with DHEA sulfate, however, fail to demonstrate the presence of estrone, estradiol, or estriol as metabolic products.

Desmolase activity in the tumors was demonstrated by the isolation of testosterone, androsterone, androst-4-ene-3,17-dione, 5α-androstane-3,17-dione, and 5α-androstane-3α,17β-diol as metabolites of cholesterol. Of special interest is the formation of androstenedione, a compound known to be readily convertible to estrone (15). The formation of known estrogen precursors from cholesterol thus lends credence to the possibility that tumors synthesize phenolic hormones in a fashion similar to that known to occur in endocrine tissue.

Thus, the results obtained by us and by Adams (chap. 8) show that human mammary cancer tissue may indeed have the ability to synthesize estrogenic hormones. At least these experiments have demonstrated that human mammary cancer tissue contains enzyme systems to aromatize and hydroxylate estrogen precursors.

The various studies on the incubations of tumor and liver tissues which are included in this paper are representative of a larger number of investigations which gave results similar to those recorded here. In all, there were, in the tumor study, twelve incubations with testosterone, seven incubations with DHEA, four incubations with DHEA sulfate, two incubations with testosterone sulfate, two incubations with estrone and one incubation with cholesterol. In the liver study, there were three incubations each with testosterone and DHEA.

In contrast to the work of Adams dealing with the metabolism of testosterone to estriol by human breast tumors, twelve separate experiments in the present study failed to support the contention that testosterone is a precursor for estriol. Our inability to obtain estriol as the final metabolic product is probably due to the small magnitude of the conversion, since it has been conclusively demonstrated that tumor tissues possess aromatase, 16α-hydroxylase, and 17β-estradiol dehydrogenase, which are essential for the conversion of testosterone to estriol (testosterone → 16α-hydroxytestosterone → 16α-hydroxyestrone → estriol).

Although there is some evidence that fetal liver possesses aromatizing enzyme systems (16), our studies with adult human liver have failed to demonstrate the presence of aromatase. The present results can at least rule out the liver as a source of estrogenic substances derivable from testosterone, DHEA, or their sulfates in the urine of oophorectomized, adrenalectomized women.

References

1. Dao, T. L. 1953. Estrogen excretion in women with mammary cancer and after adrenalectomy. *Science* 119: 21.
2. West, C. D.; Damast, B. L.; Sarro, S. D.; and Pearson, O. H. 1956. Conversion of testosterone to estrogens in castrated, adrenalectomized human females. *J. Biol. Chem.* 218: 409.
3. Dao, T., and Morreal, C. 1968. Isolation and identification of estriol in urine of castrated and adrenalectomized women receiving 4-^{14}C-testosterone. *Steroids* 12: 651.
4. Chang, E., and Dao, T. L. 1961. Adrenal estrogens. I. Conversion of 4-^{14}C-cortisone acetate to 11-oxygenated estrogens in women. *J. Clin. Endocr. Metab.* 21: 624.
5. Chang, E.; Dao, T. L.; and Mittleman, A. 1962. Adrenal estrogens. III. Conversion of 4-^{14}C-cortisone to 11β-hydroxyestrone by human breast tumor slices. In *International Congress on Hormonal Steroids*, ed. M. Connolly et al., p. 237. International Congress Series no. 51, Excerpta Med. Foundation.
6. Ryan, K. J., and Smith, O. W. 1961. Biogenesis of estrogens by the human ovary. I. Conversion of acetate 1-^{14}C to estrone and estradiol *J. Biol. Chem.* 236: 705.
7. Engel, L. L. 1950. The chemical estimation of steroid hormone metabolites. *Recent Prog. Hormone Res.* 5: 335.
8. Morreal, C. E.; Dao, T. L.; and Lonergan, P. A. 1970. A method for the separation of polar androgens from estrogens. *Anal. Biochem.* 34: 352.
9. Feher, T. 1966. Some aspects of the determination of individual urinary 17-oxosteroids: Methodology. *Clin. Chim. Acta* 14: 83.
10. Lipsett, M. 1965. Hormonal syndromes associated with cancer. *Cancer Res.* 25: 1068.
11. Liddle, G. W.; Givens, J. R.; Nicholson, W. E.; and Island, D. P. 1964. The ectopic ACTH syndrome. *Cancer Res.* 25: 1057.
12. Samuels, L. T., and Eik-Nes, K. B. 1968. Metabolism of steroid hormones. In *Metabolic pathways*, ed. P. M. Greenberg, 2: 169. New York: Academic Press.
13. Baulieu, E. E.; Corpechot, C.; Dray, F.; Emilozzi, R.; Lebean, M.; Mauvais-Jarvis, P.; and Robel, P. 1965. An adrenal-secreted "androgen": Dehydroisoandrosterone sulfate, its metabolism and a tentative generalization on the metabolism of other steroid conjugates in man. *Recent Prog. Hormone Res.* 21: 411.
14. Schubert, K. 1964. In vivo conversion of DHEA-sulfate into estrogens. *Naturwissenschaften* 51: 312.
15. MacDonald, P.; Rombaut, R.; and Siiteri, P. 1967. Plasma precursors of estrogen. *J. Clin. Endocr. Metab.* 27: 1103.
16. Slaunwhite, N. R.; Karsay, M. A.; Hollmer, A. A.; Sandberg, A. A.; and Niswander, K. 1965. Fetal liver as an endocrine system. *Steroids*, suppl. 2:211.

Thomas L. Dao and Paul R. Libby

Steroid Sulfate Formation in Human Breast Tumors and Hormone Dependency   11

Although enzymes for synthesizing steroid sulfate have been thought to be concerned mainly with catabolic inactivation of hormones, great interest has developed recently in the implication of sulfated steroids as active intermediates in steroid biosynthesis (1). These investigations showed that the metabolic conversions from cholesterol sulfate to dehydroepiandrosterone (DHEA) sulfate by the adrenal gland utilize the sulfate precursors, and that this transformation could occur without breaking the sulfate-steroid bond. Thus conjugation of steroids with sulfuric and glucuronic acids can no longer be considered only a catabolic reaction confined to the liver. In fact, many other tissues, including both endocrine and nonendocrine organs, have been shown to contain enzyme systems for conjugation of steroid hormones (2–7).

We decided to study steroid conjugation systems in mammary cancer (1) to determine whether sulfation of steroid hormones by the neoplastic tissues is related to the apparent capacity of tumors to carry out metabolic transformation of hormones and (2) to determine how liver, as the major site for steroid conjugation, may influence the responsiveness of the tumor to hormonal alterations. We did not know whether metastatic involvement of liver might increase or reduce the ability of liver to synthesize steroid conjugates.

Investigators on two continents (8, 9) independently demonstrated the presence of enzyme systems for forming steroid sulfate esters in mammary gland and mammary cancer tissues. In our earlier study,

The authors are affiliated with the Department of Breast Surgery and Endocrine Research Laboratory at the Roswell Park Memorial Institute of the New York State Department of Health at Buffalo.

we showed that breast cancer contains two populations of cells—one that lacks enzyme and one that possesses enzymes capable of forming sulfate esters with several steroid hormones (9). We also demonstrated that sulfurylation of different steroid hormones by normal human liver tissues may vary among individuals, but that the relative activity within each person is almost constant; dehydroepiandrosterone is the most efficiently sulfurylated, and the ratio of each of the other steroids such as pregnenolone, deoxycorticosterone, corticosterone, testosterone, 19-nortestosterone, estrone, 17β-estradiol, and estriol to DHEA is about the same. The pattern of conjugation of steroid hormones is not the same in breast cancer tissue, however, as in normal liver tissue, especially with respect to 17β-estradiol. Some breast cancers can conjugate estradiol more efficiently than DHEA, and others conjugate DHEA more efficiently.

These findings led to an extended study to determine whether formation of steroid sulfate in mammary cancer is related to the response to endocrine ablation in patients with disseminated cancer of the breast. We reported earlier that the conjugation of steroid hormones by breast cancer tissue may be related to the response to adrenalectomy in patients with metastatic cancer of the breast (10).

If sulfation of steroid hormones by mammary cancer is indeed related to the hormone dependency of a tumor, the biological mechanism of this relationship should be elucidated. We are particularly interested, from the clinical standpoint, in knowing (1) whether conjugation of steroid hormones by mammary cancer tissue has any value in predicting the recurrence of metastases; (2) whether the ability to conjugate steroid hormones in a primary breast cancer indicates future response to adrenalectomy or oophorectomy when metastases appear; and (3) whether recurrent lesions differ from the primary breast cancer in their ability to conjugate steroid hormones. Our experiments were designed to answer these questions.

BIOCHEMICAL STUDIES OF THE CHARACTERISTICS OF STEROID CONJUGATION SYSTEMS

All tissues were worked up within 15 min after surgery. Each was carefully cleared of fatty tissues, and a small piece of the tumor was excised for histological sections. We have described the methods for the preparation of tissues, incubation, extraction, and final estimation of steroid sulfate synthesized in detail in a previous publication (9).

Briefly, the minced tissue was homogenized in 4 volumes of 0.25 M sucrose and centrifuged (12,000 g). Aliquots of the supernatant fluid containing the enzyme were then incubated with 100 μmoles of pH 7.6 Tris buffer, 5 μmoles of ATP, 2 μmoles of $MgCl_2$, 0.1 μmole K_2SO_4, approximately 5μc (0.10 μmole) of $H_2^{35}SO_4$, and 0.5 μmole of steroid in a final volume of 1.0 ml. The steroids routinely used were dehydroepiandrosterone (DHEA), pregnenolone, deoxycorticosterone (DOC), 17β-estradiol, estrone, estriol, and testosterone. Incubation was for 1 hr at 37° C.

The reaction was stopped by chilling, and 1 ml of 2 N NH_4OH saturated with $(NH_4)_2SO_4$ was added to the incubation mixture, which was then extracted 3 times with 3 ml of ethyl acetate. The ethyl acetate extract was brought up to 10 ml, and was backwashed with 7/8 saturated $(NH_4)_2SO_4$. Aliquots were counted in a scintillation counter with 10 ml of a scintillation fluid. Steroid sulfate synthesized by all tissues was calculated in pmoles (10^{-12} moles) per mg of protein per hr. Total protein content was estimated by the biuret reaction.

Studies of the characteristics of the system (9) showed that ATP and magnesium ions were required, as would be expected for a sulfate-activating system. The overall reaction was linear with both time and enzyme concentration under the conditions employed and had a pH optimum of 7.6. The enzyme was saturated with DHEA at approximately 10^{-6}M, but was not inhibited by excess substrate concentration at 5×10^{-5}M, the routine concentration for the assay.

To demonstrate that the synthesized and isolated radioactive material was the steroid sulfate corresponding to the steroid added to the incubation system, we chemically synthesized authentic steroid sulfates. Chromatography of extracted radioactive material plus chemically synthesized markers was carried out in five systems: n-butyl acetate:n-butanol:10% acetic acid (80:20:100); n-butyl acetate:n-butanol:10% formic acid (80:20:100); n-butyl acetate:methanol:0.1 M sodium barbital buffer, pH 8.2, in 50% aqueous methanol (150:50: 50); ethyl acetate:n-butanol:0.2% NH_4OH (175:25:200); and water. In all cases involving alcoholic steroids, the radioactive material cochromatographed with the marker in all five systems. In the estradiol sulfates, the radioactivity coincided with the 3-sulfate in the systems ethyl acetate:n-butanol:0.2% NH_4OH (175:25:200) and water. In these systems, the radioactive material separated from the marker 17β-sulfate. No evidence was seen for any disulfate product.

In addition to the preceding chromatographic evidence, the radioactive DHEA sulfate was cocrystallized with authentic DHEA sulfate to constant specific activity (9).

To test the stability of our preparations, we assayed several each day for three days, storing them in the freezer overnight between assays. Table 1 shows the results of one such assay. Short-term storage in the frozen state (ca. 48 hr), as well as the associated freezing and thawing, had no appreciable effect on the activity of the enzymes.

TABLE 1: STEROID SULFATE SYNTHESIZED BY A METASTATIC TUMOR IN A PATIENT WITH CANCER OF THE BREAST

Number of Experiment[a]	Steroid Sulfate Synthesized (cmp)	
	DHEA	E-17β
1	111	224
	103	293
2	104	304
	112	311
3	129	292
	107	296
	111 ± 9.5	295 ± 12.4

[a] Three experiments were done on three consecutive days on the same tumor.

Other experiments suggest that the half-life of human liver DHEA sulfotransferase is about 8 to 10 mo at $-20°$ C, whereas human liver estrogen sulfotransferase has a half-life of about 2 mo under these conditions (9).

CONJUGATION OF STEROID HORMONES BY NORMAL AND NEOPLASTIC TISSUES

Synthesis of Steroid Sulfate by Normal and Neoplastic Mammary Glands

Steroid sulfate synthesis by normal mammary tissues and their neoplastic counterparts was studied in 25 patients. Table 2 shows that 19 of the 25 normal mammary tissue samples examined were inactive, whereas only 8 tumors were inactive. In this group of 8 inactive tumors, the normal mammary gland tissues were also inactive. In no case did the normal mammary gland contain enzyme activity if the tumor was inactive, and in most cases the normal glands were significantly lower in enzyme activity than their neoplastic counterparts. We believe that the absence or low level of enzyme activity may be due to the extremely low cellularity of normal mammary tissues.

Although the specific activity of different mammary tumor extracts varies widely, the ratio of activities of sulfate formation, using different steroids as precursors, is not constant, as it is in liver (9). Over

TABLE 2: SULFOKINASE ACTIVITY IN NORMAL BREAST AND BREAST CANCER TISSUES

Sulfokinase Activity	No. of Patients
Normal breast tissue—no activity Tumor tissue—active	11
Normal breast tissue—active Tumor tissue—active	6
Normal breast tissue—no activity Tumor tissue—no activity	8

NOTE: In each case, normal breast tissue and tumor tissue are from the same patient. All normal tissues are proved by histological sections to contain no neoplastic cells.

an extended series (more than 200 tumor samples), the proportion of DHEA to estradiol has been greater than one in about 30% but less than one in about 40% of all samples tested. We found no measurable sulfokinase activity in the remaining 30% of the tumor samples.

Enzymatic Sulfation of Steroids by Normal and Neoplastic Liver Tissues

Data from one earlier study (9) showed that normal liver is highly active in conjugating steroid hormones. In normal liver preparations examined, DHEA was always sulfurylated more actively than any other steroid. As a major site for steroid conjugation, the liver may be concerned with metabolic inactivation of steroids. We do not know whether replacing normal liver tissue with neoplastic cells may decrease or increase the ability to form steroid sulfate. We are particularly interested in comparing the steroid conjugation systems in mammary cancer tissue, normal liver, and metastatic liver tissues. Such comparisons may yield important information on response of liver metastases to hormonal treatment.

The synthesis of steroid sulfate by normal and metastatic liver tissues was compared in 20 patients with disseminated breast cancer. In these patients, both types of liver tissues were removed at the time of adrenalectomy and were assayed for steroid sulfotransferase activity. The results can be divided into three groups: in the majority of cases (11 patients), the ability to synthesize steroid conjugates is greatly impaired in liver metastases; in about a third (6 patients), steroid sulfate synthesis is considerably increased in the neoplastic liver tissues; and in a small number of cases (3 patients), there is a decrease in conjugation of C_{19} and C_{21} steroid hormones, but a markedly enhanced synthesis of estrogen sulfate (table 3). When the ratios of DHEA sulfate and estradiol sulfate in the normal and neoplastic livers are compared, the results can again be divided into three groups: the ratio of DHEA sulfate to estradiol sulfate is greater in neoplastic liver tissue than in the normal liver in 4 patients, lower in 11 patients, and equal in 5 patients. When the response to adrenalectomy is assessed in these 20 patients, we note that all 3 patients with remission after adrenalectomy have significantly higher ratios of DHEA sulfate to estradiol sulfate in the neoplastic liver tissue than in the normal liver tissue (table 4). In contrast, the ratios of DHEA sulfate to estradiol sulfate in the metastatic liver tissues in 16 adrenalectomy failures are either lower than those in the corresponding normal tissues or equal to them. Only one patient with a ratio lower in neoplastic liver tissue than in its normal counterpart has had an objective remission.

We can draw these conclusions: (*a*) In most cases, the capacity of the liver for conjugating steroid hormones is markedly impaired when normal cells are replaced with neoplastic cells. This suggests that neoplastic liver cells may be incapable of metabolically inactivating steroid hormones. (*b*) Some metastatic liver tissues, in contrast, contain more enzyme activity for steroid conjugation than their normal counterparts. It seems that the neoplastic livers not only retain the physiological activity, but sometimes contain more enzymes than the normal tissues. (*c*) There can be a differential in the enzymatic synthesis of sulfate for C_{19}, C_{21}, and C_{18} steroid hormones. Irrespective

TABLE 3: SYNTHESIS OF STEROID SULFATE BY NORMAL AND NEOPLASTIC LIVER TISSUES

Patients	Age	Tissues	Steroid Sulfate Synthesized ($\mu\mu$mole/mg protein/hr)						
			DHEA	Pregnenolone	E_2[a]	E_1[b]	E_3[c]	Testosterone	Ratio
J. M.	48	Normal liver	474.8	411.4	316.9	264.6	152.6	270.7	1.4
		Liver metastases	497.5	188.1	414.4	327.7	181.5	153.3	1.2
A. B.	63	Normal liver	674.0	616.0	400.0	405.0	228.0	431.0	1.6
		Liver metastases	79.1	47.9	389.0	246.0	62.5	47.9	0.2
C. V.	54	Normal liver	264.0	287.0	98.9	77.0	52.1	200.0	2.5
		Liver metastases	303.0	139.0	179.0	150.0	83.0	98.5	1.6

[a] Estradiol. [b] Estrone. [c] Estriol.

TABLE 4: SYNTHESIS OF STEROID SULFATE BY NORMAL AND NEOPLASTIC LIVER TISSUES IN ADRENALECTOMY RESPONDERS

Patients	Age	Tissues	DHEA	Pregnenolone	E_2[a]	E_1[b]	E_3[c]	Testosterone	Ratio
M. B.	65	Normal liver	1,150.0	1,082.0	709.0	668.0	377.0	732.0	1.6
		Liver metastases	1,065.0	496.0	469.0	427.0	233.0	291.0	2.2
B. M.	46	Normal liver	40.5	40.9	24.2	18.0	11.0	5.5	1.6
		Liver metastases	13.7	10.5	5.5	5.0	3.0	2.0	2.4
N. K.	57	Normal liver	46.5	30.5	24.5	21.5	10.5	24.0	1.8
		Liver metastases	87.0	70.0	39.0	30.0	18.0	28.1	2.2
T. L.	54	Normal liver	268.2	270.1	88.2	62.8	35.5	173.9	3.0
		Liver metastases	163.3	70.3	91.1	73.0	42.6	49.5	1.7

Steroid Sulfate Synthesized (μμmole/mg protein/hr)

[a] Estradiol. [b] Estrone. [c] Estriol

Steroid Sulfate Formation and Hormone Dependency

of these differences in ability to synthesize steroid sulfate, however, the most important factor controlling the response to adrenalectomy is still the ratio of DHEA sulfate to estradiol sulfate. It appears that the tumors of responders must be able to synthesize significantly more DHEA sulfate than their normal counterparts.

CLINICAL CORRELATIONS

Clinical Materials

Mammary cancer tissue was obtained from 195 patients: 53 underwent radical mastectomy for primary breast cancer; 33, simple mastectomy for locally advanced breast cancer; and 109, adrenalectomy

TABLE 5: AGE AND MENSTRUAL STATUS OF WOMEN WITH CANCER OF THE BREAST

		Age			Menstrual Status	
Groups	No. of Patients	Range	Median	Mean	Premenopausal	Postmenopausal
Radical mastectomy	56	29–74	55	56	12	44
Simple mastectomy	36	45–82	66	62	4	32
Adrenalectomy	109	36–75	54	53	—	109

for disseminated disease. The age and menstrual status of each of these patients are indicated in table 5. Tumor tissues removed for biochemical study in patients with disseminated cancer were either soft-tissue metastases or inoperable primary lesions in the breast. At the time of adrenalectomy, the abdominal cavity was explored routinely, and both normal and metastatic lesions in the liver and other sites were obtained for assay of steroid conjugation enzyme systems.

Sulfation of Steroid Hormones by Breast Cancer Tissue and Clinical Correlation with Response to Adrenalectomy

Mammary cancer tissue was obtained from 109 women with disseminated breast cancer who were scheduled to undergo bilateral adrenalectomy. All were postmenopausal. Menopause was either spontaneous or induced by surgical castration. Assessment of remission was based solely upon objective evidence of regression, and subjective improvement alone was not considered a remission. Fleeting tumor regression of less than 6 mo was scored as a failure.

In this series, mammary cancer tissues from 30 patients were found to be inactive (no measurable steroid sulfokinase). All 30 failed to respond to adrenalectomy. The ratio of DHEA sulfate to estradiol sulfate was greater than unity in 29 tumors, less than unity in 46, and equal to unity in 4. Results in table 6 show clearly that breast cancers possessing enzymes that sulfurylate DHEA more efficiently than estradiol are more likely to regress after adrenalectomy than are those that sulfurylate estradiol more efficiently than DHEA. Perhaps the most

TABLE 6: SULFOKINASE ACTIVITY IN TUMOR AND RESPONSE TO ADRENALECTOMY

No. of Patients	Sulfokinase Activity in Tumor (DHEA:E-17β Ratio)	Response to Adrenalectomy Remission	Failure
30	No activity	—	30
46	<1	6 (15%)	40
29	>1	21 (73%)	8
4	=1	3	1
Total 109		30	79

significant finding in the study is that tumors that lack demonstrable steroid sulfate synthesis uniformly fail to respond to adrenalectomy. It is most striking that all patients whose tumors were negative in enzyme activity are now dead (fig. 1). In contrast, the data clearly show that patients whose tumors form more DHEA sulfate than estradiol sulfate survive significantly longer. This strongly suggests a correlation between the results of the in vitro study and clinical response to adrenalectomy.

Steroid Sulfate Synthesis by Primary Cancer: Its Relationship to Recurrence Rate and to Response to Adrenalectomy

Although results so far provide convincing evidence that assay of enzymes for steroid conjugate synthesis by metastatic breast cancer tissue may be valuable in selecting patients for adrenalectomy, practical application of this method will be impeded because more than half

Steroid Sulfate Formation and Hormone Dependency

of all patients undergoing adrenalectomy have metastatic tumors in organs such as lungs, bones, and the central nervous system which cannot routinely be excised for assay. An important question is, "Can assay of primary breast cancer for steroid sulfotransferases predict response to adrenalectomy?" We also intend to determine whether assay of steroid-conjugating systems in primary breast cancer has any prognostic value for patients undergoing "curative" radical mastectomy.

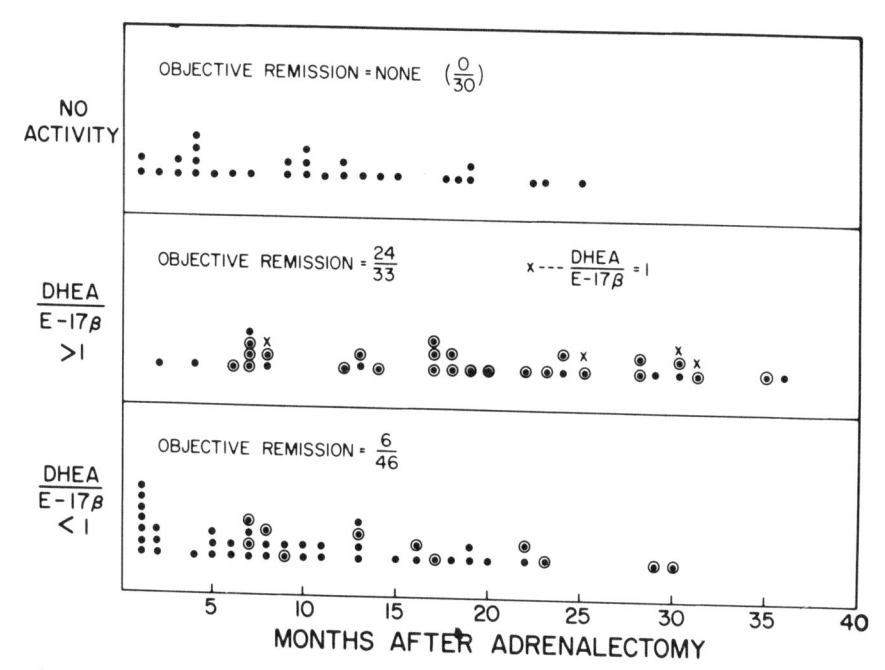

Fig. 1. Correlation between steroid sulfotransferase activity in tumor and survival after adrenalectomy (⊙ = living   ◯ = dead).

Primary breast cancers removed at the time of mastectomy were studied in 92 patients, from July 1967 through July 1969. Of these patients, 56 had radical mastectomy and 36 had simple mastectomy. In the final analysis, 3 patients in the radical mastectomy group (2 lost to follow-up and 1 with a diagnosis of melanoma) and 3 patients in the simple mastectomy group (all 3 lost to follow-up) are excluded. All patients with operable lesions satisfying the criteria for "curative" surgery (i.e., clinical stage I or II) underwent radical mastectomy. No patients in clinical stage III (those with large tumors, large axillary lymph nodes, and signs of locally advancing disease) were subjected to radical mastectomy, since they were incurable. Simple mastectomy was done in these patients and also in those with medical contraindications and in those of advanced age (over 75). Table 7 shows that the 18 patients with recurrence in the radical mastectomy group are almost equally divided between subgroups whose tumors either have no measurable sulfotransferase activity or have ratios of DHEA sulfate and estradiol sulfate equal to 1 or less than 1. In contrast, none of the 7 patients whose tumors have greater activity in forming

TABLE 7: ASSAY OF STEROID SULFATE IN THE PRIMARY BREAST CANCER AND CLINICAL CORRELATIONS WITH INCIDENCE OF RECURRENCE

Sulfokinase Activity in Tumor (DHEA:E-17β Ratio)	Radical Mastectomy		Simple Mastectomy	
	No. without Recurrence	No. with Recurrence	No. without Recurrence	No. with Recurrence
No activity	13/21	8/21	2/8	6/8
>1	7/7	0/7	3/3	0/3
<1	15/25	10/25	6/22	16/22
Total	35/53	18/53	11/33	22/33

DHEA sulfate than estradiol sulfate (ratio > 1) have shown evidence of metastases. The simple mastectomy group shows similar results.

When the capacity of breast cancer tissue for synthesizing steroid sulfate is correlated with the extent of axillary lymph node involvement and recurrence, some very interesting observations become apparent. Table 8 shows that not a single tumor in any of the 20 patients with axillary metastases involving more than four nodes had a ratio of DHEA sulfate to estradiol sulfate greater than 1. The data also clearly show that even patients whose axillary lymph nodes are negative for metastases develop early recurrence only when either their tumors contain no sulfotransferase activity or the ratio of DHEA sulfate to estradiol sulfate is less than unity. These results suggest that the capacity of tumors for synthesizing steroid conjugates may determine their capability for forming metastases. This study is too preliminary, however, to permit any definitive conclusions, since the great majority of patients in this series had mastectomy less than three years ago.

Of the 40 patients who have developed metastases, only 15 have soft-tissue lesions that can be excised for a second assay of sulfotransferase activity. Of these 15 patients, 11 underwent adrenalectomy, and the results are shown in table 9. The data show that tumors from 6 patients differ significantly in their ability to synthesize steroid sulfate. In 3 patients, L. B., B. H., and J. W., the primary tumors were

TABLE 8: SYNTHESIS OF STEROID SULFATE BY THE PRIMARY BREAST CANCER AND CORRELATION WITH METASTASES IN THE AXILLARY LYMPH NODES AND RECURRENCE

No. of Positive Lymph Nodes	Sulfokinase Activity in Tumors		
	No Activity	$\dfrac{\text{DHEA-S}}{\text{E-17}\beta\text{-S}^a} > 1$	$\dfrac{\text{DHEA-S}}{\text{E-17}\beta\text{-S}} < 1$
0	2/9[b]	0/5	1/6
1–3	0/4	0/2	1/7
4 and more	7/9	—	7/11
Total	9/22	0/7	9/24

[a] Estradiol-17β-sulfate.
[b] Number of patients with recurrence/Total number of patients.

inactive, whereas the recurrent lesions acquired the ability to conjugate steroid hormones. In contrast, the recurrent tumors in 2 patients, L. L. and T. A., seemed to have lost their ability to synthesize steroid sulfate, since the primary tumors in both patients contained enzymes to catalyze the formation of steroid sulfate. In only 1 patient, E. B., the ratio of DHEA sulfate to estradiol sulfate rose from less than unity in the primary tumor to greater than 1 in the recurrent tumor. In the remaining patients, the primary tumors and their metastatic lesions showed no difference in conjugating ability. These results demonstrate that the capacity of tumor tissue for forming steroid sulfate may indeed change in some tumors.

Of the 40 patients developing metastases, 9 underwent bilateral adrenalectomy without a second assay of steroid sulfokinase activity, since the metastatic lesions were in bones or in visceral organs not amenable to biopsy. Even so, the assay of the enzyme activity of the primary tumors predicted correctly that none would respond to adrenalectomy, since 5 tumors were inactive and 4 had DHEA sulfate and estradiol sulfate ratios less than 1 (0.3–0.7). If these data are combined, they disclose that assay of sulfotransferase activity in the primary tumor is highly accurate in predicting response to adrenalectomy when metastases develop.

TABLE 9: COMPARISON OF STEROID SULFATE SYNTHESIS IN THE PRIMARY AND RECURRENT TUMORS

| | Primary Tumor ||| Recurrent Tumor ||| |
Patient	DHEA-S	Estra-diol-S	Ratio	DHEA-S	Estra-diol-S	Ratio	Response to Adrenalectomy
F. J.	5.0	7.1	0.7	25.0	73.0	0.3	Good
E. B.	6.5	8.6	0.8	19.5	13.0	1.5	Good
L. L.	9.4	19.7	0.4	0	0	0	None
L. B.	0	0	0	17.5	13.8	1.2	None
B. H.	0	0	0	54.4	110.0	0.5	None
C. K.	2.1	4.7	0.4	3.9	10.3	0.3	None
T. A.	9.4	24.9	0.3	0	0	0	None
A. B.	0	0	0	0	0	0	None
F. De.	37.2	112.7	0.3	33.6	100.0	0.3	None
J. W	0	0	0	6.7	6.4	1.0	Good
D. R.	0	0	0	0	0	0	None

NOTE: Primary tumors were removed at the time of radical or simple mastectomy and recurrent tumors were removed at the time of adrenalectomy.

These results suggest that the concentration of enzyme systems for forming steroid sulfate in mammary cancer tissue is related to the hormone responsiveness of the neoplasm. Our data demonstrate a correlation between the assay in vitro and the clinical results of adrenalectomy. It appears that the assay of enzymes for synthesis of steroid conjugates by the tumor tissue is an accurate method of selecting patients for adrenalectomy.

How sulfation of steroid hormones by mammary cancer is related to the hormone dependency of the cancer cannot be readily determined. It seems that in many cases conjugation is indeed a major step in the metabolic inactivation of hormones, whereas in other instances it may be concerned with metabolic transformation of those hormones. It is conceivable that sulfation of steroids may be an intermediary step in the biosynthesis of hormones.

CONJUGATION OF STEROID HORMONES AND SULFATE METABOLISM

As we have shown, some 25–30% of our tumor samples were lacking in measurable enzyme activity under our conditions. Because these tumors were from patients who uniformly failed to respond to adrenalectomy, we wished to determine what enzyme or enzymes these preparations lacked.

The enzymes required in our systems for the sulfurylation of steroids are sulfate adenylyl transferase, adenylylsulfate kinase, and a steroid sulfotransferase. Actually, there are probably three or four sulfotransferases being studied: an estrogen sulfotransferase, 3β-hydroxytransferase, possibly a 17β-hydroxytransferase, and a 21-hydroxytransferase (11). The enzymes catalyze the following series of reactions:

$$ATP + SO_4^= = APS + PPi \qquad (1)$$
$$APS + ATP = PAPS + ADP \qquad (2)$$
$$PAPS + Steroid = steroid\ sulfate + PAP \qquad (3)$$

Before the synthesis of steroid sulfate, there must be a two-stage reaction leading to the synthesis of adenosine 3'-phosphate 5'-phosphosulfate (PAPS) (12). If a tumor lacks sulfate-activating enzymes, there will be no synthesis of PAPS, and consequently no synthesis of steroid sulfate, even in the presence of sulfotransferase. A crude sulfate-activating system (13) was prepared and added to the inactive preparations in the assay. When this was done with a series of inactive tumors (14), the results shown in table 10 were obtained. As is evident, the "inactive" tumor preparations synthesized steroid sulfates actively in the presence of the yeast activating system. This suggested that the tumors lacked one or both of the enzymes necessary for forming PAPS.

We then prepared highly purified preparations of both sulfate adenylyl transferase and adenylylsulfate kinase from yeast, resulting in the complete separation of the two activities. When each enzyme was added separately to inactive tumor preparations, no activity was found; but when both enzymes together were added to the preparations, we obtained the results recorded in table 11. Thus, both enzymes are necessary for the formation of steroid sulfates by the tumor preparations.

Examining the effect of each enzyme separately and both together showed that both estradiol sulfate and DHEA sulfate were formed in increased amounts by using active tumor preparations (14). Also, the data reveal a synergistic effect of the two enzymes, which implies

TABLE 10: SYNTHESIS OF STEROID SULFATE IN INACTIVE BREAST TUMOR PREPARATIONS AFTER THE ADDITION OF YEAST ENZYMES

Tumor Preparations	Synthesis of Steroid Sulfate ($\mu\mu$mole/mg of protein/hr)	
	DHEA-S[a]	E$_2$S[b]
M. O.	35.9	31.4
R. S.	93.8	61.8
K. B.	36.6	37.7
H. O.	22.2	34.7
H. D.	36.5	36.0
A. E.	29.6	35.5
D. Z.	18.2	22.6
J. P.	33.2	28.9
H. B.	53.1	54.3
M. M.	31.2	28.4
C. Z.	4.4	6.6
R. B.	3.6	5.0
G. W.	6.6	3.4

[a] Dehydroepiandrosterone sulfate.
[b] Estradiol sulfate.

that both have low concentrations in the tumor preparations in comparison with the sulfotransferases, and that it is the low level of synthesis of PAPS that controls the rate of synthesis of steroid sulfate. Adding each enzyme separately or both enzymes together to these preparations also had no effect on the ratio of the formation of DHEA sulfate and estradiol sulfate (table 12). This indicates, as would be expected, that the ratio is controlled by the levels of the two sulfotransferases rather than by a specific effect of one or the other steroid on the enzymes controlling the synthesis of PAPS.

It is conceivable that the phenomena observed are concerned with mucopolysaccharide and sulfate metabolism in these tumors. It is also possible that some human breast cancers do not synthesize sulfated mucopolysaccharides because they lack sulfate-activating enzymes.

TABLE 11: SYNTHESIS OF STEROID SULFATE IN INACTIVE BREAST TUMOR PREPARATIONS AFTER THE ADDITION OF YEAST SULFATE ADENYLYLTRANSFERASES AND YEAST ADENYLYLSULFATE KINASE

Tumor Preparations	Steroid	+ Both Enzymes[a]
M. F.	E_2[b]	54.2
	DHEA[c]	61.0
M. H.	E_2	28.8
	DHEA	17.0
H. D.	E_2	39.9
	DHEA	25.2
H. B.	E_2	51.3
	DHEA	29.8
C. Z.	E_2	7.2
	DHEA	6.5
H. O.	E_2	30.2
	DHEA	16.3
J. C.	E_2	24.0
	DHEA	17.9
N. S.	E_2	126.0
	DHEA	77.8

[a] Steroid sulfate ($\mu\mu$mole/mg of protein/hr).
[b] 17β-Estradiol.
[c] Dehydroepiandrosterone.

The role of ground substance in tumor invasion and metastases has been of interest for many years. It has been suggested that there is a close functional interaction between stroma and growing epithelia, whether the latter are normal or neoplastic. By chemical staining and histological examination, Sylven (15) found that the amounts of an "ester-sulfuric acid-protein complex" in the stroma could be roughly correlated with the growth rate of several human carcinomas. He showed that slow-growing tumors contained large amounts of the complex, whereas there were only small amounts in the fast-growing cancers. Although these earlier data are hard to interpret, they suggest that biosynthesis of the sulfated mucopolysaccharide components of the ground substance is a determining factor in the formation of metastases. In this respect, the results from our investigation are both interesting and significant. Our

TABLE 12: SYNERGESTIC EFFECT OF SULFATE-ACTIVATING ENZYMES FROM YEAST IN ACTIVE TUMOR PREPARATIONS

Tumor Preparations	Steroid	Without Yeast Enzymes	+Sulfate Adenylyltransferase	+Adenylylsulfate Kinase	+Both Enzymes
		Steroid Sulfate Synthesized ($\mu\mu$moles/mg of protein/hr)			
H. W.	E_2[a]	25.80	33.70	45.50	119.20
	DHEA[b]	7.30	10.10	13.10	23.90
	DHEA:E_2	0.20	0.30	0.29	0.20
E. S.	E_2	20.50	21.80	36.20	69.80
	DHEA	13.10	20.00	32.20	37.80
	DHEA:E_2	0.64	0.92	0.89	0.54
A. M.	E_2	24.80	29.80	37.40	76.70
	DHEA	8.40	12.30	15.80	20.90
	DHEA:E_2	0.34	0.34	0.41	0.27

[a] 17β-Estradiol.
[b] Dehydroepiandrosterone.

data disclose that synthesis of steroid sulfate by primary breast cancer tissue has definite biological implications, particularly for the growth of the tumor. In both the radical and the simple mastectomy groups, the overwhelming majority of early recurrences developed in patients whose tumors showed either no conjugation enzyme activity or enzyme ratios less than unity for DHEA sulfate to estradiol sulfate. Even more striking is the observation that sulfokinase activity can be correlated with lymph-node status, which is by far the most accurate clinical parameter for prognosticating the clinical course of breast cancer (16). Our results show that early recurrence after radical mastectomy occurs only in patients whose tumors are unable to either synthesize steroid sulfate or sulfurylate estradiol more efficiently than DHEA (ratio < 1). Interestingly, these are also the patients whose axillary lymph nodes contain metastases at the time of "curative" surgery (table 8). This correlation strongly suggests that the ability of the tumor to synthesize steroid sulfate is one of the determinants controlling tumor metastasis.

Acknowledgments

This investigation was supported by grant CA-08219-01-06 from the National Cancer Institute, National Institutes of Health, United States Public Health Service.

References

1. Lieberman, S. 1967. Sulfates as biosynthetic intermediates. In *Second international congress on hormonal steroids*, ed. L. Martini, F. Fraschini, and M. Motta, p. 22. International Congress Series no. 132, Excerpta Med. Foundation.
2. Holcenberg, J. S., and Rosen, S. W. 1965. Enzymatic sulfation of steroids by bovine tissues. *Arch. Biochem.* 110: 551.
3. Wallace, E., and Silberman, N. 1964. Biosynthesis of steroid sulfates by human ovarian tissue. *J. Biol. Chem.* 239: 2809.
4. Dixon, R.; Vincent, V.; and Kase, N. 1965. Biosynthesis of steroid sulfates by normal human testis. *Steroids* 6: 757.
5. Lehtinen, A.; Hartiala, K.; and Nurmikko, F. 1958. Duodenal glucuronide synthesis. II. Identification of estradiol glucuronide as a conjugation product of estradiol by the rat duodenal mucosa: Quantitative analysis. *Acta Chem. Scand.* 12: 1589.
6. Wotiz, H. H.; Ziskind, B. S.; Lemon, H. M.; and Gut, M. 1956. Studies in steroid metabolism. IV. Evidence for the formation of a water-soluble conjugate during *in vitro* incubations of human tissue with testosterone. *Biochim. Biophys. Acta* 22: 266.
7. Adams, J. B. 1964. Enzymic synthesis of steroid sulphates. I. Sulphation of steroids by human adrenal extracts. *Biochim. Biophys. Acta* 82: 572.
8. ———. 1964. Enzymic synthesis of steroid sulfates. II. Presence of steroid sulfokinase in human mammary carcinoma extracts. *J. Clin. Endocr. Metab.* 24: 988.
9. Dao, T. L., and Libby, P. R. 1968. Conjugation of steroid hormones by normal and neoplastic tissues. *J. Clin. Endocr. Metab.* 28: 1431.
10. ———. 1969. Conjugation of steroid hormones by breast cancer tissue and selection of patients for adrenalectomy. *Surgery* 66: 162.
11. Adams, J. B., and Poulos, A. 1967. Enzymic synthesis of steroid sul-

phates. III. Isolation and properties of estrogen sulphotransferase of bovine adrenal glands. *Biochim. Biophys. Acta* 146: 493.
12. Robbins, P. W., and Lipmann, F. 1957. Isolation and identification of active sulfate. *J. Biol. Chem.* 229: 837.
13. Robbins, P. W. 1962. Sulfate-activating enzymes. In *Methods in enzymology*, ed. S. P. Colowick and N. O. Kaplan, 5: 964. New York: Academic Press.
14. Libby, P. R., and Dao, T. L. 1970. Lack of sulfate-activating enzymes in human breast tumors. *Proc. Soc. Exp. Biol. Med.* 133: 1409.
15. Sylven, B. 1949. Ester sulphuric acids in stroma connective tissue. *Acta Radiol.* 32: 11.

John B. Adams, Roger K. Ellyard, and Joyce Low

Studies on Adrenal Estrogen Sulfotransferase 12

INTRODUCTION

Great interest has developed in the last few years in the idea that sulfurylated forms of steroids may be intermediates in steroid biosynthesis (1). If further experiments prove that this is true, an analogy will exist with the metabolism of carbohydrates via their ionized phosphate esters. We already know that at least eleven separate enzymatic transformations of steroids can occur with steroid sulfates as substrates (1). In addition, of course, dehydroepiandrosterone (DHEA) sulfate and cortisol are quantitatively the most important secretions of the human adrenal cortex. The steroid sulfokinases, or transferases, have been under study in my laboratory for several years. We isolated estrogen sulfotransferase from bovine adrenals free of steroid alcohol or phenol sulfotransferase activities (2). It exhibited unusual kinetic properties (3) which suggested that the sulfotransferase responsible for the sulfurylation of DHEA in the human adrenal (4) would be worth examining in depth. This latter enzyme also exhibited most unusual kinetic properties, with peaks and troughs in the velocity-substrate curves (5). A number of active enzyme species with different molecular weights were demonstrated by gel filtration and sucrose gradient centrifugation. We found evidence of a slowly reversible association-dissociation equilibrium. It was possible to isolate individual species by density-gradient centrifugation, and changes in activity which accompanied the slow return to equilibrium indicated that such activity was related to the state of association. Both substrates, adenosine-3'-phosphate-5'-

The authors are affiliated with the School of Biochemistry at the University of New South Wales.

phosphosulfate (PAPS) and DHEA, affected the state of association, PAPS causing dissociation and the steroid tending to cause association. It was suggested that the unusual kinetics could be explained by the effect of the ratio of substrates on the position of the association-dissociation equilibrium. Such properties indicated that the enzyme could possibly enter into some form of control mechanism (5). ACTH elevates DHEA adrenal venous levels twenty- to one-hundred-fold but has no effect on DHEA sulfate adrenal venous levels (6). One interpretation of this is that the sulfurylation step is rate limiting in the overall formation of DHEA sulfate (6).

Because of the restricted supply of human adrenals we could not isolate reasonable amounts of pure enzyme for chemical and biochemical studies. Bovine estrogen sulfotransferase, which, as was mentioned previously, exhibits kinetics similar to those of the DHEA sulfotransferase, has now been isolated pure as a model for studies on this class of enzyme.

Properties of the Enzyme Isolated by DEAE-Cellulose Chromatography

Initially, estrogen sulfotransferase was isolated in two forms, A and B, by DEAE-cellulose chromatography of the 60% ammonium sulfate fraction derived from the supernatant fluid of bovine adrenal gland homogenates (2). Evidence suggested that these forms represented a monomer (A) and a higher associated form, probably a trimer (8). Form B gave nonlinear double reciprocal plots on varying estrogen in the presence of fixed concentrations of PAPS (3). Form A was thought to give normal Michaelis-Menten kinetics, but insufficient points were used to construct the curves and it is now established that form A also gives nonlinear double reciprocal plots. The enzyme was sensitive to heavy metal ions, especially Zn^{2+} and Ni^{2+}. Mg^{2+} and Ca^{2+} caused some activation, but EDTA had no effect on enzyme activity. Sulfhydryl blocking agents were inhibitory at relatively high concentrations (e.g., p-chloromecuribenzoate inhibited by 43% at 1 mM and 80% at 10 mM) suggesting that one or more SH groups were near the active site or perhaps were involved in maintaining an active conformation (2).

The effect on the enzyme kinetics of adding different thiols, using a lyophilized preparation of the combined enzymically active fractions from a DEAE-cellulose column, is shown in figures 1 and 2. The

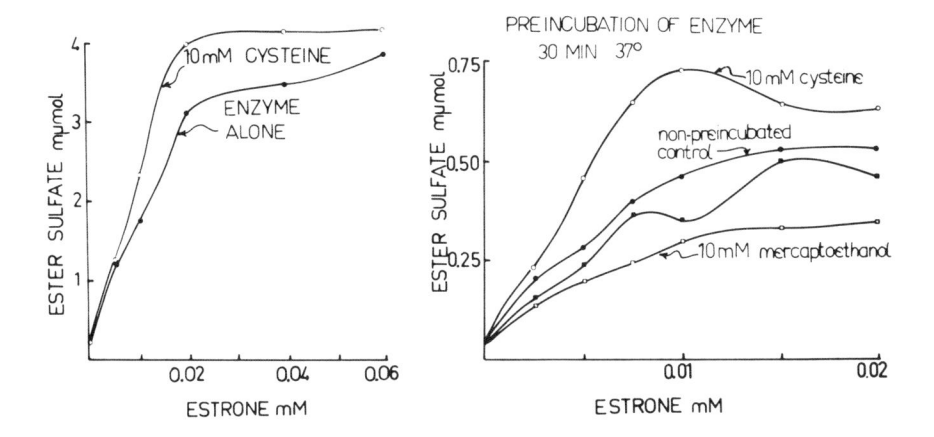

Fig. 1. Kinetics of "intact" enzyme isolated from DEAE cellulose column. *Left,* protein 100 μg; ^{35}S PAPS, 0.07 mM; MgCl$_2$, 20 mM. *Right,* protein 50 μg; ^{35}S PAPS, 0.07 mM; MgCl$_2$, 20 mM. Preincubation was carried out in 0.1 M Tris/HCl, pH 8.1, with or without thiol, and reaction was started by adding substrates plus Mg^{2+}.

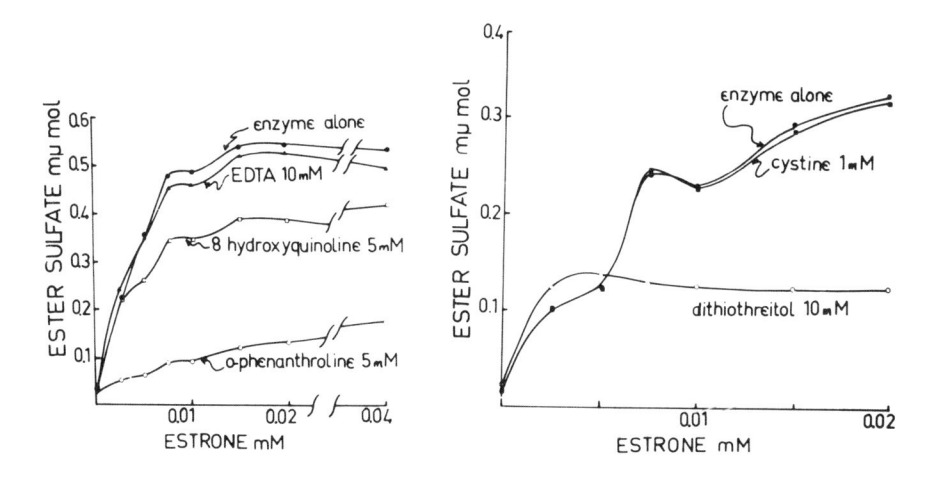

Fig. 2. Left, effect of chelating agents on kinetics. Protein 50 μg; ^{35}S PAPS, 0.05 mM. Mg^{2+} absent. *Right,* effect of cysteine and dithiothreitol on kinetics. As above, but MgCl$_2$, 20 mM. Preincubation of enzyme at 37° C for 30 min was carried out in the presence or absence of chelating agent or thiocompound and reaction was started by adding substrate.

exaggeration of the "wavelike" function caused by preincubating the enzyme is noteworthy (fig. 1). Cysteine activated this, whereas mercaptoethanol and dithiothreitol inhibited it. Cystine had no effect. In addition, the inhibition caused by mercaptoethanol, and more especially by dithiothreitol, was accompanied by a smoothing out of the curve into one resembling a normal rectangular hyperbole. Effects of metal chelating agents are shown in figure 2. EDTA had very little, if any, effect, but 8-hydroxyquinoline caused some inhibition. The marked inhibition by o-phenanthroline appeared to be competitive as judged by double-reciprocal plots, suggesting that its

TABLE 1: SULFATION OF SYNTHETIC ESTROGENS

Substrate	"Ester-Sulfate"[a] (cpm)
Propylene glycol control	2,200
Stilbestrol	4,830
Dienestrol	2,670
Hexestrol	1,790
Estrone	201,600

[a] The soluble fraction remaining after removal of ^{35}S sulfate and ^{35}S PAPS by addition of H_2SO_4 and $Ba(OH)_2$.

structural resemblance to the steroid ring system was responsible.

No enzyme activity was detected using DHEA, phenol, p-nitrophenol, α-naphthol, β-naphthol, β-naphthylamine and 17β-estradiol-3-methyl ether as substrates at 1.5 mM concentration (2). Only monosulfated products were obtained with 17β-estradiol and estriol. Stilbestrol and hexestrol gave low but reproducible rates of sulfation (table 1). Stilbestrol exists in a *trans*configuration in which the hydroxyl groups are separated by a distance like that in 17β-estradiol, as shown by x-ray crystallography (7). That this configuration is present in solution is suggested by its ability to act as substrate for the enzyme. Comparative rates of sulfation of the natural estrogens, compared with estriol taken as unity, are estratriene-3-17β-diol-16-one, 0.62, 17β-estradiol, 0.60, estrone, 0.53, 17α-estradiol, 0.45, and equilenin, 0.42. There was no sulfation of estradiol-17β-3-methyl ether. Estrone was bound to the enzyme and released as estrone ^{35}S

sulfate on prolonged incubation with ^{35}S PAPS of high specific activity (8). This provides some evidence that estrone may be the natural substrate in the adrenal gland.

One other most interesting feature of the enzyme was that four closely migrating bands, as revealed by acrylamide gel electrophoresis, were always present during each of the purification steps (3). These bands were associated with enzyme activity, thus providing evidence for the existence of isoenzyme forms. The four isoenzymes have been numbered 1-4 beginning at the cathode end.

Isolation of Pure Enzyme by CM-Sephadex and DEAE-Sephadex Chromatography

We investigated procedures for isolating the enzyme in amounts sufficient for chemical and biochemical studies. The final procedure adopted involved initial chromatography of the 55-70% saturated ammonium sulfate fraction on a CM-Sephadex column which abstracted hemo proteins. The latter proved difficult to remove by other chromatographic means (fig. 3). The enzymatically active fraction was dialyzed, concentrated, and chromatographed on a column of DEAE-Sephadex (fig. 4). Three peaks of enzyme activity were obtained, and fractions throughout these peaks were analyzed by acrylamide gel electrophoresis. Protein patterns obtained by staining with amido black are shown. The initial enzyme peak seems to be an associated form of isoenzyme 3, since after this enzyme peak the isoenzymes, including isoenzyme 3, were eluted roughly in order of their apparent negative charge, although we achieved only partial resolution of the four isoenzymes. This initial enzyme peak alone showed evidence of association when examined by sucrose gradient ultracentrifugation (fig. 5). Individual isoenzymes could not be isolated using pH gradients in place of the salt gradients. By combining the enzymatically active peaks and rerunning through a second DEAE-Sephadex column, we isolated pure enzyme containing the four isoenzyme components ("intact" enzyme) (fig. 6). This preparation was used to study the following chemical properties.

Molecular Weight. The molecular weight was determined at three different pH values by sucrose gradient centrifugation, using the method of Martin and Ames (9). Alcohol dehydrogenase (yeast) was used as reference protein. Results are shown in table 2. Only one species of enzyme was evident at each of the three pH values chosen. The average value of 74,000 is in fair agreement with the value of

67,000 previously reported for the monomer determined by thin-layer chromatography on Sephadex G-200 (3).

Amino Acid Analysis. Table 3 shows the amino acid analysis determined on reduced, carboxymethylated protein. Corrections were made for destruction of threonine and serine but not for possible destruction of part of the *s*-carboxymethylcysteine.

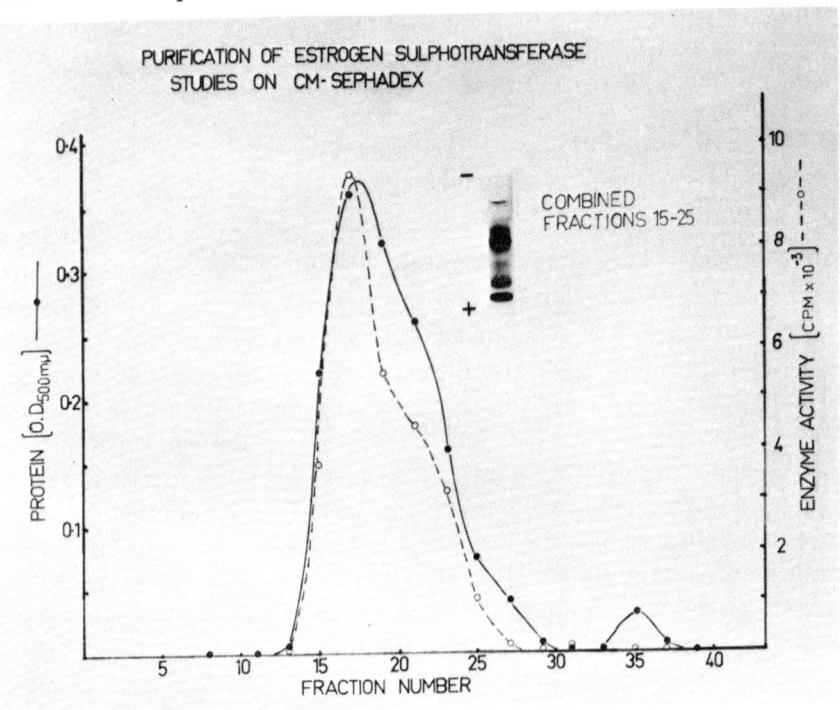

Fig. 3. The column (4.4 × 20 cm) was equilibrated with 0.05 M phosphate buffer, pH 6.2. An ammonium sulfate fraction (55–70% saturation, 3 g protein) was exhaustively dialyzed against the above buffer and the same buffer was used for elution. Flow rate was 35 ml/hr and fractions (12 ml) were assayed for enzyme activity and protein (Lowry).

Sulfhydryl and Disulfide Determinations. Cysteine and cysteic acid were absent in the above amino acid analysis; so presumably all the disulfide bonds had been reduced and stabilized by carboxymethylation. Only one SH group per mole of protein was shown to be present by titration employing two different methods, and this single SH group was revealed only upon adding detergent or preincubating with cysteine (tables 4 and 5). The very low value obtained by the Ellman method in the absence of detergent was not increased in the presence of ATP, estriol, or PAPS at the concentrations shown. If we assume the presence of only one sulfhydryl group, at least ten disulfide bonds would be present to account for the amino acid analysis. Only three of these could be titrated using the method of Zahler and Cleland (10), which involves reduction with dithiothreitol and complexing of excess reagent with sodium arsenite.

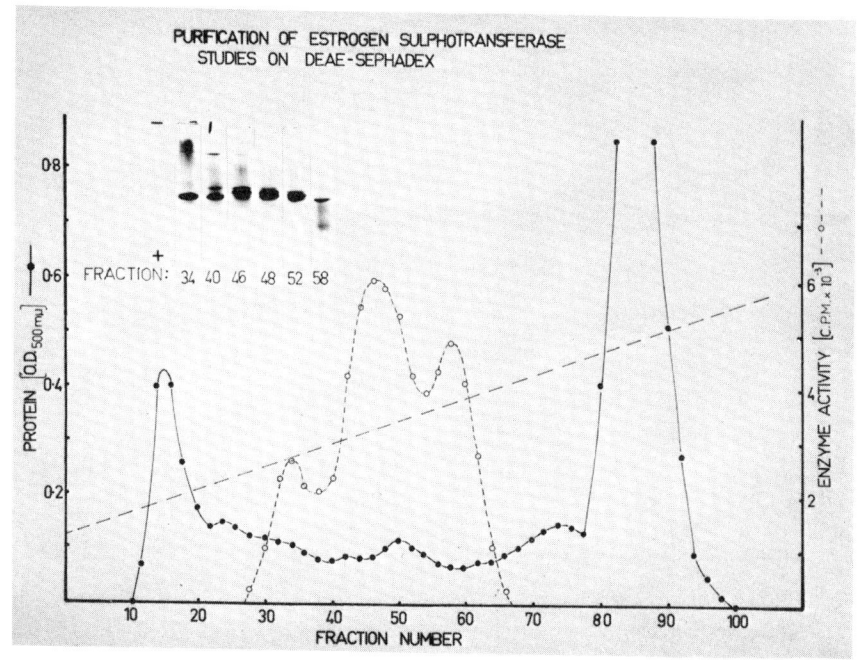

Fig. 4. The combined enzyme from CM-Sephadex was dialyzed against 0.02 M Tris-HCl, pH 8.0, and concentrated by vacuum dialysis. Enzyme protein (1.5 g) was placed on a column of DEAE-Sephadex (4.4 × 30 cm) equilibrated with 0.025 M Tris-HCl, pH 8.0, containing 0.06 M NaCl. A linear gradient of NaCl (0.06–0.3 M in same buffer) was applied. Flow rate was 30 ml/hr and fractions (10 ml) assayed as above. Samples were analyzed on 6% acrylamide gels.

Studies on the Isoenzymes

Isolation. Preparative gel electrophoresis on a Shandon apparatus gave only partial separation. Failure of column chromatography to separate the isoenzymes completely (fig. 4) has forced us to fall back on isolating small amounts of the individual isoenzymes 1–4 by acrylamide gel electrophoresis on 7 × 7 × 0.3 cm slabs. Ten mg can be run on gels of this size, but the recovery of protein and enzyme units has been poor. Strips of gel on each side were cut out, fixed in 2 N HCl for 1 min, and exposed to a solution of anilino-8-naphthalene sulfonic acid for 5 min (11). Under ultraviolet light, the separated protein bands could be seen and served as guides for cutting out the areas of gel containing the remaining protein. After maceration, the gel was shaken overnight at 5° C with 0.05 M

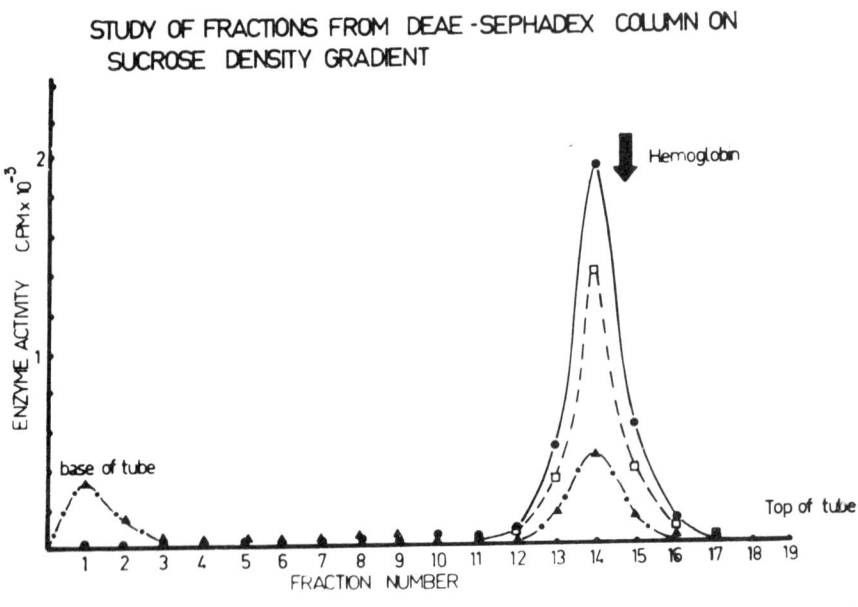

STUDY OF FRACTIONS FROM DEAE-SEPHADEX COLUMN ON SUCROSE DENSITY GRADIENT

Fig. 5. Sucrose gradients (5–20%) were prepared in 0.025 M Tris-HCl, pH 8.2. Aliquots (0.2 ml) of fractions 34, 47, and 58 from the DEAE-Sephadex column (fig. 5) were layered on the gradients and hemoglobin was added as reference protein. Time of run at 0° C was 20 hr at 40,000 rpm (Beckman model L2-65B instrument, using swinging bucket rotor). Fraction 34 ——▲——●——   Fraction 47 ——●——
Fraction 58 ----□----

Tris-HCl buffer, pH 8.1. The gel particles were removed by filtration and the filtrate was concentrated by vacuum dialysis through collodion membranes.

The isolated isoenzymes, when rerun on acrylamide gels, behaved like single protein species. Thus, if any equilibrium exists between these species it must normally be a very slow process.

Testing for Subunits. Subunits in the protein were detected by the method of Weber and Osborn (12). The intact enzyme composed of all four isoenzymes was incubated in 1% sodium dodecyl sulfate

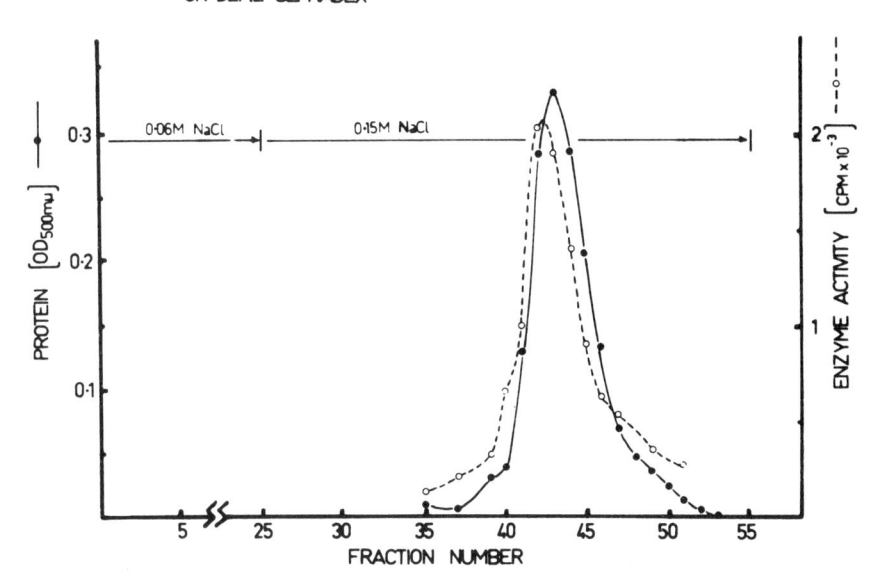

Fig. 6. Combined enzyme from DEAE-Sephadex was dialyzed against 0.025 M Tris-HCl, pH 8.0, and concentrated to 30 ml by vacuum dialysis. NaCl was added to reach a concentration of 0.06 M and the solution was chromatographed on a column (2.2 × 30 cm) of DEAE-Sephadex. Stepwise elution was carried out as shown. Fractions were 6 ml.

TABLE 2: MOLECULAR WEIGHT DETERMINATION OF ESTROGEN SULFOTRANSFERASE BY SUCROSE GRADIENT CENTRIFUGATION

Buffer	Mol. Wt.	Mean
Tris-HCl 0.05M., pH 9.0	74,000	
Sodium phosphate 0.05M, pH 7.0	74,500	74,800
Sodium phosphate 0.05M, pH 5.8	76,000	

SOURCE: Method of Martin and Ames (9).
NOTE: Reference protein: yeast alcohol dehydrogenase.

TABLE 3: AMINO ACID COMPOSITION OF ESTROGEN SULFOTRANSFERASE AND BOVINE SERUM ALBUMIN

Amino Acid	Estrogen Sulfotransferase Residues per Mole	Bovin Albumin
Lysine	60	61
Histidine	16	18
Arginine	24	24
Cysteine	22[a]	38
Aspartic acid	81	57
Threonine	39	34
Serine	46	28
Glutamic acid	68	79
Proline	30	29
Glycine	52	17
Alanine	50	49
Methionine	6	4
Isoleucine	25	14
Leucine	54	65
Tyrosine	21	20
Phenylalanine	28	28
Valine	41	35

NOTE: Values are given to the nearest integer.

[a] As s-carboxymethyl cysteine after reduction of protein with mercaptoethanol in urea and alkylation with iodoacetate. Cysteine or cysteic acid did not appear in the hydrolysate after this treatment.

TABLE 4: SULFHYDRYL BONDS

Buffer	Method	Sodium Dodecyl Sulfate	SHGroup/ Mole Enzyme
0.3 M Acetate, pH 4.6	p-hydroxymercuribenzoate (Boyer)	—	0.0
		+	1.03
0.05 M Tris-HCl, pH 8.2	5.5'-dithiobis-(2-nitrobenzoic acid) (Ellman)	—	0.17*
		+	0.91
Pretreatment with 10 mM cysteine**	Ellman	—	0.80
		+	1.03

* Not increased in the presence of estriol (5×10^{-5} M) ATP ($5 \times 10^{-6} - 1 \times 10^{-4}$ M) or 3'-phosphoadenosine-5'-phosphosulfate ($3 \times 10^{-6} \times 5 - 10^{-5}$ M).

** Enzyme incubated with 10 mM cysteine in 0.05 M Tris/HCl, pH, 8.2 at 37° C for 30 min and reagent removed by filtration on a Sephadex G-25 column.

containing 1% mercaptoethanol, subsequently dialyzed and then subjected to electrophoresis on 10% gels containing 0.1% sodium dodecyl sulfate. Two closely migrating bands were formed (fig. 7). Harsher treatment (1% dodecyl sulfate at 60° C for 1 hr) did not alter this result. Intact enzyme which was reduced and s-carboxymethylated behaved identically. Each isoenzyme when similarly treated gave the same result as that obtained with intact enzyme (fig. 7). When migration rates relative to standard proteins were measured under the above conditions (12, 13), the molecular weights of the two closely migrating species were calculated to be 72,000 and 76,000 (fig. 8).

TABLE 5: DISULPHIDE BONDS

Reducing Agent	Method	Denaturant	SH Group/Mole Enzyme
Dithiothreitol	Ellman	—	2.7
		8M Urea	4.6
		4M Guanidine hydrochloride	7.0

The double band illustrated in figure 7 appears to be an artifact, however, rather than two distinct protein species, since the relative concentration of the two bands varied considerably from run to run. Furthermore, when the test was run in 8% gel, and the gel disk was split lengthwise and one half used to define the position of the protein bands by staining, then the eluted unstained bands were each again split into two when run once more. We therefore concluded that each of the isoenzymes had the same, or very nearly the same, molecular weight of about 74,000 and that no subunits were present.

When the electrophoretic mobility of the isoenzymes in gels of increasing concentration was examined by the method of Hedrick and Smith (14), the result was approximately parallel lines on plotting relative mobility against concentration of gel (fig. 9). This evidence also rules against the possibility that the difference between the isoenzymes is related only to molecular weight. In such cases intersecting lines instead of parallel lines are obtained (14).

Effect of Urea. Urea at concentrations above 2 M caused inactivation of the enzyme, apparently by forming aggregates (fig. 10). Aggregation, resulting from intermolecular disulfide bond formation, could occur following initiation by the free sulfhydryl group. Such a mechanism has been proposed to account for the aggregation of bovine serum albumin on treatment with urea (15).

Kinetics of Isolated Isoenzymes. It has been difficult to retain sufficient enzyme activity after eluting isoenzymes from the gel to

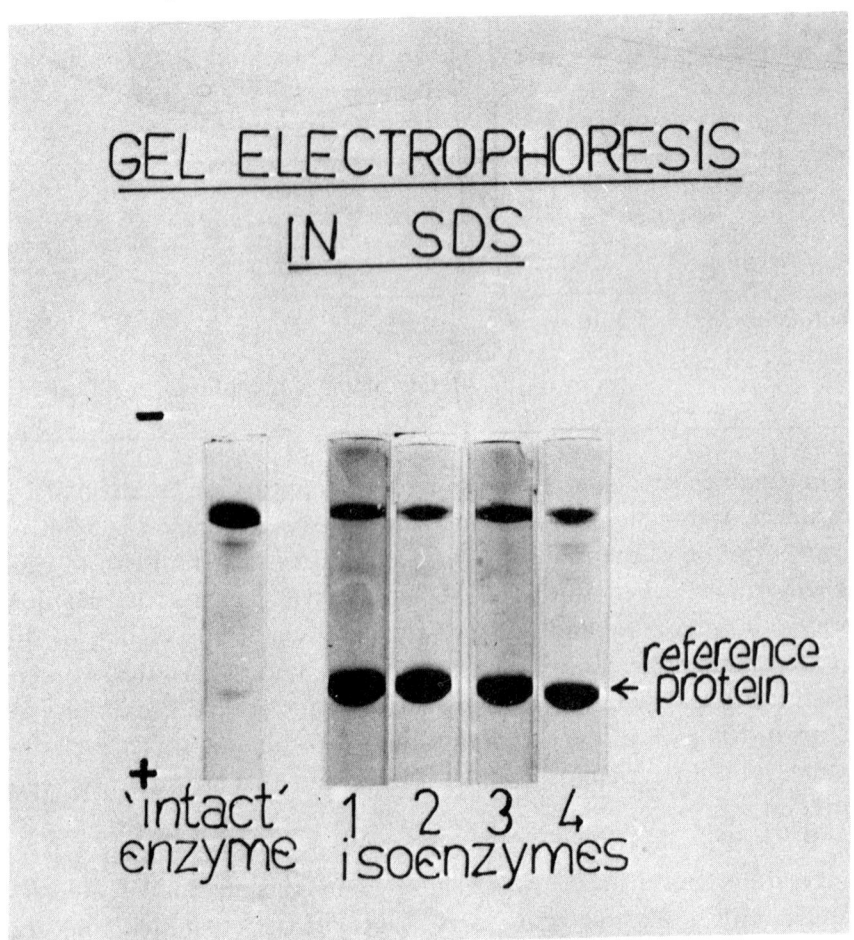

Fig. 7. Acrylamide gel electrophoresis was carried out in 10% gels containing 0.1% sodium dodecyl sulfate (SDS). Both "intact" enzyme and isoenzymes were incubated in 1% SDS at 37° C for 1 hr (12). Reference protein was chymotrypsinogen.

carry out kinetic studies. Nevertheless, preliminary results show that each isoenzyme exhibits the characteristic "wavelike" function on plotting initial velocities against varied estrogen, at constant levels of PAPS. This was also a feature of the protein in fraction 58 of figure 4, which, by analytical gel electrophoresis, appeared to be isoenzyme 4. A kinetic run using this fraction is shown in figure 11.

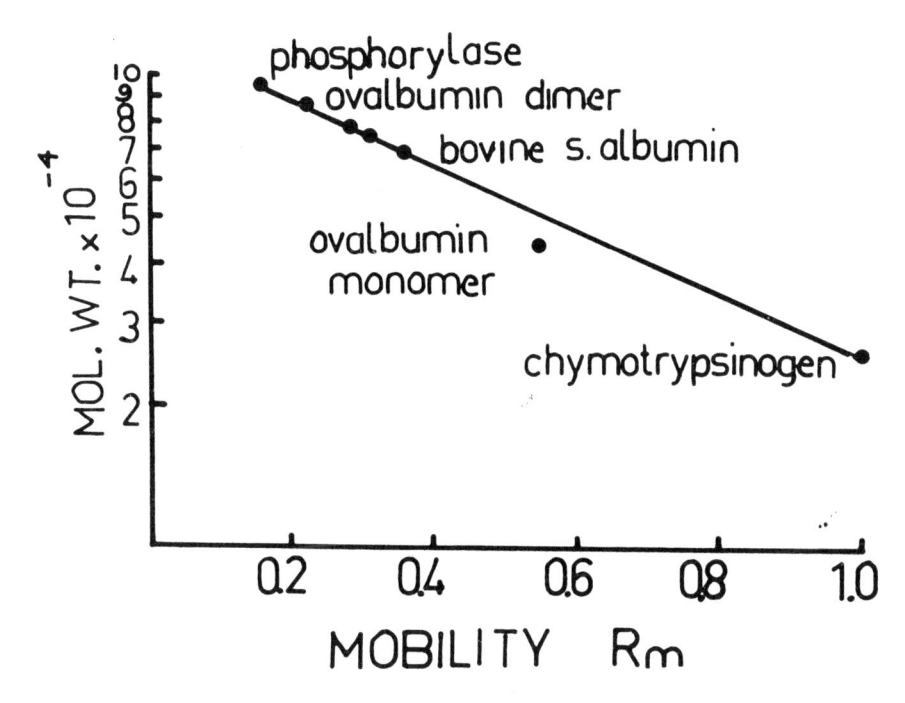

Fig. 8. Molecular weight estimation by comparison of electrophoretic mobility with standard proteins. The method of Dunker and Rueckert (13) was used, the samples being prepared in 4 M urea, 0.1% sodium dodecyl sulfate (SDS) in the absence of thiol. Electrophoresis was carried out in 10% gels containing 0.1% SDS.

Thus the unusual kinetics, obtained using intact enzyme, cannot be explained solely on the basis of an interplay between the constituent isoenzymes, but seem to be due to intrinsic properties of the individual protein species. The close similarity between the shape of this curve and that obtained using a crude high-speed supernatant fluid from human adrenals and DHEA as variable substrate (5) is shown for comparison in figure 12.

DISCUSSION

The chemical studies carried out so far point to a protein with a single polypeptide chain of molecular weight 74,000, whose structure is maintained by intradisulphide bonds and which contains possibly only one sulfhydryl group. Enzyme activity is moderated by changes which very likely occur on this group as is indicated by sensitivity

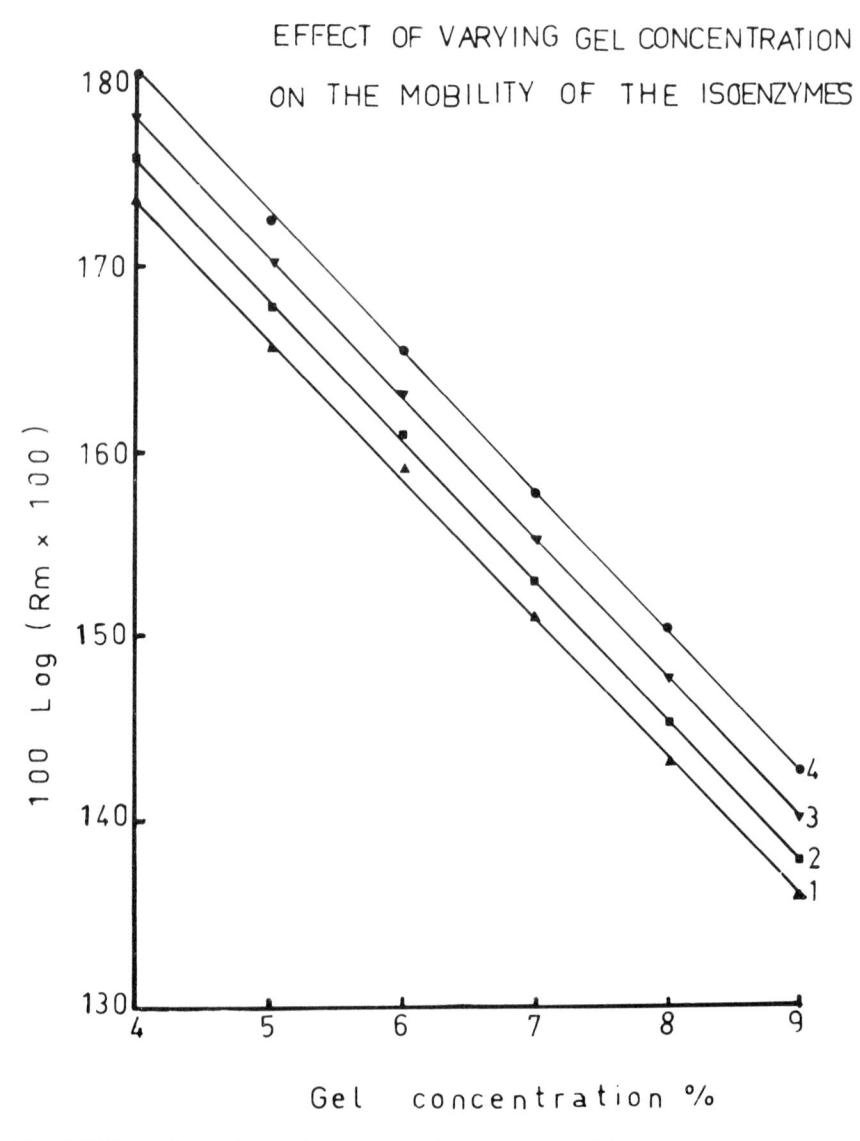

Fig. 9. Effect of varying gel concentration on the mobility of the isoenzyme.

Studies on Adrenal Estrogen Sulfotransferase

to heavy metal ions and to SH blocking agents. Structurally the enzyme greatly resembles bovine serum albumin, with a molecular weight of 69,000, 17 disulfide bonds, and one SH group. Subunits are not present in either protein, although association can occur in both cases. The amino acid compositions of the two proteins are also very similar (table 3), suggesting that they may derive from a common ancestral gene.

The nature of the isoenzymes is of great interest. As far as can be ascertained at this time, these do not appear to be artifacts, since

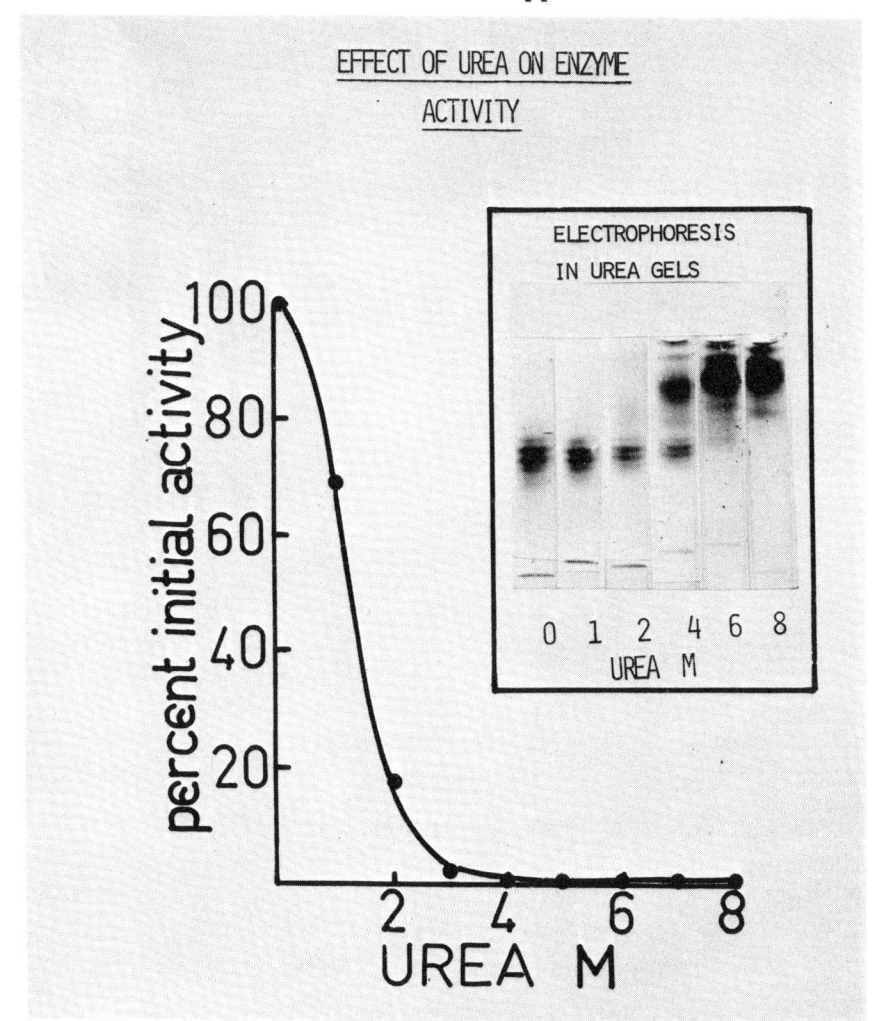

Fig. 10. Enzyme assay conditions: ^{35}S PAPS, 0.25 mM; $MgCl_2$, 20 mM; estrone, 0.1 mM; protein, 50 µg, and urea concentrations as shown.

(1) incubation with PAPS, estrone, estrone sulfate, phosphate, lipase, or protein phosphate phosphorylase did not alter the pattern; (2) they are present at every stage of the purification procedure; and (3) the pattern (determined by protein staining of the 60–70% ammonium sulfate fraction) obtained from individual bovine adrenal glands, although similar in most cases, does exhibit differences; for example, isoenzyme 3 may be greatly diminished. Although

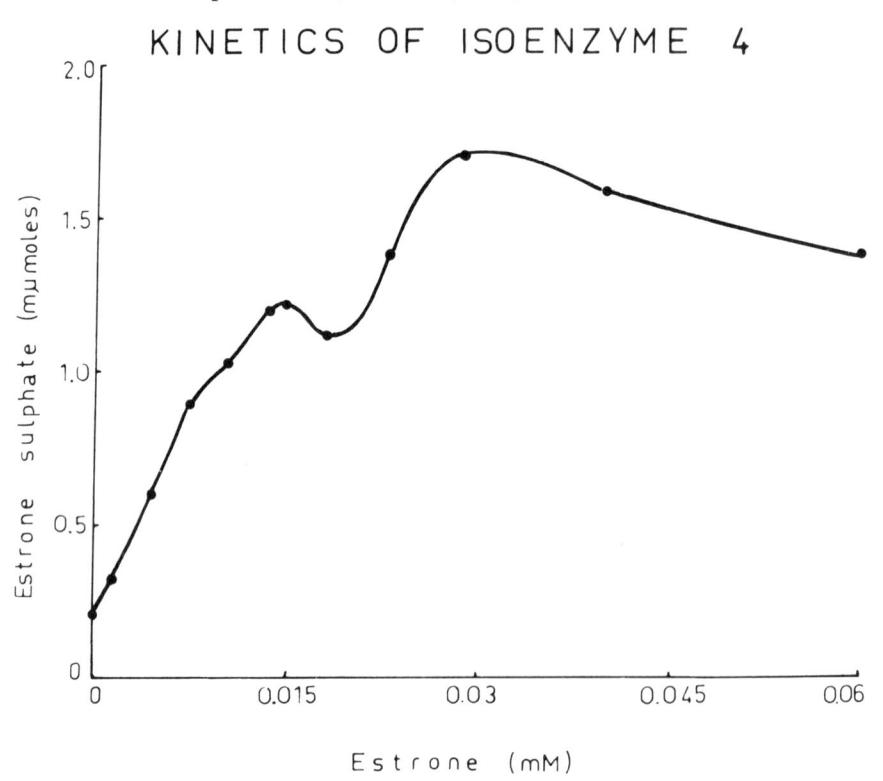

Fig. 11. Kinetics obtained with isoenzyme 4 isolated from DEAE-Sephadex as shown in fig. 5. ^{35}S PAPS, 0.25 mM; MgCl$_2$, 20 mM; protein, 17 μg.

amino acid analyses have not as yet been carried out on the individual isoenzymes, the molecular weights appear to be very close, if not identical, as indicated by gel electrophoresis in sodium dodecyl sulfate. Cross reactivity with antisera and amino acid composition need to be determined to see if structural differences are present. Because the "wavelike" kinetics is due primarily to the intrinsic properties of the individual isoenzymes, it seems that substrate may cause perturbation in conformation which can dramatically alter

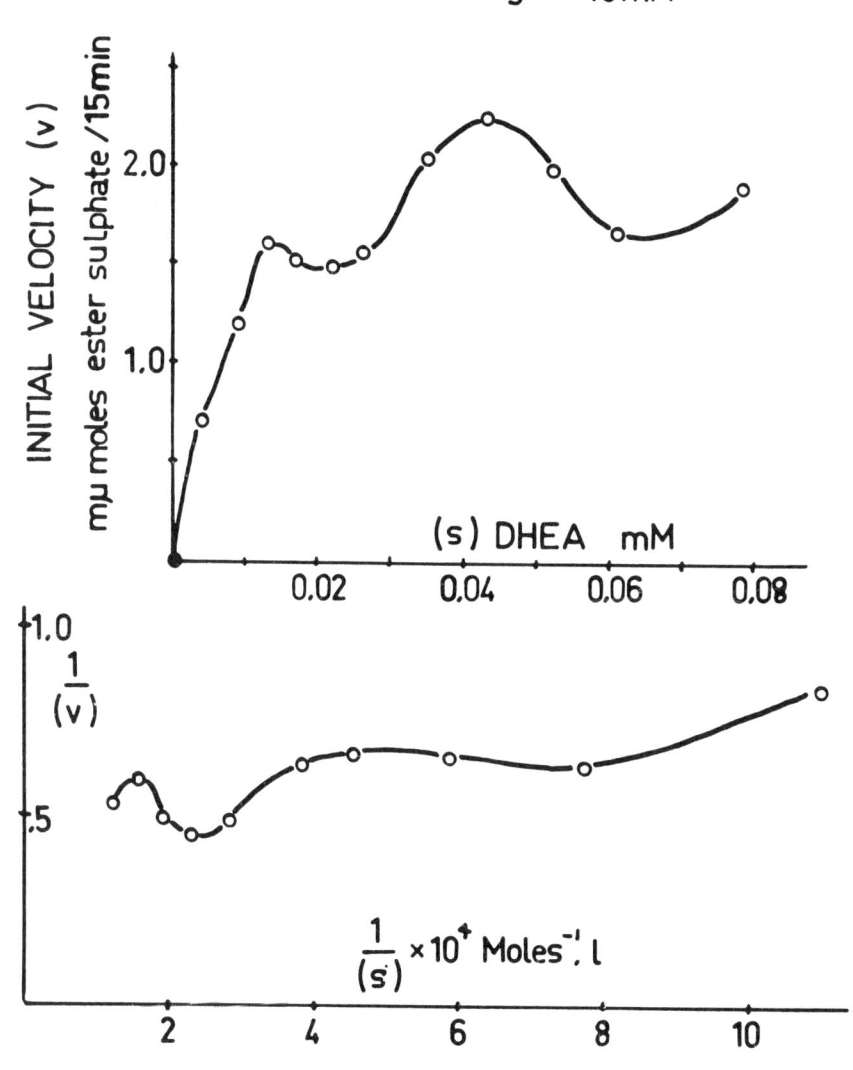

Fig. 12. Kinetics obtained with human adrenal high-speed supernatant fluid and DHEA as variable substrate (5). ^{35}S PAPS, 0.05 mM; MgCl$_2$, 10 mM.

catalytic activity in a positive or negative sense. This may or may not be linked to changes in state of association (5).

The differences recorded for cysteine, on one hand, and mercaptoethanol and dithiothreitol on the other in their effects on enzyme activity appear confusing at first sight. However, various sulfhydryl compounds of similar oxidation-reduction potential vary in their rates of reducing disulfide bonds in proteins (16). Because of its charged groups, cysteine may be unable to penetrate rapidly to disulfide linkages, and the activation—rather than the inhibition found by neutral thiols—appears to be due to liberation of the SH from its involvement in an intramolecular association with some other group (tables 4 and 5). This single group is the one normally rendered titratable in the presence of detergent, since adding detergent to protein previously activated by cysteine did not increase the number of SH groups beyond one. Releasing the SH from its involvement in an intramolecular association upon addition of cysteine presumably would alter conformation, and in this case the change in conformation is accompanied by an increase in catalytic activity (fig. 1). Mere removal of a metal ion by complexing with the added cysteine is most unlikely, since adding chelating agents did not activate the enzyme (fig. 2). Jensen has discussed the properties of the single "masked" sulfhydryl group of bovine plasma albumin and has proposed that it is also normally involved in a stable but reversible intramolecular association (17). The tendency toward normalized Michaelis-Menten kinetics in the presence of mercaptoethanol or dithiothreitol (figs. 1, 2) could be explained by reduction of one or more disulfide bonds during the incubation, forming a structure which is catalytically less active and incapable of undergoing subtle perturbations in conformation in the presence of the substrates.

The adrenal steroid sulfotransferases possess many unusual features. Whether these features are utilized in vivo in control of steroid metabolism is unknown at the moment and must await further understanding of the significance of steroid sulfate formation and secretion.

References

1. Lieberman, S. 1967. Sulfates as biosynthetic intermediates. In *Second International Congress on Hormonal Steroids,* ed. L. Martini, F. Fraschini, and M. Motta, p. 22. International Congress Series no. 132. Excerpta Med. Foundation.

2. Adams, J. B., and Poulos, A. 1967. Enzymic synthesis of steroid sulphates. III. Isolation and properties of estrogen sulphotransferase of bovine adrenal glands. *Biochim. Biophys. Acta* 146: 493.
3. Adams, J. B., and Chulavatnatol, M. 1967. Enzymic synthesis of steroid sulphates. IV. The nature of the two forms of estrogen sulphotransferase of bovine adrenals. *Biochim. Biophys. Acta* 146: 509.
4. Adams, J. B. 1964. Enzymic synthesis of steroid sulphates. I. Sulfation of steroids by human adrenal extracts. *Biochim. Biophys. Acta* 82: 572.
5. Adams, J. B., and Edwards, A. M. 1968. Enzymic synthesis of steroid sulphates. *Biochim. Biophys. Acta* 167: 122.
6. Vaitukaitis, J. L.; Dale, S. L.; and Melby, J. C. 1969. Role of ACTH in the secretion of free dehydroepiandrosterone and its sulfate ester in man. *J. Clin. Endocr.* 29: 1443.
7. Jacques, J. 1949. Molecular structure and estrogenic activity. *Soc. Chim. France Bull.* 16: 411.
8. Adams, J. B. 1967. Enzymic synthesis of steroid sulphates. V. On the binding of estrogens to estrogen sulphotransferase. *Biochim. Biophys. Acta* 146: 522.
9. Martin, R. G., and Ames, B. N. 1961. A method for determining the sedimentation behavior of enzymes: Application to protein mixtures. *J. Biol. Chem.* 236: 1372.
10. Zahier, W. L., and Cleland, W. W. 1968. A specific and sensitive assay for disulfides. *J. Biol. Chem.* 243: 716.
11. Hartman, B. K., and Udenfriend, S. A. 1969. A method for immediate visualization of proteins in acrylamide gels and its use for preparation of antibodies to enzymes. *Anal. Biochem.* 30: 391.
12. Weber, K., and Osborn, M. 1969. The reliability of molecular weight determinations by dodecyl sulfate-polyacrylamide gel electrophoresis. *J. Biol. Chem.* 244: 4406.
13. Dunker, A. K., and Rueckert, R. R. 1969. Observations on molecular weight determinations on polyacrylamide gel. *J. Biol. Chem.* 244: 5074.
14. Hedrick, J. L., and Smith, A. J. 1969. Size and charge isomer separation and estimation of molecular weights of proteins by disc gel electrophoresis. *Arch. Biochem. Biophys.* 126: 155.
15. Harmsen, B. J. M., and Braam, W. G. M. 1969. On the conformation of bovine serum albumin after alkaline or thermal denaturation. *Int. J. Protein Res.* 1: 225.
16. Boyer, P. D. 1959. Sulfhydryl and disulfide groups of enzymes. In *The enzymes,* ed. P. D. Boyer, H. Lardy, and K. Myrback, 1: 511. New York: Academic Press.
17. Jensen, E. V. 1959. Some chemical properties of the sulfhydryl group in bovine plasma albumin. In *Sulfur in proteins,* ed. R. Benesch, et al., p. 75. New York: Academic Press.

Samuel C. Brooks, B. A. Pack, and L. Horn

The Influence of Sulfation on Estrogen Metabolism and Activities   13

INTRODUCTION

Recently steroid sulfates have been implicated in biological functions other than transport, deactivation, or excretion. Lieberman (1) has shown that in the adrenal cortex the pathway from cholesterol to dehydroepiandrosterone can utilize sulfated steroids without hydrolytic products as intermediates. Furthermore, it has been reported that dehydroepiandrosterone sulfate may be the preferred precursor of estrogens in certain systems (2, 3). Also, 3β-hydroxyandrost-5-en-17-one-3-sulfate has been shown to be a better substrate of 17β-hydroxy steroid dehydrogenase than the unconjugated steroid (4). These results and other data (5, 6) indicate that the overall metabolism of a steroid may be influenced by sulfate conjugation.

Several recent studies also indicate that sulfate conjugation may have an essential role in the metabolism of the estrogens. Creange and Szego (7) have reported that 17β-estradiol-3-sulfate is an intermediate in the biosynthesis of 17β-estradiol in the sea urchin. Dahm and Breuer (8) demonstrated that liver homogenates catalyzed the reduction of estrone sulfate, at the C-17 position, to a greater extent than that observed when unconjugated estrone was the substrate. Also, it has been reported that the reduction of estrone sulfate to 17β-estradiol-3-sulfate occurs in hen liver homogenate without hydrolysis (9).

A more direct involvement of sulfate conjugation in hepatic metabolism of estrogens has been suggested by Miyazaki, Yoshizawa,

The authors are affiliated with the Detroit Institute of Cancer Research Division of the Michigan Cancer Foundation and the Department of Biochemistry, School of Medicine, at Wayne State University.

and Fishman (10). Their studies indicate that the 3-hydroxy group must be conjugated to sulfate before the 2-position of the estrogen can be hydroxylated and further metabolized to 2-methoxyestrogen (10, 11).

INFLUENCE OF SULFATION ON HEPATIC METABOLISM OF ESTROGENS

Recent investigations in our laboratory have added support to the concept that sulfation directs hepatic hydroxylation of estrogens. An example of sulfate involvement in hepatic hydroxylation of estrogens is presented in table 1. Isolated rat liver microsomes readily

TABLE 1: METABOLISM OF ESTROGENS AND THEIR SULFATE CONJUGATES BY RAT LIVER MICROSOMES

Substrate	Percentage Hydrolyzed	Product
Estradiol	—	Estrone, 48%
Estradiol-3-SO$_4$	100	Estrone, 47%
Estrone	—	Estradiol, 2.9%
Estrone sulfate	100	Estradiol, 2.3%
Estradiol-3, 17β-di-SO$_4$	100[a]	6α-OH-Estradiol-17β-SO$_4$, 14%
Estradiol-17β-SO$_4$	0	6α-OH-Estradiol-17β-SO$_4$, 29%

NOTE: The microsomes from 2 g rat liver were incubated under air at 37° C for 30 min with the various estrogens (5–15 μg) in 0.1 M Tris buffer (2 ml, pH 7.4). The reaction mixtures contained 0.1 μmole NADPH, 2.5 μmole tetrahydrofolic acid, and 5 μmole of ATP. Estrogens were isolated and identified as described in reference 12.

[a] Only the 3-sulfate was removed.

hydroxylated microgram quantities of estradiol-17β-sulfate to 6α-hydroxyestradiol-17β-sulfate. The same cell fraction, which contained arylsulfatase, metabolized 17β-estradiol or 17β-estradiol-3-sulfate only to estrone. Only a small portion of substrate estrone was reduced to estradiol. The physiological significance of this 6α-directed hydroxylation of estrogens is suggested by the isolation of 6α-hydroxyestrogens from human urine (13) and the demonstration of the unique capacity of liver to synthesize estradiol-17β-sulfate (14).

Although data have been accumulating for nearly ten years which document the influence of steroid sulfates on steroid metabolism by endocrine or hepatic tissue, little is known of the effect or fate of these conjugated hormones in target tissues. Several chapters in this volume document the capacity of mammary tumor tissue to sulfate and metabolize steroids (Adams; Dao and Libby).

PLASMA ESTROGEN SULFATES

It should also be pointed out that estrone sulfate has been shown to be a major constituent of the total plasma estrogens (15). Most of the analyses of plasma estrogens in normal human subjects were done after hydrolysis of the estrogen conjugates. Touchstone and Murawec (16) have established that 64% of the total estrogen in human pregnancy plasma is present in the form of sulfates. Wotiz, Charransol, and Smith (17) recently reported that plasma estrogens are conjugated in 65% of premenopausal women examined; however, they did not differentiate between the glucosiduronates and sulfates. Experiments carried out in our laboratories have shown that in premenopausal women 33% of the labeled estrogen administered intravenously is conjugated to sulfate within 2 hr (fig. 1). Estrone, estriol, and 2-methoxyestrone were also found in the sulfate fraction. (The presence of the latter compound in the plasma sulfate fraction indicates that the liver is the source of part of the circulating estrogen sulfates.)[1] It is interesting that the level of sulfates of estrogens sharply decreased in the plasma of postmenopausal women (fig. 1). Thus target tissues such as the uterus and mammary gland would be exposed not only to free plasma estrogens but to their sulfates as well.

FATE OF ESTROGENS AND THEIR SULFATES IN THE UTERUS

In an effort to learn more about the interaction of a target tissue with estrogens and their sulfates, we carried out a series of experiments utilizing rat uterus (12). 17β-estradiol-3-sulfate underwent extensive hydrolysis (75%) after 2 hr of incubation (fig. 2). At the same time, uptake of 3-sulfated estrogen by the uterus was nearly twice as great as for the unconjugated estradiol, regardless of the initial concentration. The 17β-sulfate group was not removed from the disulfate, and only 9% of disulfate was taken up by the tissue.

[1] The involvement of the liver in the oxidation and sulfation of circulating estrogens is an intriguing discovery in itself. This concept brings to mind the experiments of Szego and Roberts which were carried out some twenty-five years ago. In this work these investigators showed a direct correlation between the uterotrophic activity of injected 17β-estradiol and the amount of liver remaining after partial hepatectomy of previously ovariectomized rats (18).

The only metabolism of this molecule we observed was a partial (23%) hydrolysis of the 3-sulfate.

A comparison of the uterine uptake of estrone and estrone sulfate again demonstrated the tissue preference for the sulfated molecule (fig. 3). The simultaneous incubation of estrone-4-^{14}C and estrone-6,

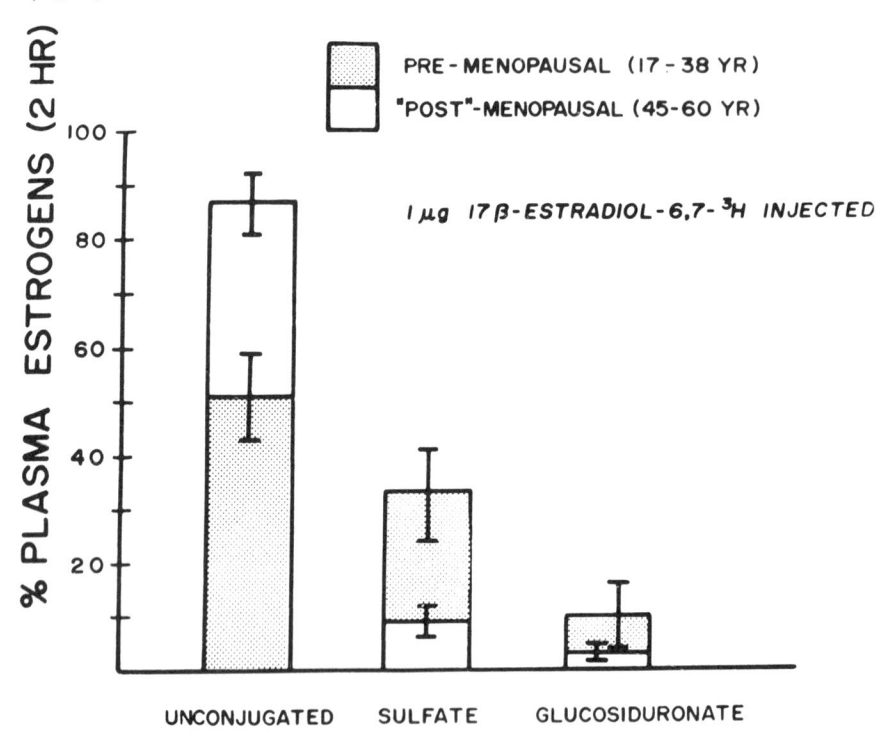

Fig. 1. Conjugation of labeled estrogens in the plasma of women 2 hr after the injection of 1 μg of 17β-estradiol-6, 7-^{3}H (100 μC/μg). Each bar represents the average of four patients, with the average deviation indicated. Conjugates were separated on neutral alumina columns (12).

7-^{3}H-3-sulfate showed that the presence of an estrogen-3-sulfate facilitated the uptake of the unconjugated molecule (fig. 3).

The difference in uptake between the 3-sulfated and unconjugated estrogen was greatest in pooled mature uteri; it was diminished by ovariectomy and was insignificant in immature uteri (fig. 4). Mature esophagus displayed some preference for the sulfated hormone, but this was not true for esophagus from immature rats. Although not restricted to estrogen target tissues, the preferential hormone concen-

Influence of Sulfation on Estrogen Metabolism

tration in the presence of the 3-sulfated estrogen was most significant in the mature animal.

Throughout the estrous cycle the sulfated estrogen was taken up by uterine minces to the same extent (40%) (fig. 5). The unconjugated molecule, however, was concentrated to the greatest degree just before histological evidence of estrus.

The only metabolism of the estrogen molecule we observed in these experiments was oxidation (or reduction) at C-17. The percentage of oxidation of 17β-estradiol or its 3-sulfate to estrone increased in the experiment with mature rat uterine minces as the

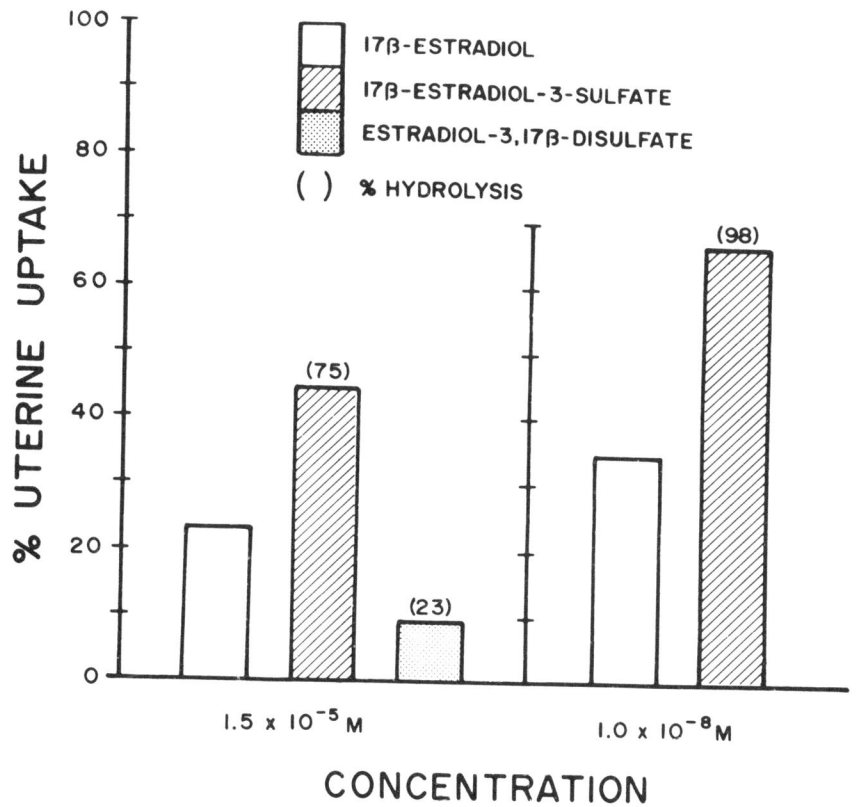

Fig. 2. The uterine uptake of 17β-estradiol-6, 7-³H, 17β-estradiol- 6, 7-³H-3-sulfate, and estradiol-6, 7-³H-3, 17β-disulfate. Incubations were carried out with 400 mg of pooled rat uterine minces in 2.5 ml of Krebs-Ringer bicarbonate buffer (pH 7.4) for 2 hr at 37° C under 95% O_2–5% CO_2. The percentage of hydrolysis of the 3-sulfate moiety is indicated. No hydrolysis of the 17β-sulfate was observed.

concentration of the substrate decreased. The estrone formed was found only in the unconjugated fraction (table 2). On the other hand, estrone was reduced only at the higher concentrations of substrate, and there was evidence that the reduction might occur in the sulfated form as well. We could find no evidence that sulfates were formed by rat uterine minces.

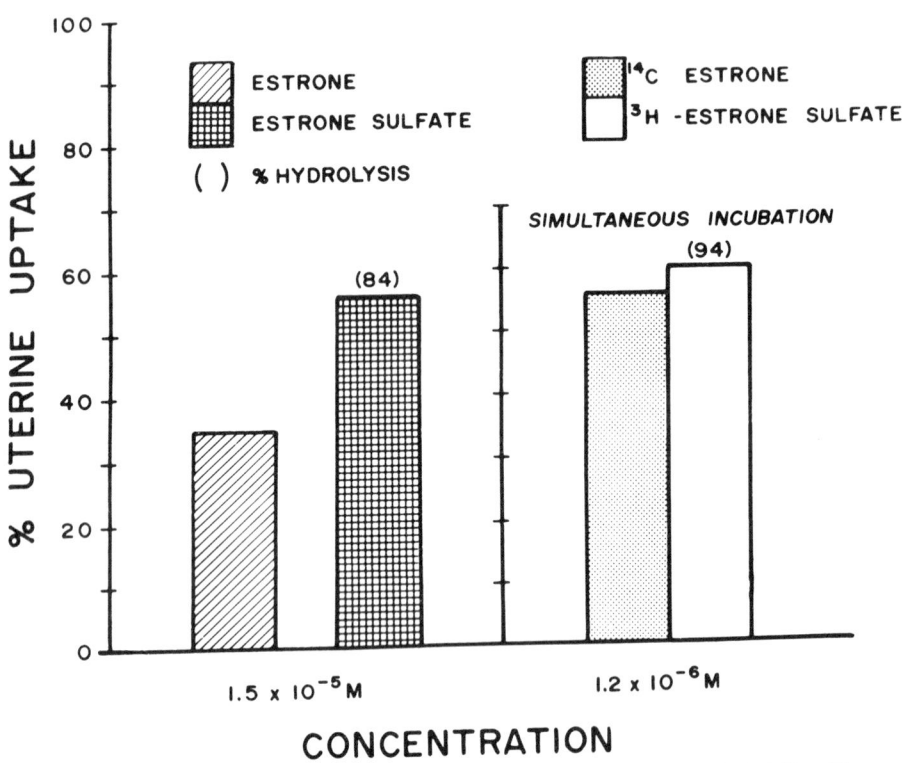

Fig. 3. The uterine uptake of estrone-6, 7-^{3}H and estrone-6, 7-^{3}H-sulfate in separate incubations and in the simultaneous incubation of estrone-4-^{14}C with estrone-6, 7-^{3}H-sulfate. Incubations were carried out as described in figure 2.

Uterine minces from immature rats (24 days) were not able to oxidize 17β-estradiol to estrone (fig. 6). This function was also lost in the uteri from mature ovariectomized rats (12 days after ovariectomy). It is interesting that a "nontarget" smooth muscle tissue such as esophagus does not require the hormone environment of maturity to maintain activity similar to 17β-estradiol-dehydrogenase.

An even greater dependence of this uterine oxidative function on the endogenous hormone environment is shown in figure 7. The amount of unconjugated estrone formed in the incubation of uterine minces with 17β-estradiol or 17β-estradiol-3-sulfate depends on the estrous state of the animal, the greatest oxidation occurring at estrus and the least at diestrus. Since an earlier report by Jensen et al. (19) has shown that immature uteri, primed by 17β-estradiol injection, do not show 17β-estradiol-dehydrogenase activity, it now seems that

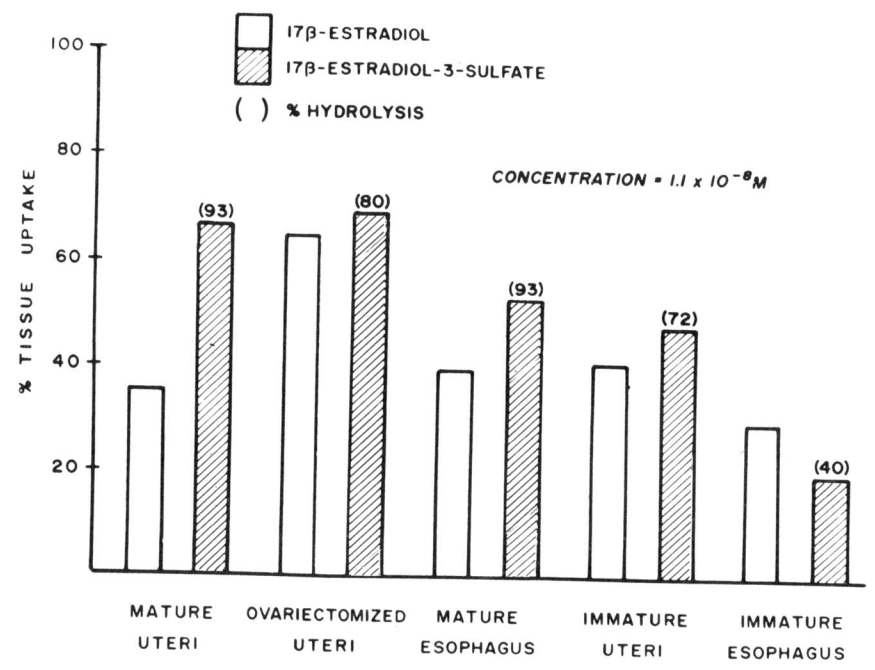

Fig. 4. Tissue uptake of 17β-estradiol-6, 7-³H and 17β-estradiol-6, 7-³H-3-sulfate by 400 mg of mature rat uteri, 480 mg uteri from ovariectomized rats, 400 mg of mature rat esophagus, 90 mg of immature rat uteri, and 90 mg of immature esophageal minces. Incubations were carried out as described in figure 2.

exposure of the uterus to the hormones involved in the full estrous cycle is necessary for the development of this oxidative function.

In expanding the scope of this work to include another species, we carried out investigations on porcine uterus. In this study, we attempted to correlate the stimulation of cytoplasmic protein synthesis with the appearance of 17β-estradiol-dehydrogenase activity. The data from a preliminary experiment (table 3) indicate that, like rat uteri, immature porcine uterine minces are incapable of oxidizing 17β-estradiol to estrone. Likewise, uteri which have been influenced by the initial tide of plasma estrogens (only one mature follicle in the ovaries) do not display this oxidative function. These uteri, however, show a great increase in microsomal peptide synthesis. On the other hand, mature uteri (which had undergone one or more estrous cycles as indicated by the presence of corpora lutea in the ovaries) showed significant oxidation of 17β-estradiol (55%). Protein was synthesized in the microsomes from these uteri at the same accelerated rate as those first exposed to estrogens. Furthermore, for the first time we have observed a substantial sulfation (35%) of estrogens by porcine uterine tissue.

Thus the 17β-estradiol-dehydrogenase activity in porcine uteri is not related to the initial stimulation of uterine protein synthesis by the hormone. However, the influence of the enzyme appears in the

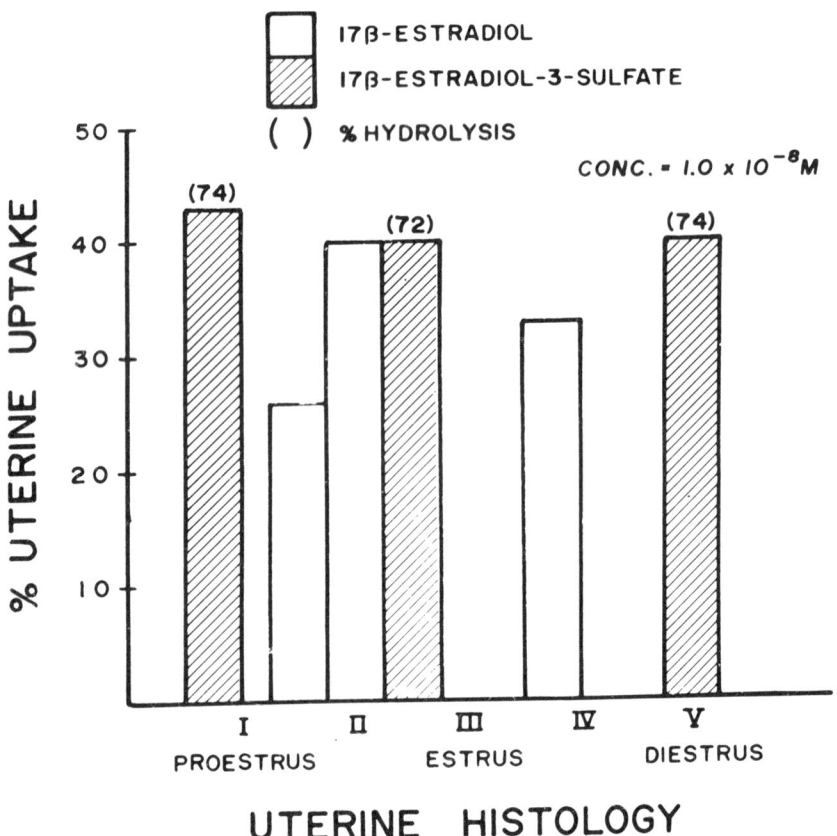

Fig. 5. Tissue uptake of 17β-estradiol-6, 7-³H and 17β-estradiol-6, 7-³H-3-sulfate by 250 mg of rat uterine minces obtained in the various stages of the estrous cycle. Incubations were carried out as described in figure 2.

TABLE 2: METABOLISM OF ESTROGENS AND THEIR SULFATES BY MATURE RAT UTERINE MINCES

| | | Estrogen Analysis ||||
| | | Unconjugated || Monosulfate ||
Labeled Estrogen	Concentration (M)	E_2 (%)	E_1 (%)	E_2 (%)	E_1 (%)
E_2	1.5×10^{-5}	86	11	—	—
	1.0×10^{-8}	49	46	—	—
E_2-3S	1.5×10^{-5}	67	8	25	0
	1.0×10^{-8}	71	27	2	0
E_1	1.5×10^{-5}	7	91	—	—
	1.2×10^{-6}	0	94	—	—
E_1S	1.5×10^{-5}	11	77	1	11
	1.2×10^{-6}	0	94	0	6

NOTE: Pooled mature rat uterine minces (400 mg) were incubated with 17β-estradiol-6, 7-³H (E_2), 17β-estradiol-6, 7-³H-3-sulfate (E_2-3S), estrone-6, 7-³H (E_1), and estrone-6, 7-³H-sulfate (E_1S). Incubations were carried out as described in figure 2.

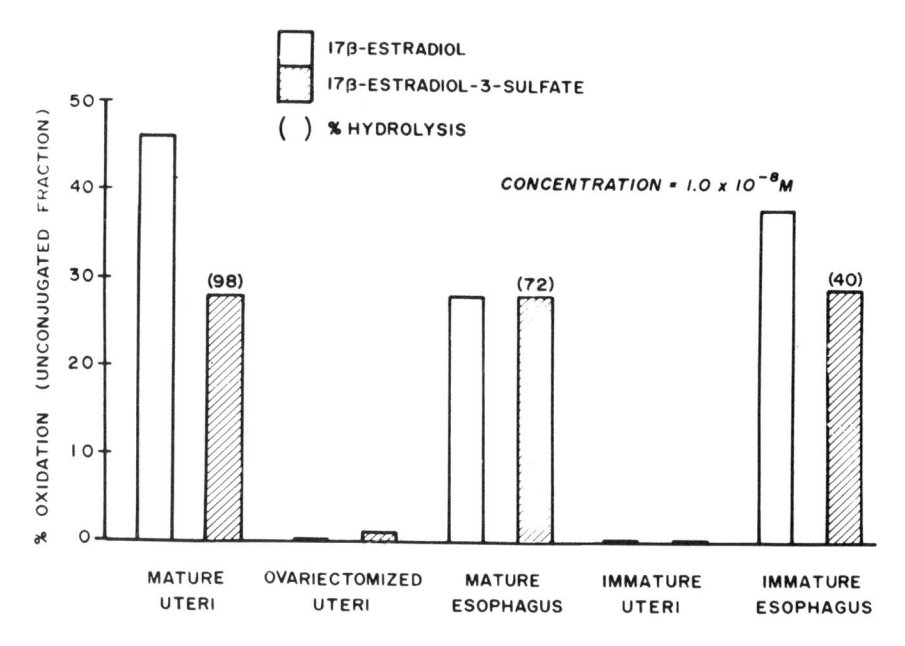

Fig. 6. Oxidation of 17β-estradiol-6, 7-³H and the hydrolyzed portion of 17β-estradiol-6, 7-³H-3-sulfate by various rat tissues. Incubations were carried out as described in figure 4.

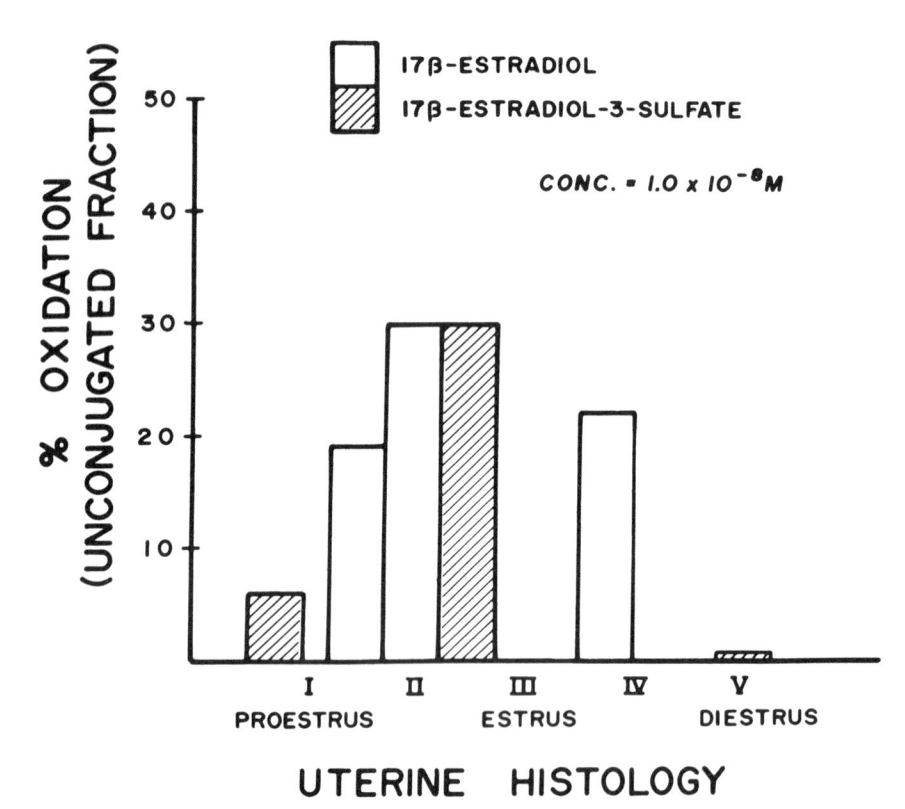

Fig. 7. Oxidation of 17β-estradiol-6, 7-³H and the hydrolyzed portion of the 17β-estradiol-6, 7-³H-3-sulfate by rat uteri obtained in the various stages of the estrous cycle. Incubations were carried out as described in Fig. 5.

TABLE 3: THE EFFECT OF PORCINE UTERINE MATURITY ON PROTEIN SYNTHESIS AND THE OXIDATION AND SULFATION OF ESTROGENS BY MINCES

State of Porcine Uteri	Microsomal Protein Synthesis[a] (dpm/mg RNA/min)	Oxidation $E_2 \rightarrow E_1$ (%)	Sulfation of Estrogens (%)
Immature	140	0	0
First estrogen exposure	350	0	0
Mature	310	55	35

NOTE: Porcine uterine minces (400 mg) were incubated with 17β-estradiol-6, 7-³H. Experiments were carried out for 2 hr at 37° C in 2 ml of Krebs-Ringer bicarbonate buffer (pH 7.4) under 95% O_2–5% CO_2.

[a] From l-leucyl-¹⁴C-tRNA.

Influence of Sulfation on Estrogen Metabolism

mature cycling uteri. Concurrent with the enhancement of dehydrogenase activity in porcine uteri is the appearance of estrogen sulfotransferase activity.

INFLUENCE OF ESTROGEN SULFATE ON UTERINE PROTEIN SYNTHESIS

The question arises of the importance of estrogen sulfates in stimulating metabolic processes in target tissue. In previously published experiments (20, 21) we reported that rat uterine cytoplasmic protein synthesis can be stimulated by low levels of estrone sulfate (75.0 mµmole/ml; fig. 8). Stimulation was not shown by similar concentra-

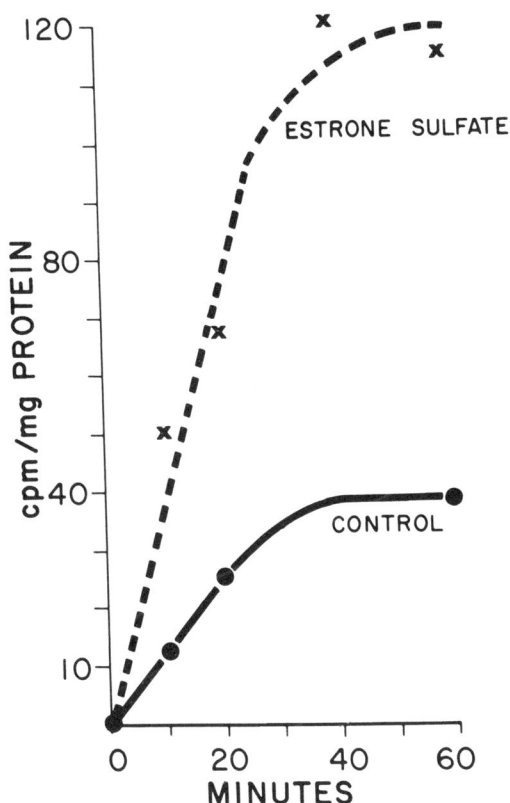

Fig. 8. Incorporation of 2-^{14}C-glycine (0.5) µC, 20 mC/mmole) into the proteins of the 15,000 g supernatant fluid of rat uteri. Incubations were carried out at 37° C in fortified 0.05 M Tris buffer (21). The experimental tubes contained 0.075 µmole/ml of estrone sulfate. Each point is the mean of three tubes. The counts present in the washed proteins at zero time were subtracted from each point. The microsomal supernatant fluid (2.1 mg protein/ml) was obtained from the pooled tissue of 60 ovariectomized rats.

tions of estrone, 17β-estradiol, or any of its sulfates. The crude supernatant fluid containing microsomes (15,000 g) utilized in these experiments was capable of hydrolysis of the sulfate moiety; but reduction of the 17-keto group was not detected.

Recent investigation which employed isolated porcine uterine ribosomes and microsomal transferases have shown that these purified systems respond to levels of 17β-estradiol (0.037 mμmole/ml), far

TABLE 4: STIMULATION OF PROTEIN SYNTHESIS IN VITRO BY VARIOUS ESTROGENS

Estrogen Concentration (mμmole/ml)	Percentage of Control Protein Synthesis		
	E_2	E_1S	E_3
None	100	100	100
0.037	138	—	—
0.18	162	—	79
0.37	186	90	101
1.8	155	—	79
3.7	109	188	38
37.0	—	138	—

NOTE: Incubations included isolated immature porcine uterine ribosomes (0.07 mg RNA), microsomal transferase enzymes (0.27 mg protein), and 1 μmole of GTP. The experiments were carried out for 20 min at 37° C in 1 ml of 0.1 M Tris buffer (pH 7.4) containing 16 μg of l-leucyl-^{14}C-tRNA. The estrogens were added in 0.02 ml ethanol or water. See table 2 for the compounds designated E_2, E_1S, and E_3.

below the active concentration of estrone sulfate (3.7 mμmole/ml; table 4). This apparent effect of estrogens on protein synthesis may be somewhat controversial in light of the established transcriptional effect (22–24) of this hormone; it should be pointed out that latter experiments were carried out in vivo. It is also possible that the many-faceted effects of estrogens on the uterus originate from separate metabolic processes. It has been shown, for example, that a small but significant level of the estrogen stimulated uterine protein synthesis is not dependent on nuclear production of RNA (25). Nevertheless,

Influence of Sulfation on Estrogen Metabolism 233

it appears that although the sulfated estrogen is not essential for the in vitro stimulation of immature uterine cytoplasmic protein synthesis, this conjugated hormone has an indirect role in stimulating protein synthesis in crude homogenates and in facilitating the uterine uptake of the estrogens.

CONCLUSIONS

It has now been established in many laboratories that only free 17β-estradiol is capable of entering the immature or unstimulated

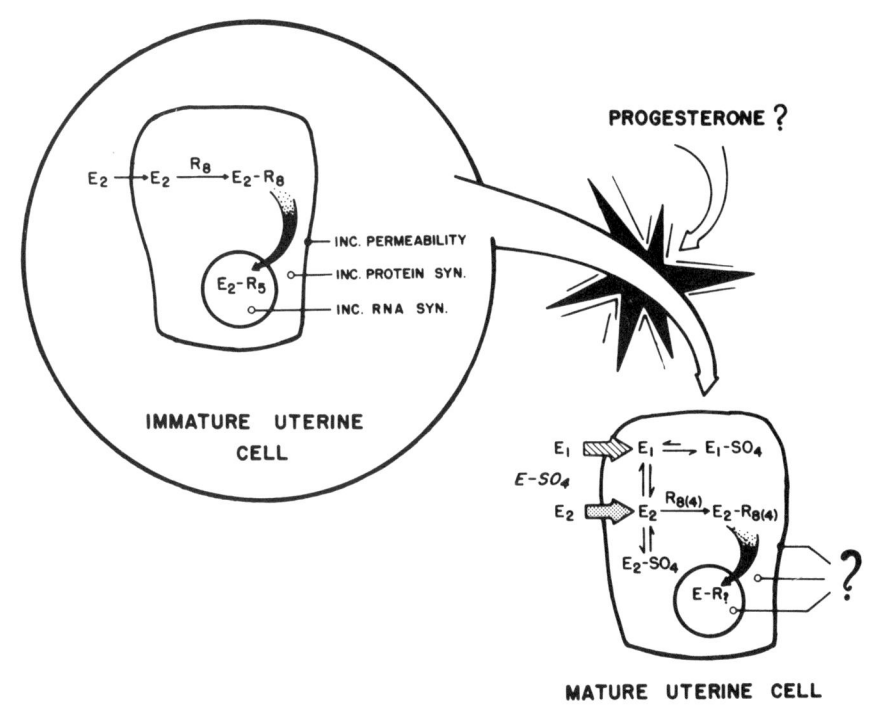

Fig. 9. Schematic representation of the changing fate of estrogens in the uterus of immature and mature rats.

uterine cell. The steroid is not metabolized by this tissue. However, it is tightly bound by an 8S receptor protein which may transport the hormone to the nucleus where the receptor is altered to form a 5S protein (fig. 9).

Once the uterus has undergone a full estrous cycle, marked changes occur; at present it may be assumed that the fate of estrogens in the mature uterus has been influenced by enzymatic changes brought about by the activity of progesterone within the estrogen-primed "target" tissue (26).

Mature uterine tissue has been demonstrated to contain an estrogen receptor protein (27) in addition to 17β-estradiol dehydrogenase and estrogen sulfotransferase. The significance of the last two enzymes in the uterus of normal cycling animals is unknown, but their dependence on the mature endocrine environment suggests that they may be important. A better understanding of the interrelationship of these metabolic functions and their controls is essential, since cancer most often develops in mature estrogen responsive tissue.

Acknowledgments

This work was supported in part by grant CA-04519 from the National Cancer Institute, by contract NIH-69-2210 with the National Institutes of Health, and by an institutional grant to the Michigan Cancer Foundation from the United Foundation of Greater Detroit.

References

1. Lieberman, S. 1967. Steroid sulfates as biosynthetic intermediates. In *Proceedings of the Second International Congress on Hormonal Steroids*, ed. L. Martini, F. Fraschini, and M. Motta, p. 22. Excerpta Med. Foundation.
2. Oertel, G. W.; Treiber, D.; Wenzel, D.; Knapstein, P.; Wendeberger, F.; and Menzel, P. 1968. Biosynthesis of steroid hormones in human gonads. In vivo perfusion of the human ovary with 4-^{14}C-dehydroepiandrosterone and 7α-^{3}H-dehydroepiandrosterone ^{35}S-sulfate: V. *Experientia* 24: 607.
3. Payne, A. H., and Mason, M. 1969. Metabolism of dehydroepiandrosterone and dehydroepiandrosterone sulfate in tissue extracts of rabbit ovaries. *Steroids* 13: 213.
4. Payne, A. H., and Mason, M. 1965. Conversion of dehydroepiandrosterone sulfate extracts of rat testis. *Steroids* 6: 323.
5. Pocklington, T., and Jeffery, J. 1969. 20β-Hydroxysteroid: NAD oxidoreductase activity towards 3β-hydroxy-pregn-5-en-20-one sulfate and related free steroids. *European J. Biochem.* 9: 142.
6. Milgrom, E., and Baulieu, E. E. 1970. C_{19}-Steroid conjugates as substrates and inhibitors of 17β-hydroxysteroid oxido-reductases. *Steroids* 15: 563.
7. Creange, J. E., and Szego, C. M. 1967. Sulfation as a metabolic pathway for oestradiol in the sea urchin Strongylocentrotus franciscanus. *Biochem. J.* 102: 898.

8. Dahm, K., and Breuer, H. 1967. Vergleichende Untersuchungen über den Stoffwechsel von Oestronsulfat und Oestron in Zellfraktionen der Rattenleber. *Biochim. Biophys. Acta* 137:196.
9. Mathur, R. S. 1969. Metabolism of steroid estrogens in the hen. III. Conversion in vitro of estrone-6, 7-^{3}H sulfate-^{35}S. *Steroids* 13: 637.
10. Miyazaki, M.; Yoshizawa, I.; and Fishman, J. 1969 Directive O methylation of estrogen catechol sulfates. *Biochemistry* 8: 1669.
11. Miyazaki, M., and Fishman, J. 1968. Acid catalyzed hydrolysis of estrogen aryl sulfates: Effects of hydroxyl substitution. *Steroids* 12: 465.
12. Pack, B. A., and Brooks, S. C. 1970. Metabolism of estrogens and their sulfate in rat uterine minces. *Endocrinology* 87: 924.
13. Knuppen, R.; Haupt, O.; and Breuer, H. 1966. The isolation of 6α-hydroxyoestrone from the urine of pregnant women. *Biochem. J.* 101: 397.
14. Payne, A. H., and Mason, M. 1963. The enzymatic synthesis of the sulfate esters of estradiol-17β and diethylstilbestrol. *Biochim. Biophys. Acta* 71: 719.
15. Purdy, R. H.; Engle, L. L.; and Oncley, J. L. 1961. The characterization of estrone sulfate from human plasma. *J. Biol. Chem.* 236: 1043.
16. Touchstone, J. C., and Murawec, T. 1965. Free and conjugated estrogens in blood plasma during human pregnancy. *Biochemistry* 4: 1612.
17. Wotiz, H. H.; Charransol, G.; and Smith, I. N. 1967. Gas chromatographic measurement of plasma estrogens using an electron captive detector. *Steroids* 10: 127.
18. Roberts, S. and Szego, C. M. 1947. The early reduction in uterine response to α-estradiol in the partially hepatectomized rat, and the subsequent enhancement during active liver regeneration. *Endocrinology* 40: 73.
19. Jensen, E. V.; Jacobson, H. I.; Flesher, J. W.; Saha, N. N.; Gupta, G. N.; Smith, S.; Colucci, V.; Shiplacoff, D.; Neumann, H. G.; DeSombre, E. R.; and Jungblut, P.W. 1966. Estrogen receptors in target tissues. In *Steroid dynamics,* ed. G. Pincus, T. Nakao, and J. F. Tait, p. 133. New York: Academic Press.
20. DeLoecker, W. C.; Brooks, S. C.; and DeWever, F. 1966. The stimulation *in vitro* of protein synthesis in muscle microsomal supernatant by estradiol-3, 17β-disulfate. *Biochim. Biophys. Acta* 119:655.
21. Brooks, S. C.; Leithauser, G.; DeLoecker, W. C.; and DeWever, F. 1969. *In vitro* stimulation of protein synthesis in uterine microsomal supernatant by estrone sulfate. *Endocrinology* 84: 901.
22. Hamilton, T. H. 1968. Control by estrogen of genetic transcription and translation. *Science* 161: 649.
23. Gorski, J. 1964. Early estrogen effects on the activity of uterine ribonucleic acid polymerase. *J. Biol. Chem.* 239: 889.

24. Ui, H., and Mueller, G. C. 1963. The role of RNA synthesis in early estrogen action. *Proc. Nat. Acad. Sci. USA* 50: 256.
25. Nicolette, J. A., and Mueller, G. C. 1966. Effect of actinomycin D on the estrogen response in the uteri of adrenalectomized rats. *Endocrinology* 79: 1162.
26. Macartney, J. C., and Thomas, G. H. 1969. NADP-linked-17β and 20α-steroid reductase activity in the rabbit uterus. *J. Endocr.* 43: 247.
27. Steggles, A. W. and King, R. J. B. 1969. Sedimentation studies on oestrogen receptors. *Acta Endocr.* suppl. 138: 36.

Mortimer Lipsett, *Chairman*

Discussion: Part II 14

DR. LIPSETT: All the speakers were careful to emphasize that what they were measuring was the capacity of the tumor tissue to carry out these transformations. This does not tell us what we really want to know; that is, What does the tumor tissue actually do in vivo in converting acetate, cholesterol, DHEA, or DHEA sulfate to estrogen? Some of Dr. Griffiths's infusion data suggest that this does occur in vivo to a certain extent.

DR. KORENMAN: Exocrine gland tissue, such as the skin, can perform considerable steroid conversion, and so it may not be evidence of a tumor's performing a function which cannot be performed by a cell of origin. It is perhaps important to study the conversion capability of normal mammary tissues.

DR. BRENNAN: Considering the embryological and evolutionary origins of the mammary gland and its relationship to those organs of the skin which metabolize cholesterol and produce steroids, I wonder whether we need hold ourselves entirely to examining the breast tissue as such, or should not also ask whether glandular skin derivatives may have the enzyme systems we're concerned with here in the normal state. One would think of using skin with hair glandular appendages of the sort that the breast is derived from, on the one hand, against glabrous skin on the other, looking for differences in these enzymes in order to get at the problem of whether the normal tissue possesses steroidogenic capacity.

DR. GRIFFITHS: The synthesis of steroid hormone by skin is certainly very interesting. In 1966 Dr. C. Cameron, our colleague in Tenovus, demonstrated the transformation in vitro of labeled DHEA to testosterone by slices of male human skin. Conversion was small,

The chairman is affiliated with the National Institutes of Health.

but there is a considerable amount of skin on a human body, and the amount of testosterone produced may be very concerned in the endocrine status of the body.

DR. WILLIAMS-ASHMAN: It is very well known that certain bacteria not only are rich in a variety of hydroxysteroid dehydrogenases, but also can readily aromatize C_{19} to C_{18} steroids. It is conceivable that some of the steroid interconversions observed to be carried out by certain nonendocrine tissues, and especially by skin, may reflect, at least in part, the activity of adventitious bacteria rather than the mammalian tissues themselves. I would like to inquire whether bacteria or other microorganisms can be ruled out as a source of steroid-transforming enzymes in the experiments discussed.

DR. LIPSETT: Dr. Williams-Ashman has made a very pertinent point. In many biochemical systems people do make a practice of taking bacteria counts after incubations.

DR. ADAMS: A point that would seem to rule out bacteria as responsible for the results obtained was that in some instances incubation with primary tumors resulted in very low conversions, and these were explainable when histological sections obtained subsequently revealed a predominance of dense fibrous tissue with scanty ductal epithelial areas. In other words, the extent of metabolism seemed dependent on the cellularity of the specimen and, furthermore, the metabolic transformation was consistent—for example, 16α-hydroxylation of DHEA.

Studies on skin show that DHEA can be converted to testosterone. More recently (G. W. Oertel and L. Treiber., *European J. Biochem.* 7:234, 1969) DHEA sulfate was used in a perfusion experiment and C_{18} compounds, double labeled with tritium and ^{35}S, were isolated from skin extracts which were different from the double-labeled C_{18} compounds in the serum. On the basis of this, the claim was made that the skin may be able to catalyze DHEA sulfate conversion into estrogen.

DR. JENSEN: In regard to Dr. Adams's suggestion that hormone independence of a breast cancer may be related to its ability to make its own hormones, it would be interesting to know whether the breast cancer which can carry out these biosynthetic transformations is indeed hormone independent.

DR. GRIFFITHS: In our work, we have not yet attempted to relate the steroid metabolic activity of breast tumor tissue to the patient's response to endocrine therapy.

DR. DAO: Contrary to what Dr. Jensen suggests, I think that mammary cancers capable of performing steroid hormone transformations are hormone-dependent tumors. It seems to me that the tumor cell types which are dependent on hormones for growth activity would also make hormones to perpetuate their propagation.

DR. JENSEN: Then that would be in complete disagreement with Dr. Adams's suggestion that they are hormone independent because they can make the hormones they need. I understood from your published studies that you found that hormone-dependent tumors did not metabolize estrogens or that the metabolic capability of the hormone-dependent tumors was less.

DR. DAO: We do not yet know whether the conjugation of steroids by the mammary cancer tissue has anything to do with synthesis of hormones.

DR. GRIFFITHS: Dr. Adams said that he did not find estradiol synthesis in his experiments. If the steroid metabolic activity is related to the requirement of the tumor cells for the steroid hormone concerned with promotion of growth, then 17β-estradiol should be synthesized.

DR. KORENMAN: We have found that the concentration of plasma estradiol in postmenopausal women is uniformly very low, in most cases close to the limits of our assay system. On the other hand, the concentration of estrone in the plasma of postmenopausal women is significant, averaging 40 pg/ml and sometimes going up to 100. We have also shown that both the normal breast tissue and the breast tumor may contain significant concentrations of estrone. Furthermore, in contrast to the rat and the rabbit—where conversion of estradiol to estrone or estrone to estradiol does not appear to occur in the uterus and by presumption probably does not occur in the breast—in the human uterus these interconversions do occur, as Sweat's group showed a number of years ago (*Endocrinology* 81:167, 1967). These three pieces of evidence suggest that in the human tumor it may not be necessary for estradiol to either be made or be present to get estrogen in action. Now if adrenalectomy is sometimes effective through eliminating an estrogen, the estrogen likely to be eliminated is estrone. It seems reasonable that the presence of estrone is not just for the synthesis of estrone sulfate by the tumors. It may be an important estrogen in itself, independent of the presence or absence of estradiol.

DR. JENSEN: MacDonald et al. (*J. Clin. Endocr. Metab.* 27:1103, 1967) have shown that the adrenal in the postmenopausal woman is not making any estrogen. What it is making is androstenedione, which is then converted to estrone somewhere in the organism. When one takes out the adrenals one is removing androstenedione, the source of estrone. In the distinction between the rat and the human in regard to being able to convert estradiol to estrone, these studies are not strictly comparable because we usually look at the immature rat and the mature human. As Dr. Brooks (chap. 13) has demonstrated, the ability of the rat uterus to convert estradiol to estrone seems to be acquired with age, so that the mature rat uterus can carry out this transformation whereas the immature rat uterus cannot. To my knowledge no one knows what happens in the immature human uterus.

DR. TORGERSEN: With regard to the differentiation between hormone-dependent and hormone-independent mammary tumors, the capacity of the tumor cells to take up hormones from the circulating blood may be a crucial point. It was shown experimentally by Mobbs (*J. Endocr.* 36:409–14, 1966) and at our institute by Sander (*Acta Path. Microbiol. Scand.* 74:169–78, 1968) that rat hormone-dependent tumors accumulate distinctly more 17β-estradiol than the hormone-independent ones. A similar difference might also be present in human mammary tumors (Sander, *Acta Path. Microbiol. Scand.* 74:301–2, 1968).

DR. BROOKS: The scheme proposed by Dr. Adams and Dr. Griffiths is not unusual; it is very much like the pathway of estriol synthesis during pregnancy. The dehydroepiandrosterone sulfate which is synthesized and secreted by the fetal adrenal is hydroxylated at position 16 in the liver of the fetus and then aromatized by the placenta to form estriol. Fetal mammalian tissue has therefore been shown to be capable of synthesizing estriol in this manner. It is not surprising that breast cancer might have a similar pathway, since cancerous tissue has often been compared metabolically to fetal (or "primitive") tissue.

DR. DAO: I wonder whether the small magnitude of these metabolic interconversions can be related to the significance of these biochemical studies. Although only a small piece of tissue is used in these experiments and in a patient with kilograms of tumor the amount of conversion may be considerable, what is the significance of such a conversion in a woman with only local primary cancer? We have heard three papers on this subject, but only Dr. Adams reported a conversion of testosterone to estriol. Why have the others failed to find a similar conversion?

DR. ADAMS: The amount of work done with the aromatase was very limited. Conversion of DHEA to estrogen could not be shown using homogenates or microsomes. Only one experiment was carried out with labeled testosterone, but formation of estriol would not be unexpected in view of the presence of a very active 16-hydroxylase. In your experiments, you have confirmed the presence of the aromatase. Although these conversions are small, it is very important to realize that DHEA sulfate, for example, is quantitatively the most important circulating 17-ketosteroid in the blood. In other words, a big flux is available and although these conversions may be taking place to a limited degree, they may nevertheless be significant for this reason.

DR. DE OME: I am disturbed about stromal-epithelial relationship in these studies. We test a tissue sample as though it were composed only of epithelial cells when in fact it may be composed mostly of stromal elements. In the rodent model system, there are ways of separating the stromal element from the epithelial elements. The use of collagenase, gentle centrifugation, and sucrose gradient centrifugation works very well. The procedure yields epithelial cell populations that are relatively free from fat cells and most of the stromal elements. The isolated epithelial cells are metabolically active and have been used instead of tissue slices in a number of biochemical studies.

DR. TORGERSEN: I wish to point out a potential source of error in the philosophy of some biochemists who seem to look upon cancer as a single disease entity. This is not necessarily true. In breast cancer, there may be a world of difference between the relatively benign intraductal ("comedo") type and the rapidly metastasizing, undifferentiated form. And these may again be biologically very different from other well-defined histological entities such as the colloid carcinoma or the medullary carcinoma with amyloid. If all of these types are lumped together as "breast cancer," no pathologist would expect uniform results from biochemical investigations.

DR. BRENNAN: There is another caution that we all must keep in mind in comparing the so-called nontumorous breast with the tumorous breast. In many cancerous breasts, at wide distances from seemingly well-circumscribed primary tumor sites, columns of tumor cells are invading ducts. Consequently, it is really not accurate to say that the grossly uninvolved portion of the breast does not contain neoplastic cells. It might well contain enzymes of cancerous origin also. It perhaps is wise to insist that every biochemical study be properly controlled with morphological observation.

We know that the sebaceous and apocrine glands in the axilla also mature with age and vary their activity according to sex hormone secretion. Dr. Adams's observations are largely on secondary tumors taken from the axillary region. If these glandular elements in the axillary region are part of the same embryological system which in the mammary line differentiates specifically to form the breast, then again we have the question whether some of the features of metabolism recorded for mammary tumors should be looked for in these related skin appendages, and whether they might be entering the picture of his observations unknown to us.

DR. WILLIAMS-ASHMAN: In Dr. Adams's experiments on sulfurylating enzymes, it seems to me that some of the rather anomalous effects of varying the steroid concentrations were obtained at levels close to the limits of solubility of the steroids in water or dilute salt solutions. Is it possible that under these conditions the concentration and activity of the steroids may not be the same? Perhaps the steroids could stack or form micelles under these conditions.

DR. ADAMS: Enzyme activity was measured in solutions containing propylene glycol. That we get the same type of curve with DHEA as with the estrogen—considering that DHEA is much more soluble in water than estrogens, which are notoriously insoluble—makes me think that probably we don't have this complication. In addition the curves approached the normal rectangular hyperbole in the presence of certain thiols.

DR. LIBBY: The human ovarian enzyme exhibits similar kinetics. In the presence of estradiol, the plot of substrate concentration versus velocity shows a sharp peak at 5×10^{-7} M. After a fall-off, the rate smoothly rises up to 5×10^{-5} M, which is the maximum concentration employed. At the lower concentrations there can be no solubility effects. DHEA, on the other hand, shows a typical rectangular hyperbolic curve, and the plot of reciprocal concentration versus reciprocal velocity shows a straight line. We calculate the K_m for DHEA to be 2×10^{-6} M.

DR. WILLIAMS-ASHMAN: It seems potentially very important if Dr. Dao can correlate some clinical conditions with the absence of a particular enzyme; however, is it possible that the apparent absence of PAPS-forming enzymes might really reflect the presence of adventitious enzymes which actually destroy PAPS?

DR. LIBBY: This is certainly a possibility. We have started to examine some tumor incubations for the presence of APS, which could imply the presence of 3'-nucleotidase, but we cannot find evidence for this enzyme. Hydrolysis of the phosphatosulfate bond has been described, but the enzyme or enzymes is lysosomol, which has a pH optimum of about 6, and requires cobalt for activation, conditions which are not present in incubations.

DR. ADAMS: One point in reference to PAPS breakdown. A PAPS sulfatase is widely distributed in tissues and is also present in serum (J. B. Adams, *Biochim. Biophys. Acta* 83: 127, 1964). In the early experiments of Strominger on the biosynthesis of sulfated mucopolysaccharides, sulfate was not incorporated into the polysaccharides unless the incubation was performed in the presence of

Discussion

0.1 M phosphate and 0.05 M fluoride. This effectively inhibited the PAPS sulfatase (S. Suzuki and J. L. Strominger, *J. Biol. Chem.* 235:257, 1960).

DR. WILLIAMS-ASHMAN: I would like to ask if Dr. Jensen has reasonably pure preparations of the uterine estradiol acceptor proteins. Do they show any affinity for conjugates of estradiol or other steroids, such as the corresponding sulfates or glucuronides?

DR. JENSEN: I can't answer this question because we haven't tried it. We do know that in vivo there doesn't seem to be any tendency to take up the conjugates, even though, as has been pointed out, most of the estrogens circulating are in this form.

DR. KORENMAN: At zero degrees, where binding is at its maximum, estradiol glucuronide does not bind, and estrone sulfate does not compete for estradiol receptor sites even at high concentrations.

DR. BROOKS: In our incubations of uterine tissue with sulfates, so far as we can determine, the entire estrogen taken up by the tissue was unconjugated. Therefore, hydrolysis probably occurred before or during uptake of the hormone by uterine slices.

DR. JENSEN: In regard to Dr. Brooks's demonstration that uteri from either immature or ovariectomized rats lack the ability to oxidize estradiol, I wonder whether these are animals that are ovariectomized when they are immature or mature animals whose uteri once had the capacity to oxidize estradiol and then lost it.

DR. BROOKS: The animals used in these experiments were mature rats that had the ability to oxidize 17β-estradiol to estrone and lost this function after ovariectomy. Macartney and Thomas (*J. Endocr.* 43:247, 1968) showed that the ability to reduce estrone to 17β-estradiol in rabbit uterus depends on the ovarian hormones. Furthermore, your experiments carried out a few years ago (*Steroid Dynamics*, New York: Academic Press, 1966, p. 133) demonstrated that the uteri from immature rats injected for 3 days with physiological levels of 17β-estradiol were unable to oxidize 17β-estradiol to estrone. These experiments indicate that progesterone plays a role in the induction of the 17β-estradiol-estrone oxidoreductase capability in the uterus. Once the source of progesterone is removed (ovariectomy), the 17β-estradiol oxidating capability is lost.

DR. LIPSETT: Dr. Brooks mentioned that in a mature uterus E_1 and E_2 are taken up much better if conjugates are present. Is this due to the effect of E-sulfate or a sulfate?

DR. BROOKS: In the experiment where ^{14}C-labeled estrone was incubated with mature uterine slices in the presence of ^{3}H-labeled estrone sulfate, the ^{14}C-labeled molecule entered the uterine tissue at the same rate as the ^{3}H-labeled hormone, or at approximately twice the rate of uptake of estrone alone incubated with uterine tissue. It is the presence of the estrogen sulfate in the system which aids the uptake of other estrogens. This finding is not too unusual, since estrogen sulfates have been shown to increase the uptake of amino acids in Ehrlich ascites cells (Riggs and Walker, *Endocrinology* 74:483, 1964).

DR. MASARACCHIA: Dr. Brooks's data suggest that sulfate conjugates may be primary intermediates in estrogen stimulation of target tissue. This proposed role of sulfate conjugates in estradiol metabolism and target tissue stimulation is supported by studies with the synthetic estrogen diethylstilbestrol.

TABLE 1: METABOLISM OF 25 μG ^{3}H-DIETHYLSTILBESTROL BY RAT LIVER MICROSOMES

Incubation Time (hr)	Ether Fraction	Sulfate Fraction	Glucuronide Fraction	Water Fraction	Protein Fraction
0.25	69,000	20,850	1,610	15,240	1,020
0.50	59,500	18,600	2,020	17,800	1,090
1.00	49,000	9,700	3,910	22,000	1,840
1.50	36,100	9,600	4,150	26,000	3,050
2.00	29,100	9,230	4,030	33,800	3,135
3.00	22,500	8,600	3,850	46,500	3,982

NOTE: The microsomes were incubated with 0.5 mM magnesium chloride, 1.0 mM ATP, and 1mM NADPH in 0.1 M sodium phosphate buffer, pH 7.4, at 37.5° C.

^{3}H-Diethylstilbestrol was incubated with rat liver microsomes and supernatant, and the metabolites were isolated and identified by chromatography, spectroscopy, and derivative synthesis. At short incubation times the ether-soluble and sulfate-conjugated metabolites of diethylstilbestrol predominated (table 1). The levels of these metabolites gradually decreased with incubation time, and the levels of water-soluble metabolites, excluding the sulfate and glucuronic acid conjugates, increased.

When NADPH was omitted from the incubations or replaced with NADH, large quantities of the sulfate conjugates were accumulated during the incubation (table 2). Estradiol and diethylstilbestrol disulfate decreased the rate of synthesis of water-soluble diethylstilbestrol metabolites.

Discussion

These data suggest that the sulfate conjugates of diethylstilbestrol play an important role in the estrogen's metabolism (fig. 1). It appears that the sulfate conjugate is easily formed in vitro and is a prerequisite for further oxidative metabolism.

It is not yet possible to evaluate the role of the diethylstilbestrol-sulfate conjugate in uterine stimulation. However, it does appear that the synthetic estrogen is metabolized by the same pathway as the natural estrogen.

Finally, it appears that the "pool" of estrogen-sulfate metabolites increases as the size of the animal increases (table 3). The physio-

TABLE 2: EFFECT OF NADPH AND NADH ON THE METABOLISM OF ^{3}H-DIETHYL-STILBESTROL

Cofactor	DES	Ether Fraction DES-OH	DES-OMe	Sulfate Fraction	Glucuronide Fraction	Water Fraction
Blank	84,000	0	325	20,500	4,350	0
NADPH	24,000	680	11,200	9,230	4,030	33,800
NADH	53,300	283	1,720	27,000	4,350	16,200

NOTE: 1 mM NADPH and 1 mM NADH were used; 25 µg ^{3}H-diethylstilbestrol was incubated for 2 hr with rat liver microsomes, 1 mM magnesium chloride, 1 mM ATP, and sodium phosphate buffer, pH 7.4, at 37.5° C.

logical significance of this increased level of sulfate conjugates is not yet known.

DR. HORWITZ: I would like to emphasize the importance of conducting comparison studies on mucopolysaccharides to achieve a better understanding of the significance of steroid sulfates relative to such sugar sulfates as heparin, the chondroitins, mucoitins, and so on. This is particularly important since the sulfate group also plays an effective role in determining the physiological, as well as the chemical and physical, properties of the polysaccharides.

The proposed investigation presents an entirely new spectrum of problems in isolation and identifying relatively complex products. The elucidation of structures, however, can be effected by controlled alkaline or enzymatic degradation. Such studies would provide a greater understanding of the total role of PAPS in mammalian metabolism.

DR. LIPSETT: In Dr. Adams's discussion about the isolation of estriol, some people would not consider recrystallization of estriol in only one system as proof. It would require one or two derivatives with recrystallization to constant specific activities.

DR. ADAMS: The only thing I am sure of is that the testosterone metabolite wasn't α-triol. It is my experience that the latter just does not cocrystallize with estriol or 16-epiestriol. I will admit that it could be some compound other than estriol which hangs on during crystallization, but I am sorry to say we haven't done more on this.

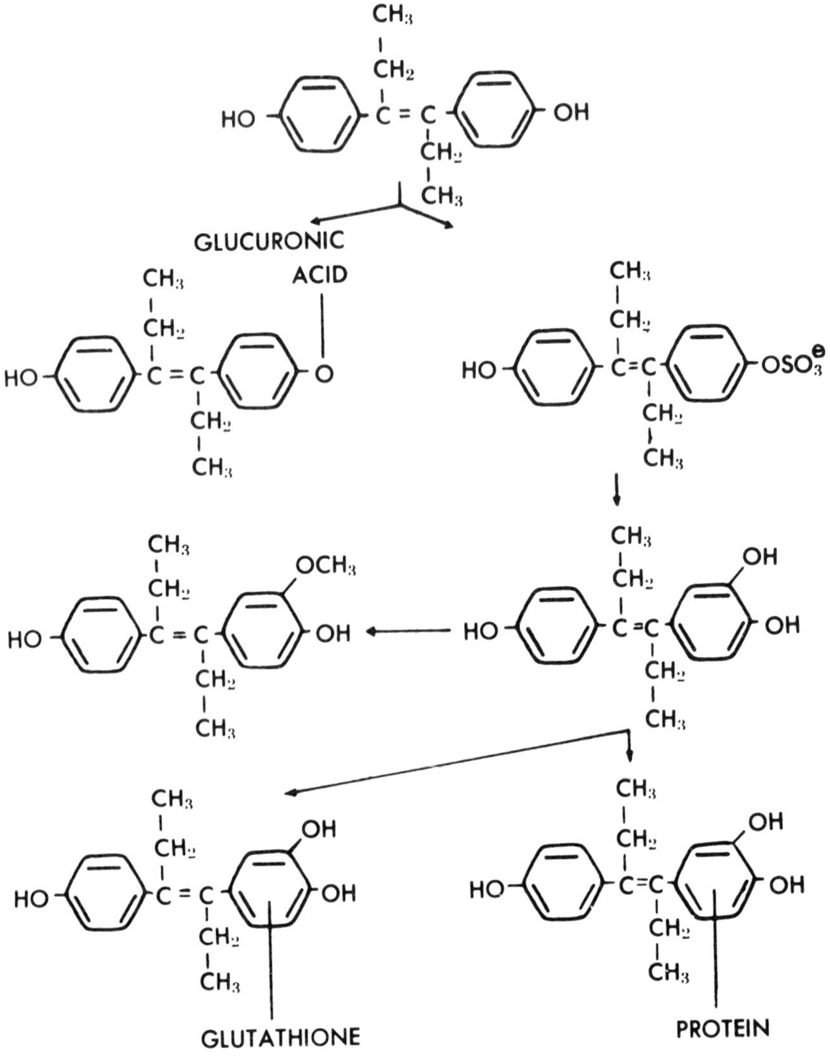

Fig. 1. The proposed metabolic pathway of diethylstilbestrol

Discussion

However, in the work we did on metabolism of ^{14}C-estradiol, two tumors formed estriol; one was accompanied by 17-epiestriol and the other by 16-epiestriol. An additional tumor formed 17-epiestriol without detectable estriol, and another yielded a "tetrol" and a compound chromatographically identical to 2-methoxyestrone. Estrone was formed in every case. Dr. Dao and Dr. Morreal have shown the formation of 16α-hydroxyestrone from testosterone. We are not very far off. I think the aromatase seems to be there.

DR. KORENMAN: With regard to the question of the positive identification of estriol, I recommend that one use the ability to bind the

TABLE 3: METABOLISM OF 25μG ^{3}H-DIETHYLSTILBESTROL BY LIVER MICROSOMES

Animal	Ether Fraction	Radioactivity (dpm) Sulfate Fraction	Glucuronide Fraction	Water Fraction
Rat, male	29,100	9,230	4,030	33,800
Rat, female	30,800	8,380	4,470	35,300
Hamster, male	18,800	5,500	5,100	54,000
Guinea pig, male	63,300	26,400	14,000	20,800
Rabbit, male	66,500	21,400	8,210	24,000
Steer	64,600	28,300	9,200	6,380

NOTE: Liver microsomes were incubated for 2 hr with 0.5 mM magnesium chloride, 1.0 mM ATP, and 1mM NADPH in 0.1 M sodium phosphate buffer, pH 7.4, at 37.5° C.

cytosol receptor as a form of recrystallization. It may be possible to obtain a very substantial purification biologically by selecting the appropriate receptor and incubating it with partially purified material and then extracting it. You may very rapidly find that if it is not an estrogen.

DR. ADAMS: I'd like to suggest a similar approach by the use of purified bovine estrogen sulfotransferase, which possesses a high specificity for estrogens.

DR. LIPSETT: I think it would be interesting if Dr. Adams found estriol from 16α-hydroxy DHEA, because one would then have a tumor forming an impeded estrogen, which might be exactly what it ought to do to prevent its growing very fast. One ought to try to find out which pathway of biosynthesis to estriol is being used.

DR. GRIFFITHS: I think that would be very interesting. There is a reasonable amount of evidence that estradiol may in some way control the metabolism of testosterone by the prostate gland, and I wonder if 5α-dihydrotestosterone could affect the binding or the uptake of estradiol by the breast tumor tissue.

DR. JENSEN: We don't know about the breast tissue, but the dihydrotestosterone doesn't compete very strongly for uptake by uterine tissue in vitro. It does compete a little when it is present in 1,000 times the concentrations of estradiol. Dihydrotestosterone at 10^{-7} M will reduce the uptake of 10^{-10} M estradiol by the immature rat uterus by a factor of some 20%. Testosterone in the same concentration has no effect at all.

DR. KORENMAN: The ratio of association constants (RAC) of dihydrotestosterone to estradiol for the estradiol binding site in uterus is about 0.0003. In certain of the breast tumors we studied it was a little higher, about 0.0006. Testosterone was never found to be active. We also studied the effect of estradiol on dihydrotestosterone binding in prostate, and it does not compete at that site. The effect of estradiol in inhibiting androgen effect in the prostate is due to another unknown influence.

DR. SARFATY: A comment seems pertinent concerning human breast tumor regression following ovarion or adrenal ablation. In relation to this response, I would like to put forward the idea that although there appear to be several different factors associated with tumor regression, they all reflect a similar process; that is, the ability of the host to produce and metabolize steroids.

We know that responders have higher levels of urinary androgenic steroid metabolites than nonresponders, that they are more able to sulfate steroids than nonresponders, and that their tumors have an estradiol binding protein.

I think figure 2 gives some evidence in further support of this idea. This is the probability of remission after adrenalectomy based on urinary steroid metabolite discriminants shown. Each of the curves represents probabilities at different ages, 25 to 65 years, based on discriminants of the urinary steroids shown in the figure. Women at age 65 have considerably lower probabilities of remitting as a result of ablation than women at age 25. The probabilities depend on levels of urinary steroids, and these metabolites decrease with increasing age, so that older women may be unresponsive because of lowered steroid production rate. In other words, parallel these younger counterparts with lower response rates.

It would be interesting to know if a similar relationship exists for steroid sulfation and the estradiol binding protein of the tumor.

Discussion

DR. PEARSON: Has it been shown now that there is ectopic hormone production by mammary cancer? And what criteria are necessary to prove that breast cancer is a paraendocrine organ?

DR. LIPSETT: We consider the hormone production ectopic if the normal tissue does not have this capacity. We don't yet know whether normal breast tissue has these enzymes. Until normal breast tissue is studied using the same numbers of cells and the same amount of cellular protein as in the carcinoma tissue, we can't really say that breast cancer is an example of paraendocrine production of steroid hormones.

DR. ADAMS: I've tried to look for this cholesterol-cleaving enzyme (C^{27} desmolase) in lactating mammary glands of animals, but I haven't been able to demonstrate its presence. I think what we need is lactating mammary tissue from humans.

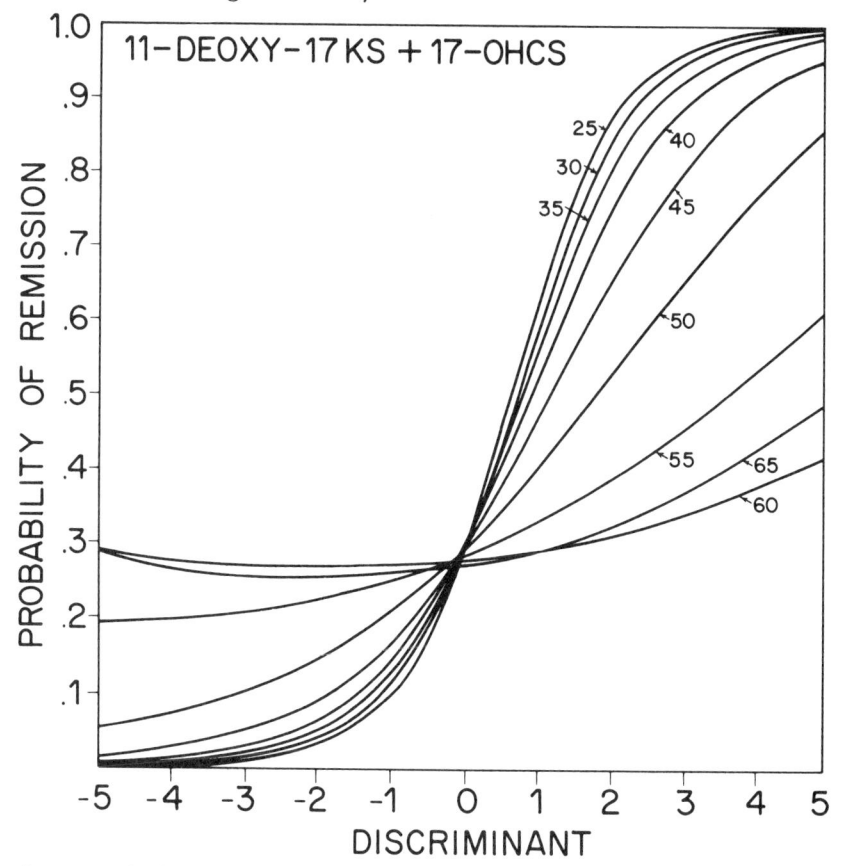

Fig. 2. Probability of remission after adrenalectomy

Mortimer Lipsett, *Chairman*

Summary: Part II 15

Of the three people summarizing, I am the only physician, and so I will take the prerogative of looking at the data from a physician's point of view. For many years investigators have been trying to define the hormonal milieu in which breast cancer develops. We now have increasingly refined methods so that we can measure estrogens and androgens in blood. As has been shown in this meeting, prolactin can be measured in a number of species other than man, and perhaps within the next several years we shall be able to measure human blood prolactin levels as well. Thus, in the immediate future we should be able to define the hormonal milieu in patients with and without breast cancer, in patients who respond to therapy and in those who do not. But the work presented here has raised the extremely important point that assessing the plasma hormonal milieu may not be sufficient. We may have to define the microenvironment in which the breast cancer develops and grows. I am convinced by the studies Dr. Adams and Dr. Griffiths have reported that breast cancer cells can, in fact, synthesize steroids and that most probably they do have an aromatizing system to synthesize estrogens. Since there are now several studies from Jensen, Korenman, and McGuire showing that breast tumors in animals and human breast cancers have the estrogen receptor, it is clear that breast cancer may in a sense be a self-contained system; that is, the cancer cell not only has the mechanism for synthesizing estrogen but also has the receptor giving it the capacity to respond to the estrogen.

Demonstrating a capacity to synthesize estrogen, however, doesn't tell us anything about what the cells are doing in vitro. Thus, in the postmenopausal woman with breast cancer we must determine

The chairman is affiliated with the National Institutes of Health.

the relative contributions of the breast cancer and of the liver and other tissues which synthesize estrogen from a variety of nonestrogenic precursors.

We should accept Dr. Torgerson's strictures about the characterization of the tissue we must deal with. Certainly it will be important not only to characterize the type of breast cancer but to make some attempt to separate the cells from the stroma to see what role each of these structures has within a particular cancer and to determine the relative significance of each. However, if breast cancer doesn't vary too much around the world, it is likely that we are dealing with intraductal carcinoma and there is probably a fair degree of uniformity among all the studies in this regard.

Dr. Pearson asked if breast cancers are examples of paraendocrine neoplasms. This is of interest in another context, of course, but in terms of the cancer cell making estrogens, it is not terribly important whether the normal breast cell can do this. From the theoretical point of view, we must determine whether enzymes of steroid biosynthesis are present in normal breast tissue. This information should help to structure our concept of the carcinogenic process.

If we accept that breast cancer can, in fact, synthesize estrogens, it will then be important to determine the pathways of biosynthesis. Dr. Jungmann has shown that cholesterol can be converted directly to dehydroepiandrosterone. Since there is an active 16α-hydroxylase in cancer tissue, one could easily envision that dehydroepiandrosterone is converted to 16α-hydroxydehydroepiandrosterone and that this compound is then metabolized to estriol. This takes us back to the early observations by Jensen and Huggins in the 1950s, when they showed that estriol, an impeded estrogen, can actually act as an antiestrogen in several biological systems. Thus the intriguing possibility appears that the breast cancer cell could synthesize an antiestrogen by one pathway and at the same time perhaps synthesize biologically active estrogens by the pathways of biosynthesis, proceeding through cholesterol, pregnenolone, and androstenedione. Thus in this particular instance it will be important to define the relative significance of each possible pathway of biosynthesis.

There was surprisingly little discussion about the urinary excretion of the 16-hydroxylated intermediates measured by Dr. Adams. Since he demonstrated first that breast tissue could 16-hydroxylate steroids and second that there was an increase in some of these steroids in the urine of women with breast tumors, it would seem that those of us who are interested in urinary discriminants would do well to examine this more closely. One might guess that the larger fraction of the 16-hydroxysteroids is derived from metabolism by the liver

Summary

and that cancer tissue would play a relatively small part. This is only a guess, however, and the direct contribution of the breast cancer tissue shoud certainly be examined closely.

We come now to consideration of the very interesting work that Dr. Dao presented. For reasons which are not entirely clear to me, Dr. Dao studied the sulfokinases of human breast cancer. He did this using steroid substrates because of the obvious relationship between steroid hormones and the growth of breast cancer. It is not certain that he would have obtained the same data using other substrates for the sulfokinase enzyme. But the data he presented gave the best discriminant of response to adrenalectomy that I have yet seen. Thus, when there was no sulfokinase present there was no response to adrenalectomy; and when the sulfation of dehydroepiandrosterone was more efficient than the sulfation of estradiol, there was more than 70% response. Similarly, the data presented by Dr. Jensen (chap. 2). on response to adrenalectomy and the presence or absence of the estradiol receptor were almost as efficient in predicting response to adrenalectomy. Here we have two examples of what appear to be excellent discriminants for at least one ablative procedure for breast cancer, and at the moment give much better discrimination than any measurement of urinary steroids. I hope that it will be possible for somebody to look at both the receptor and the sulfokinase to see if these two indexes will complement each other.

Predicting response to adrenalectomy and hypophysectomy has, of course, clinical interest, but to me it has even greater theoretical implications. Adrenalectomy and hypophysectomy are still short-term palliative procedures. But if these techniques will allow us to predict more successfully something about the biological nature of breast cancer at the time of mastectomy, we will have taken a great step forward. We may then attempt to alter the disease very early, based on a high probability of recurrence, or we may be able at the time of mastectomy to show that a particular breast cancer is either hormonally responsive or autonomous.

I would like to come back to the studies of estradiol binding which were initiated by Dr. Jensen and his collaborators over ten years ago and which now provide the focus for much important investigation of the action of the steroid hormones as well as of breast cancer. If it is true that the first step in the action of estrogen in the cancer cell is binding to a cytoplasmic receptor, this may be a vulnerable point for the chemotherapist. When I was still a postdoctoral fellow with Dr. Pearson, we discussed ways of trying to remove estrogens from the diet because we knew that adrenalectomized women still had biological estrogens in their urine. The problem is even harder now, since we have seen that the cancer cell itself can synthesize estrogen. Thus, what is needed at the moment is a way either to antagonize the binding of estrogen using a competitor which is not estrogenic or to destroy the binding protein. We now have neither capacity, but given some time and ingenuity one approach or another should prove satisfactory.

This meeting signifies the recognition of significant progress in the endocrinology of breast cancer. The discoveries that breast cancer can synthesize steroids and contain estrogen receptors and that the presence of these receptors or certain enzymes can categorize responsiveness will be focuses for future research.

III

The Relation of Estrogens and Prolactin to Tumorigenesis of the Mammary Gland

Leonard J. Beuving and Howard A. Bern

Hormonal Influence upon Normal, Preneoplastic, and Neoplastic Mammary Gland
16

The growth and development of mammary tissue are regulated by complex integration of the products of a large part of the mammalian endocrine system. Under the appropriate hormonal stimuli, mammary gland cells divide, giving rise to daughter cells capable of producing specialized structures and secretory materials (1, 2). Mammary gland tumorigenesis also requires and is affected by endocrine function (3, 4). Hormones can be used as tools for studying normal mammary growth and development, because mammary gland–specific structures and products can be elicited in vivo and in vitro by hormones. Similarly, the process of mammary tumorigenesis is affected when the normal hormonal milieu is altered. Its preliminary stages in the mouse have well-defined hormonal requirements. These stages result in mammary tumors which are relatively hormone independent. The growth and maintenance of rat mammary tumors, on the other hand, are characterized by hormone dependence similar to that of many human breast tumors. Therefore it is particularly important to understand under what hormonal conditions the progressive stages of mammary tumorigenesis in the rat occur and how hormones affect their development.

THE HYPERPLASTIC ALVEOLAR NODULE AS A
PRENEOPLASTIC LESION

Our particular interest has been in delineating the progressive alterations in the mammary gland before carcinoma formation and

L. Beuving is affiliated with Department of Biology, Western Michigan University at Kalamazoo, and H. Bern is affiliated with the Department of Zoology and Cancer Research Genetics Laboratory at the University of California at Berkeley.

determining how endocrine function affects these processes. We have found in both the mouse and at least one strain of rats that mammary neoplasms arise within discrete lobuloalveolar structures, called hyperplastic alveolar nodules, which appear in the mammary gland before tumor formation. An increase in the number of these lesions is associated with increased risk of tumor formation (5, 6). They occur in small numbers in old mice of low mammary-tumor strains and in rats not treated with carcinogenic agents. By the mammary fat pad transplantation technique, we were able to demonstrate that hyperplastic nodules give rise to tumors displaying characteristic histologic features sooner and more frequently than normal mammary tissue.

The tumor-producing capability of nodules from inbred mice and rats shows considerable variability. For example, 69% of the nodules from mammary-tumor virus-infected $C_3H/Crgl$ mice, which have a high tumor incidence in virgin animals, produce tumors in less than 6 mo, whereas only 13% of nodules from low tumor incidence $C_3Hf/Crgl$ mice, which lack the mammary tumor virus, produce tumors by about 12 mo after transplantation (5). No carcinogen-induced nodules from Fischer strain rats formed tumors (7), but 25% of the nodule transplants in the Lewis strain gave rise to tumors within a year after transplantation (8). Even though not all nodules from a variety of strains give rise to tumors when tested, they are in all cases distinguishable from normal mammary gland in outgrowth morphology and increased tumor-producing capabilities. This observation, combined with the occurrence of large numbers of nodules in relation to numbers of tumors, shows a causal relationship between nodule formation and tumorigenesis. We can therefore designate hyperplastic alveolar nodules as preneoplastic in the sense that neoplastic transformation occurs within the nodule cell population.

Hyperplastic alveolar nodules represent, however, only one type in a family of hyperplastic lesions. These can be produced by a variety of carcinogenic agents in mice (9, 10) and rats (7, 11) and have varying tumor-producing capabilities in these two species; attempts are being made to categorize an even more diverse group of hyperplastic lesions in the mammary glands of women and dogs to determine whether mammary carcinogenesis in long-lived species is similar to the process in rodents.

Hyperplastic alveolar nodules are not neoplasms, because they more closely resemble normal pregnant mammary gland by histologic, cytologic (12), and metabolic criteria (13), and they, unlike mammary neoplasms, respond to mammary gland growth regulatory mechanisms (14, 15). When nodules from inbred mice or rats are transplanted into subcutaneous areas away from mammary fat or among mammary gland elements, they are maintained but do not grow. Mammary tumors grow progressively when transplanted into these areas. Hyperplastic alveolar nodules or normal mammary gland placed in the gland-free portion of the mammary fat pad of young mice or rats produce hyperplastic and normal outgrowths, respectively, which fill the unoccupied portion of the mammary fat pad. Transplanted mammary tumors, on the other hand, grow progressively despite encroaching autochthonous mammary ducts. Hyperplastic nodules, therefore, can be distinguished from normal mammary gland by their morphology, their ability to produce and retain nodular outgrowth characteristics upon transplantation, and their tumor-producing capabilities. They can be distinguished from neoplastic mammary gland by their responsiveness to growth regulatory mechanisms. They are an identifiable stage in a continuum of progressive changes in mammary cells leading to tumor formation.

Defining the biologic significance of these lesions permits separation of the process of mammary tumorigenesis into two experimentally identifiable steps: the alteration of normal mammary cells to preneoplastic nodule cells and the transformation of nodule cells to neoplastic cells. By appropriate experimental procedures one step can be isolated from the other and analyzed independently.

LOCI OF HORMONAL INFLUENCES IN MAMMARY TUMORIGENESIS

The influence of hormones on mammary tumorigenesis can be analyzed at several points during the progression of normal cells to hyperplastic cells and then to neoplastic cells. Hormones may render normal mammary tissue susceptible to a variety of carcinogens. They may promote or permit the development and maintenance of hyperplastic lesions. They may affect neoplastic transformation within the nodule cell population, and finally, they may promote multiplication of neoplastic cells.

Mice

Analysis of the hormonal influences on these several steps of mammary tumorigenesis in the rat is incomplete. However, excellent analysis of the ovarian, adrenocortical, and adenohypophyseal hormonal influences upon noduligenesis and tumorigenesis in several strains of mice has been performed (3). It was possible to define the hormonal combinations supporting formation and maintenance of hyperplastic alveolar nodules and the transformation to tumors in ovariectomized, adrenalectomized, hypophysectomized C₃H/Crgl mice. A summary of these results is given in table 1.

TABLE 1: SUMMARY OF MINIMUM EXPERIMENTAL HORMONAL COMBINATIONS FOR MAMMARY DEVELOPMENT IN THE C₃H/crgl MOUSE

	Estradiol	Progesterone	Deoxycorticosterone	Cortisol	Mammotropin	Somatotropin
Normal mammary gland:						
Ductal development	+	+ or	+		+ or	+
Lobuloalveolar development	+	+ or	+		+ or	+
Lactation				+	+ or	+
Hyperplastic alveolar nodules:						
Induction	+	+ or	+		+[a] or	+
Maintenance			+ or	+	+ or	+
Adenocarcinomatous change			+		+ or	+

SOURCE: Bern and Nandi (3).

[a] Only estradiol-progesterone-deoxycorticosterone-mammotropin combination has been tested to date.

Normal development of the mammary ducts as well as nodule formation occurs in the presence of estrogen in combination with a corticoid or luteoid and with prolactin or somatotropin. Among the hormones from the adenohypophysis, combinations containing prolactin are effective in all strains of mice tested, whereas combinations containing somatotropin as the only adenohypophyseal hormone are effective only in the strains of mice with a high incidence of tumors in virgin females. In these strains, the mammary tumor virus increases the sensitivity of the mammary gland to somatotropin-containing combinations of hormones. As a consequence the same hormonal combinations supporting normal ductal growth also support lobuloalveolar differentiation and therefore are effective for noduligenesis. In those strains of mice lacking the mammary tumor virus, prolactin in combination with estrogen and a C_{21} steroid, luteoid, or corticoid, is required for both normal lobuloalveolar development and noduligenesis. One of the primary reasons for low tumor incidence in virgin animals of these strains is that the mammary gland cannot produce normal lobules or nodules in response to somatotropin.

Experiments in older, nodule-bearing female mice have shown that the hormonal combination maintaining nodules differs from the milieu essential for nodule formation. Although both ovariectomy and adrenalectomy inhibit nodule formation, neither procedure affects nodule maintenance. Combining ovariectomy and adrenalectomy or hypophysectomy results in the atrophy of most hyperplastic nodules. These differences between nodule formation and nodule maintenance are reflected in the essential hormonal combination required for these processes in triply operated mice. Nodules can be maintained by combinations containing a C_{21} steroid such as cortisol or deoxycorticosterone in combination with either prolactin or somatotropin, whereas nodule formation requires estrogen as well as corticoids and adenohypophyseal hormones. A parallel situation exists in normal mammary gland development. Once lobuloalveolar development has occurred in the presence of estrogen, corticoid, and prolactin, estrogen is no longer essential for maintenance and lactation.

Inasmuch as nodules are maintained in nonpregnant animals whereas normal lobules are not, it is clear that the hormonal sensitivity of nodules differs from that of normal lobules. Qualitatively they differ in that some nodules will lactate in vivo in response to deoxycorticosterone and prolactin, whereas normal lobules require cortisol or corticosterone and prolactin. There are also quantitative differences; Elias and Rivera (16) observed that less hormone is required for maintaining organ-cultured hyperplastic nodules than morphologically similar normal lobules.

To determine the hormonal requirements for nodule growth and for the nodule-to-tumor transformation, we transplanted hyperplastic alveolar nodules into gland-free mammary fat pads of isologous mice from which endocrine organs had been removed. By examining nodule outgrowth morphology and tumor incidence among these transplants in response to a variety of hormone combinations, we determined the essential requirements for these processes. Nodules transplanted to normal hosts produce hyperplastic outgrowths which fill the mammary fat pads within 10 wk. Removing the ovaries or the adrenals fails to alter the ability of transplants to produce outgrowth or tumors. But when the host mice lack both adrenals and ovaries or the adenohypophysis, neither nodule outgrowths nor tumors appear. Administering corticoid with either prolactin or somatotropin to triply operated mice bearing nodule transplants was sufficient to permit nodule outgrowth and tumor formation in some of the animals. Simultaneous administration of estrogen enhanced tumor formation, indicating a probable interaction between estrogen, corticoids, and pituitary hormones in normal nodule-bearing mice. Estrogen therefore is a component of the normal hormonal milieu affecting noduligenesis and tumor formation but is not essential beyond its contribution to nodule formation.

When the essential hormonal requirements for normal mammary gland development are compared with the hormonal requirements for nodule formation and maintenance and for the nodule-to-tumor transformation, it is apparent that abnormal mammary development occurs in the same hormonal conditions that support normal mammary development. Continuous administration of minimum effective combinations of estrogen, corticoids, and somatotropin to triply operated mice assures normal mammary gland lobuloalveolar development as well as nodule and tumor formation in mammary tumor virus infected C_3H/Crgl mice. No special hormonal combination is essential. Once nodules have appeared, the same hormonal milieu that supports their formation is adequate for their maintenance and for tumor formation. No single hormone is especially important for mammary tumorigenesis. Each essential hormone is important only to the extent that it contributes to the minimum effective hormonal milieu. Therefore we view the role of hormones in mouse mammary tumorigenesis as supportive or permissive rather than inductive. In genetically susceptible mice infected with the mammary tumor virus, the normal hormonal conditions provide the mammary substrate necessary for noduligenesis and tumor formation.

Rats

Carcinogen-induced mammary tumorigenesis in the rat also requires hormonal support (3). Ovariectomy decreases tumorigenesis and combined ovariectomy and adrenalectomy or hypophysectomy completely inhibits this process. In addition, carcinogen-induced mammary tumors in the rat, unlike mammary tumors in the mouse, are usually hormone dependent. They diminish in size after ovariectomy, adrenalectomy, or hyphysectomy as well as in response to exogenous estrogens and androgens.

With the demonstration that carcinogen-induced hyperplastic alveolar nodules in rats were preneoplastic, we became interested in where ovariectomy had its primary effect in the sequence of steps leading to mammary tumor formation. It was possible that ovariectomy at the time carcinogen was administered would decrease the responsiveness of the rat mammary gland to the carcinogenic effects of polycyclic aromatic hydrocarbons. Alternatively, it was possible that carcinogen-induced mammary cell alterations occurred in ovariectomized rats, but that nodule formation from these progenitors was inhibited. Finally, ovariectomy could cause nodules to regress or prevent the nodule-to-tumor transformation and thereby prevent tumor formation. By utilizing a nodule assay to measure the effectiveness of ovariectomy upon noduligenesis induced by 7, 12-dimethylbenz(a)anthracene (DMBA) treatment, and by employing the mammary fat pad transplantation technique, we were able to determine at what stage ovariectomy interfered with mammary tumorigenesis (17).

Noduligenic Response of Mammary Gland to DMBA in Ovariectomized Rats. We found that ovariectomy performed as much as 30 days before carcinogen was administered did not inhibit the ability of the mammary gland to produce nodules in response to DMBA. This experiment was designed along the lines of experiments performed by Dao (18) for testing whether ovariectomy inhibited the responsiveness of the mammary gland to the tumor-initiating effects of DMBA. We ovariectomized female rats of the inbred Lewis strain 10, 20, and 30 days before administering 20 mg of DMBA at 60 days of age. An ovary was transplanted under each kidney capsule 20 days after carcinogen was administered to provide an essentially normal hormonal milieu for nodule formation. The animals were killed 60 or 80 days after ovary transplantation, a time sufficient for tumor formation in this strain of rats. Animals ovariectomized 10 days before DMBA treatment, but without ovary transplants, had neither nodules nor tumors (table 2). The mammary glands of animals sham-operated 10 days before DMBA treatment had 96 nodules per animal, and 8 out of 13 of these animals developed mammary tumors. In the test groups, ovariectomy 10 days before DMBA treatment had no effect on noduligenesis, although tumor formation was half that in controls. The mammary glands of animals ovariectomized 20 or 30 days before carcinogen treatment also contained nodules and, in the group ovariectomized 20 days before treatment, contained mammary tumors 60 days after treatment. Dao also observed mammary tumorigenesis in rats ovariectomized 10 and 20 days but not 30 days before DMBA treatment. He concluded that ovarian hormones were required for carcinogen-induced alterations. This conclusion was supported by the observation that mammary

TABLE 2: EFFECT OF OVARIECTOMY ON RESPONSIVENESS OF RAT MAMMARY GLAND TO DMBA

Ovariectomy	Days of Age at Ovarian Transplantation	Termination	Number of Rats	Number of Nodules per Rat ± SE
50 (Sham)	—	140	13	96 ± 6.3
50	—	140	20	0
50	80	160	12	94 ± 7.1
40	80	140	10	31 ± 5.8
30	80	140	10	33 ± 5.4

Source: Data from Beuving (17).
ᵃ 20 mg of DMBA was administered to all groups at 60 days of age.

glands in castrated male rats failed to develop mammary cancer unless hormonal stimulation in the form of ovarian grafts was present at the time of carcinogen treatment. Our experiments show that carcinogen-induced alterations occurred in the mammary glands of rats whether ovariectomy was performed 10, 20, or 30 days before DMBA treatment. It was only necessary to supply the hormonal conditions required for the expression of these carcinogen-induced lesions. That the mammary glands of castrated rats are unresponsive to DMBA treatment unless given concomitant ovarian stimulation suggests that a hormonal milieu containing the necessary ovarian or pituitary hormones or both may be necessary for the appearance of the target cells susceptible to the carcinogenic effects of DMBA. Once carcinogen-altered cells are present in a mammary gland, they survive in the absence of ovarian hormones and can give rise to nodules under the appropriate hormonal conditions.

Inhibition of Nodule Formation in Carcinogen-treated Rats. Inasmuch as ovariectomy did not inhibit tumorigenesis by preventing the carcinogen-induced lesions, it was possible that ovariectomy prevented these altered cells from becoming preneoplastic hyperplastic nodules. To test this possibility, we ovariectomized nodule-bearing rats 80 days after carcinogen treatment and determined the incidence of nodules 50 days later (fig. 1). This value was compared with the

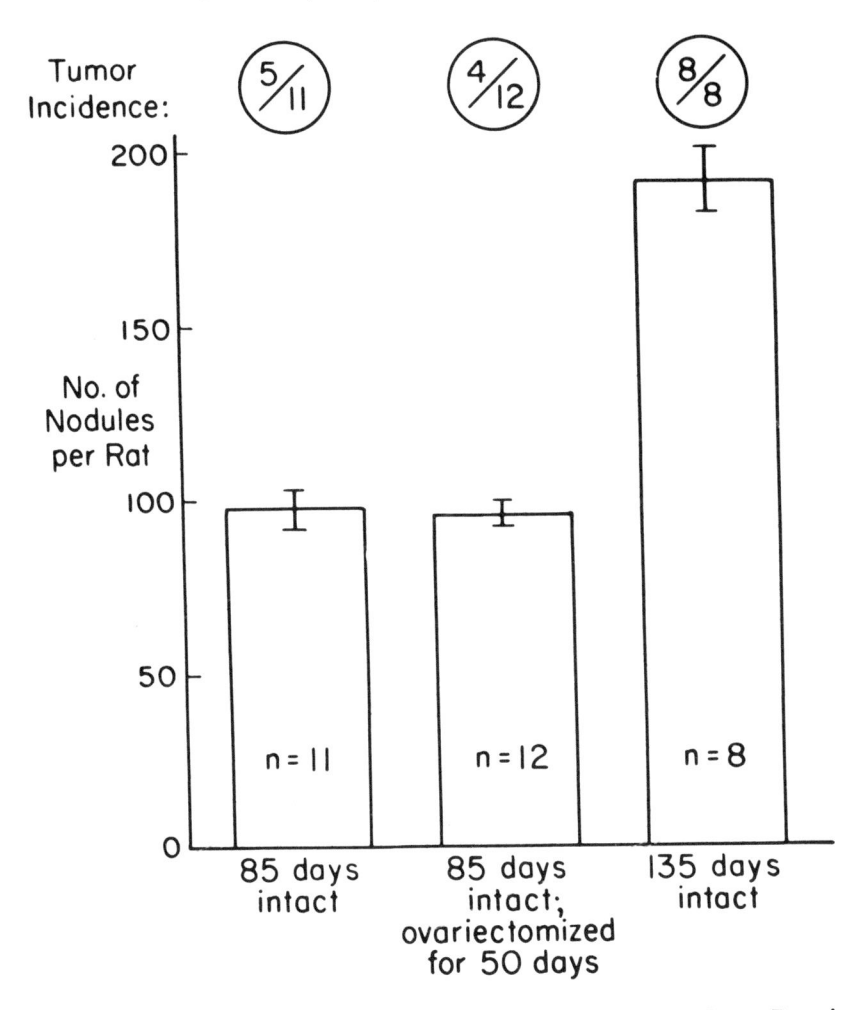

Fig. 1. Inhibition of noduligenesis by ovariectomy. (Data from Beuving [17])

nodule incidence in rats killed at the time of ovariectomy and in sham-operated rats killed 50 days later. We found approximately 100 nodules per animal both in the ovariectomized rats and in the rats killed at the time of ovariectomy. The sham-operated groups, however, showed approximately 200 nodules per rat. Clearly, ovariectomy inhibited continued nodule formation even though carcinogen-induced nodule cell progenitors were present in the mammary glands of the ovariectomized rats. We confirmed the essential conclusion that the multiplication of nodule cells requires ovarian stimulation by showing that transplanted nodules were incapable of producing outgrowths in ovariectomized hosts. Under these conditions, transplanted nodules, which fill the gland-free mammary fat pads of intact hosts with hyperplastic outgrowths within 8 wk, either failed to grow or filled less than 5% of the mammary fat pad.

Maintenance of Nodules in Ovariectomized Rats. In these experiments nodules and nodule transplants were maintained in ovariectomized rats. Mammary tumors in carcinogen-treated rats regressed after ovariectomy. Thus the hormonal conditions supporting nodule and tumor growth differed from the hormonal milieu required for nodule maintenance. We corroborated this by testing the effects of ovariectomy upon nodule-progenitor cells. We found that nodules appeared in animals ovariectomized 20 days after carcinogen treatment if ovaries were reimplanted after a period of 30 days (fig. 2). The carcinogen-altered cells, capable of forming hyperplastic nodules, survived for 30 days without ovarian stimulation and then multiplied, forming nodules, when provided with the appropriate hormonal conditions. In addition to this, the hyperplastic nodule outgrowths derived from nodules transplanted into gland-free mammary-fat pads did not regress during the 35 days following ovariectomy. Alveoli in the lobules of these outgrowths contained less secretory material, making the outgrowths appear less dense, but the numbers of lobules in most outgrowths appeared to be the same as before ovariectomy. It is possible, therefore, that the secretory activity of lobules in hyperplastic outgrowths depends upon a hormonal milieu which is incomplete in the absence of ovarian hormones. However, alveolar cells in nodules and their hyperplastic outgrowths survive in the absence of ovarian stimulation.

These results show that the primary inhibiting effect of ovariectomy is on the multiplication of carcinogen-altered cells which are the progenitors of hyperplastic nodules. Ovariectomy did not prevent carcinogen-induced alterations of mammary cells and did not affect the maintenance of hyperplastic nodule cells. But it did prevent the appearance of preneoplastic nodules and therefore of tumors. The effect of ovariectomy on the nodule-to-tumor transformation is not yet known, but it is likely that ovariectomy inhibits this stage of

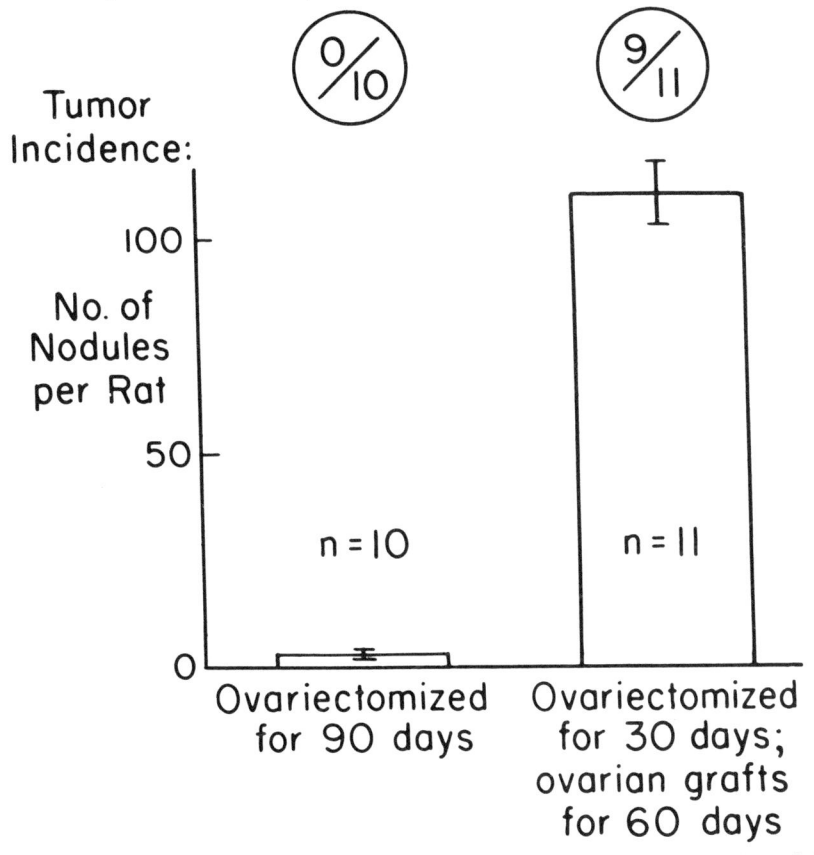

Fig. 2. Nodule formation after ovariectomy. (Data from Beuving [17])

tumorigenesis, inasmuch as carcinogen-induced tumors in rats are usually ovary dependent.

The observation that preneoplastic nodules were maintained after ovariectomy whereas carcinogen-induced mammary tumors regressed was unexpected. This suggests the unlikely possibility that the acquisition of ovary dependence is associated with the nodule-to-tumor transformation. In mouse mammary tumorigenesis, the formation but not the maintenance of nodules is ovary dependent. Nodule-to-tumor transformation occurs in ovariectomized mice and the tumors grow independently of ovarian stimulation. Once nodules have formed in mammary tumor virus infected mice, all subsequent steps are ovary independent. In rat mammary tumorigenesis the formation of nodules and possibly the nodule-to-tumor transformation are ovary-dependent but nodule maintenance is ovary independent. Because of these differences it is difficult to explain ovary-dependent rat mammary tumors arising within ovary-independent hyperplastic nodules. But it is possible that the preneoplastic cells within nodules with tumor-producing capability are ovary dependent. If they constitute only a small proportion of the nodule-cell population, no change would be observed by morphologic examination of nodules after ovariectomy. This possibility has yet to be tested by determining the tumor-producing capabilities of hyperplastic nodules from ovariectomized rats.

POSSIBLE HORMONAL DEFICIENCIES AFFECTING NODULIGENESIS IN OVARIECTOMIZED RATS

Although it is possible to show that ovariectomy dramatically inhibits noduligenesis and tumorigenesis in the rat, it is not yet clear exactly what hormonal deficiencies cause these inhibitory effects. Ovariectomy reduces circulating blood levels of estrogens and progesterone. Progesterone, however, continues to be secreted in significant amounts from the adrenal glands of ovarietomized rats (19, 20) and therefore is not likely to limit tumorigenesis in ovariectomized rats. In addition to reducing blood levels of ovarian steroids, ovariectomy decreases serum titers of prolactin (21), as measured directly and as inferred from experiments showing direct effects of estrogen upon adenohypophyseal secretion of prolactin (22). On the basis of this information, one would predict that the absence of effective concentrations of estrogen and prolactin inhibits mammary tumorigenesis in ovariectomized rats.

In the mouse, and probably in the rat, both estrogen and prolactin in combination with other hormones are essential for some steps leading to mammary tumorigenesis, but both hormones may not be necessary for the remaining steps. The normal mammary gland substrate, which is obviously necessary for tumorigenesis in both the mouse and rat, is formed in the presence of estrogen, corticoid, and somatotropin or prolactin (23, 24). By implication, estrogen is at least a synergist for this process in rats, inasmuch as estrogen is a component of the essential hormonal conditions supporting ductal growth and estrogen specifically binds to normal mouse and rat mammary gland (25). The same hormonal combinations are essential for lobule formation in the mouse and, by inference from the data on the effects of ovariectomy on noduligenesis, in the rat. On the other hand, the hormonal requirements for nodule maintenance in the mouse and rat differ from those supporting normal ductal and alveolar development. Estrogen is not essential for maintaining these lesions in mammary tumor virus infected mice, inasmuch as neither DNA synthesis nor nodule morphology is altered under estrogen-deficient conditions (26). The lack of morphological change after ovariectomy suggests that the same is true for carcinogen-induced nodules in rats.

The steps leading to tumor formation within the nodule cell population of the mouse can occur in the absence of ovarian steroids, although estrogen makes this process possible and therefore normally synergizes with corticoids and adenohypophyseal hormones. There is now considerable evidence suggesting that at least the terminal steps in carcinogen-induced rat mammary tumorigenesis can occur in the absence of estrogen. Estrogen administered to ovariectomized and adrenalectomized or hypophysectomized rats bearing carcinogen-induced mammary tumors reinstated tumor growth after combined ovariectomy and adrenalectomy, but not after hypophysectomy (27). This suggests that estrogen exerts its primary effects on tumor growth by mediating adenohypophyseal tropic hormone secretion. Supporting this conclusion are the observations that mammary tumors have been produced in ovariectomized-adrenalectomized rats treated with DMBA and given injections of prolactin and somatotropin and that normal mammary lobule formation can be induced in vivo (28) and in vitro (29) by greater than normal amounts of prolactin and somatotropin. Although these experiments show that somatotropin and prolactin have direct effects upon normal and abnormal mammary development, they do not rule out possibly important synergistic effects of estrogen on these processes in intact rats. They also do not rule out the possibility that these procedures select and stimulate the growth of tumor cells having a pattern of hormone sensitivity unlike that of most tumors elicited by DMBA in intact rats. Certainly the estrogen-binding capability of DMBA-induced mammary tumors (30, 31, 32), as well as the profound responsiveness of rat mammary tumors to steroids, suggests that ovarian hormones, adenohypophyseal hormones, and corticoids act synergistically upon the latter stages of mammary tumor formation in rats, as in mice.

It is now possible by both in vivo and in vitro techniques to determine the hormonal requirements for the identifiable stages of mammary tumorigenesis in the rat, as has been accomplished in the mouse. The acute toxicity of chemical carcinogens in triply operated rats can be avoided by transplanting the whole mammary gland (33, 34). This technique would allow us to define the minimum hormonal combinations necessary for responsiveness of the mammary gland to the noduligenic effects of carcinogens in triply operated rats which had not been treated with carcinogens. The gland-free mammary transplantation technique would let us determine the hormonal requirements for nodule maintenance and nodule-to-tumor transformation. Finally, either transplantation methods or direct in vitro tests would let us define the essential effective hormonal conditions necessary for tumor growth and maintenance. Once we know the minimum hormonal requirements for these identifiable steps in mammary tumorigenesis, we can begin to explain the precise role of hormones in rat mammary tumorigenesis.

Summary and Expectations

The formation of mammary tumors in both the mouse and the rat is the result of a series of sequential alterations in mammary cells. Regardless of the eliciting stimulus, similar morphogenetic events precede tumor formation. One identifiable stage in mammary tumorigenesis is the formation of preneoplastic hyperplastic nodules, which can be experimentally distinguished from normal and neoplastic mammary gland by their tumor-producing capability, growth-regulatory responses, morphology, and hormone responsiveness.

Growth and development of normal and abnormal mammary gland occur under specific hormonal conditions. In mammary tumor virus infected mice, the same ovarian, adrenocortical, and adenohypophyseal hormones that support normal mammary gland ductal growth are essential for noduligenesis. Inasmuch as nodules occur in virgin carcinogen-treated rats, but not in ovariectomized rats, it is likely that estrogen, corticoid, and somatotropin or prolactin, or both, which are required for normal virgin mammogenesis, are also essential for noduligenesis in the rat.

Estrogen is not required for nodule maintenance or the nodule-to-tumor transformation in the mouse. This is also probably true for nodule maintenance in the rat, inasmuch as ovariectomy does not alter nodule morphology.

It is increasingly apparent that one of the primary effects of estrogen on rat mammary tumor formation is to mediate the secretion of prolactin, which is one of the essential adenohypophyseal hormones for both rat and mouse tumorigenesis. Estrogen, however, probably also acts synergistically at the tissue level to make possible the nodule-to-tumor transformation and tumor growth in both species. If this is true, the essential hormonal requirements for the stages of mammary tumorigenesis in the mouse and rat will be very similar. The apparent endocrine autonomy of mammary tumors in the mouse as compared with the rat may then be viewed more as a difference in the control of adenohypophyseal hormone secretion than as a difference in tumor-cell hormonal requirement.

Owing to the recent development of many in vivo and in vitro techniques that can now be utilized with mammary tissues, it is possible to determine the significance of hyperplastic lesions in the breast tissue of the human and the dog, to define the essential hormonal conditions necessary for noduligenesis and tumorigenesis in the rat, and to begin a precise analysis of the role of hormones in abnormal mammary gland development.

Acknowledgments

This research was aided by National Institutes of Health grants CA-05388 and 2T1 CA-5045 to the Cancer Research Genetics Laboratory and grant GM-00142-11 to the Wistar Institute.

References

1. Lockwood, D. H.; Stockdale, F. E.; and Topper, Y. J. 1967. Hormone-dependent differentiation of mammary gland: Sequence of action of hormones in relation to cell cycle. *Science* 156: 945.
2. Turkington, R. W. 1968. Induction of milk protein synthesis by placental lactogen and prolactin *in vivo*. *Endocrinology* 82: 575.
3. Bern, H. A., and Nandi, S. 1961. Recent studies of the hormonal influence in mouse mammary tumorigenesis. *Progr. Exp. Tumor Res.* 2: 90.
4. Dao, T. L. 1967. Endocrine environment and neoplasia. In *Endogenous factors influencing host tumor balance,* ed. R. W. Wissler, T. L. Dao, and S. Wood, Jr., p. 75. Chicago: University of Chicago press.
5. Blair, P. B., and DeOme, K. B., 1961. Mammary tumor development

in transplanted hyperplastic alveolar nodules of the mouse. *Proc. Soc. Exp. Biol. Med.* 108: 289.

6. Beuving, L. J. 1967. Hyperplastic lesions in the mammary glands of Sprague-Dawley rats after 7, 12-dimethylbenz(a)anthracene treatment. *J. Nat. Cancer Inst.* 39: 423.

7. ———. 1967. Occurrence and transplantation of carcinogen-induced hyperplastic nodules in Fischer rats. *J. Nat. Cancer Inst.* 39: 431.

8. ———. 1968. Mammary tumor formation within outgrowths of transplanted hyperplastic nodules from carcinogen-treated rats. *J. Nat. Cancer Inst.* 40: 1287.

9. Bern, H. A.; DeOme, K. B.; Alfert, M.; and Pitelka, D. R., 1957. Morphologic and physiologic characterization of hyperplastic nodules in the mammary gland of C_3H/He Crgl mouse. In *Proceedings of the Second International Symposium on Mammary Cancer*, Perugia, p. 565.

10. Faulkin, L. J., Jr. 1966. Hyperplastic lesions of mouse mammary glands after treatment with 3-methylcholanthracene. *J. Nat. Cancer Inst.* 36: 289.

11. Faulkin, L. J., Jr; Shellabarger, C. J.; and DeOme, K. B. 1967. Hyperplastic lesions of Sprague-Dawley rat mammary glands after x-irradiation. *J. Nat. Cancer Inst.* 39: 449.

12. Harkness, M. N.; Bern, H. A.; Alfert, M.; and Goldstein, N. O. 1957. Cytochemical studies of hyperlastic alveolar nodules in the mammary gland of the C_3H/He Crgl mouse. *J. Nat. Cancer Inst.* 19: 1023.

13. Moretti, R. L., and DeOme, K. B. 1962. Effect of insulin on glucose uptake by normal and neoplastic mouse mammary tissues in organ culture. *J. Nat Cancer Inst.* 29: 321.

14. Faulkin, L. J., Jr. 1960. Regulation of growth and spacing of gland elements in the mammary fat pad of the C_3H mouse. *J. Nat. Cancer Inst.* 24: 953.

15. Beuving, L. J. 1969. Responsiveness of carcinogen-induced hyperplastic alveolar nodules in Lewis rats to mammary gland growth-regulatory mechanism. *J. Nat. Cancer Inst.* 43: 1191.

16. Elias, J. J., and Rivera, E. M. 1959. Comparison of the responses of normal, precancerous and neoplastic mouse mammary tissues to hormones *in vitro*. *Cancer Res.* 19: 505.

17. Beuving, L. J. 1969. Effects of ovariectomy on preneoplastic nodule formation and maintenance in the mammary glands of carcinogen-treated rats. *J. Nat. Cancer Inst.* 43: 1181.

18. Dao, T. L. 1962. The role of ovarian hormones in initiating the induction of mammary cancer in rats by polynuclear hydrocarbons. *Cancer Res.* 22: 973.

19. Holzbauer, M.; Newport, H. N.; Birmingham, M. K.; and Traihov, H. T. 1969. Secretion of pregn-4-ene-3, 20-dione (progesterone) *in vivo* by the adrenal gland of the rat. *Nature* (Lond.) 221: 572.

20. Resko, J. A. 1969. Endocrine control of adrenal progesterone secretion in the ovariectomized rat. *Science* 164: 70.
21. Niswender, G. D.; Chen, C. L.; Midgley, A. R.; Meites, J.; and Ellis, S. 1969. Radioimmunoassay for rat prolactin. *Proc. Soc. Exp. Biol. Med.* 130: 793:
22. Meites, J., and Nicoll, C. S. 1966. Adenohypophysis: Prolactin. *Ann. Rev. Physiol.* 28: 57.
23. Nandi, S. 1959. Hormonal control of mammogenesis and lactogenesis in the C$_3$H/He Crgl mouse. *Univ. Calif. Publ. Zool.* 65: 1.
24. Lyons, W. R.; Li, C. H.; and Johnson, R. E. 1958. The hormonal control of mammary growth and lactation. *Rec. Progr. Hormone Res.* 14: 219.
25. Puca, G. A., and Bresciani, F. 1969. Interactions of 6, 7-^{3}H-17β-estradiol with mammary gland and other organs of the C$_3$H mouse *in vivo*. *Endocrinology* 85: 1.
26. Banarjee, M. R. 1969. Hormonal control of DNA synthesis: Altered responsiveness of hyperplastic alveolar nodules of mouse mammary gland. *J. Nat. Cancer Inst.* 42: 227.
27. Sterental, A.; Dominquez, J. M.; Weissman, C.; and Pearson, O. H. 1963. Pituitary role in the estrogen dependency of experimental mammary cancer. *Cancer Res.* 23: 481.
28. Talwalker, P. K., and Meites, J. 1961. Mammary lobulo-alveolar growth induced by anterior pituitary hormones in adreno-ovariectomized rats. *Proc. Soc. Exp. Biol. Med.* 107: 880.
29. Dilley, W. G., and Nandi, S. 1968. Rat mammary gland differentiation *in vitro* in the absence of steroids. *Science* 161:59.
30. King, R. J. B.; Cowan, D. M.; and Inman, D. R. 1965. The uptake of (6, 7-^{3}H) oestradiol by dimethylbenzanthracene-induced rat mammary tumors. *J. Endocr.* 32: 83.
31. Mobbs, B. G. 1966. The uptake of tritiated oestradiol by dimethylbenzanthracene-induced mammary tumors of the rat. *J. Endocr.* 36: 409.
32. Jensen, E. V.; DeSombre, E. R.; and Jungblut, P. W. 1967. In *Endogenous factors influencing host-tumor balance*, ed. R. W. Wissler, T. L. Dao, and S. Wood, Jr., p. 15. Chicago: University of Chicago Press.
33. Dao, T. L. 1963. Tumor induction in transplanted mammary glands in rats. *J. Nat. Cancer Inst.* 32: 1259.
34. Dao, T. L.; King, C.; and Gowlak, D. 1968. Mammary gland transplantation and tumorigenesis. I. Concentration and clearance of 7, 12-dimethylbenz(a)anthracene in the graft. *J. Nat. Cancer Inst.* 40: 157.

Joseph Meites

The Relation of Estrogen and Prolactin to Mammary Tumorigenesis in the Rat 17

Introduction

Both anterior pituitary and ovarian hormones, particularly prolactin and estrogen, are important for development and growth of mammary tumors in rats. Long-term treatment with estrogen alone can result in mammary tumors in intact rats (1). I shall present evidence that long-term exposure of intact rats to high blood levels of prolactin and growth hormone from a transplanted pituitary tumor may evoke mammary tumors. Pituitary transplants or prolonged injections of prolactin also can elicit tumorigenesis in mice (2). If the pituitary is removed, estrogen can no longer induce mammary tumors in rats or mice, nor is there any evidence that anterior pituitary hormones alone can produce mammary tumors in rats or mice without the presence of ovarian hormones.

Carcinogen-induced mammary tumors in rats appear to require both ovarian and anterior pituitary hormones (3), although under some experimental conditions, carcinogens can induce mammary tumors in ovariectomized rats (4). At least temporary growth of established mammary tumors can be maintained after ovariectomy (5, 6) or ovariectomy-adrenalectomy (7) by increasing the blood levels of prolactin. Although estrogens per se are believed to act directly on the mammary gland to evoke tumorigenesis, there is no conclusive evidence to support this. Estrogens have certain similarities in structure to some of the natural and synthetic carcinogens, and their direct biochemical effects on the mammary gland, reproductive tract, and

The author is affiliated with the Department of Physiology at Michigan State University.

other tissues have been studied extensively. Jensen has recently demonstrated that these tissues produce specific binding proteins to estrogens (chap. 2).

Although the importance of estrogen in mammary tumorigenesis appears to be well documented, the role of anterior pituitary hormones, particularly prolactin, has been recognized only in recent years. In intact mice, transplanting extra pituitaries from other mice to provide an additional source of prolactin (and some growth hormone) induces mammary tumors even in animals free of mammary tumor virus (2). Prolonged injections of prolactin have also been reported to produce mammary tumors in intact female mice (2). In intact Sprague-Dawley female rats, elevations of blood prolactin levels by pituitary transplants or by placing bilateral lesions in the median eminence were recently found to markedly hasten the onset of spontaneous mammary tumors, which do not ordinarily appear in these rats until they reach old age (8). Similarly, elevations of blood prolactin levels induced by pituitary transplants (9), median eminence lesions (5, 6), injections of Enovid (10), or implantation of estrogen in median eminence (11) increased the growth of carcinogen-induced mammary tumors.

HORMONE DEPENDENCY OF A MAMMARY TUMOR PRODUCED IN A RAT BEARING PITUITARY TUMOR TRANSPLANT

Earlier work by Dr. Dilip Sinha and I. Weber in our laboratory indicates that prolonged stimulation of the mammary gland of inbred Wistar-Furth female rats by high prolactin and growth hormone secretion from pituitary tumor transplants may occasionally result in development of hormone-dependent tumors.

Thirteen female albino rats approximately 55 days of age, of the inbred Wistar-Furth strain, were grafted subcutaneously on the back of the neck with a mammosomatotropic tumor (MtT.W_{15}, 10th passage) obtained through the courtesy of Dr. Jacob Furth. The pituitary tumors could be palpated within 28 days and were allowed to develop further. During the next 2.5–3.5 mo a few of the rats developed palpable mammary tumors (MT). We have since observed similar development of mammary tumors in several inbred Wistar-Furth rats carrying MtT.W_{15} or MtT.W_5 pituitary tumors. These mammary tumors appeared to be adenocarcinomas.

Two weeks after development of a mammary tumor in one of the rats, both the MT (passage 1) and MtT.W_{15} were transplanted on the same day into 9 intact mature female Wistar-Furth rats. The MT was placed in the left inguinal region and the MtT.W$_{15}$ was implanted subcutaneously on the back of the neck. All grafts were made by first mincing the tumor tissue in sterile medium 199 and then injecting 0.1–0.2 ml of the mixture into each rat. The mammary tumors became palpable in all 9 rats after a mean latency period of about 28 days (fig. 1).

In a second group of mature female rats, 10 rats were first grafted with MtT.W$_{15}$ (groups II and IV). Fourteen days later, each rat

MT ORIGINALLY FOUND IN MtT.W$_{15}$ BEARING RATS
av. latency, approx. 80 d
↓
PASSAGE I

9 INTACT RATS, MtT.W$_{15}$ TRANSPLANTED ON SAME DAY
↓
9/9 tumors
latency, approx. 28 d
↓
PASSAGE II

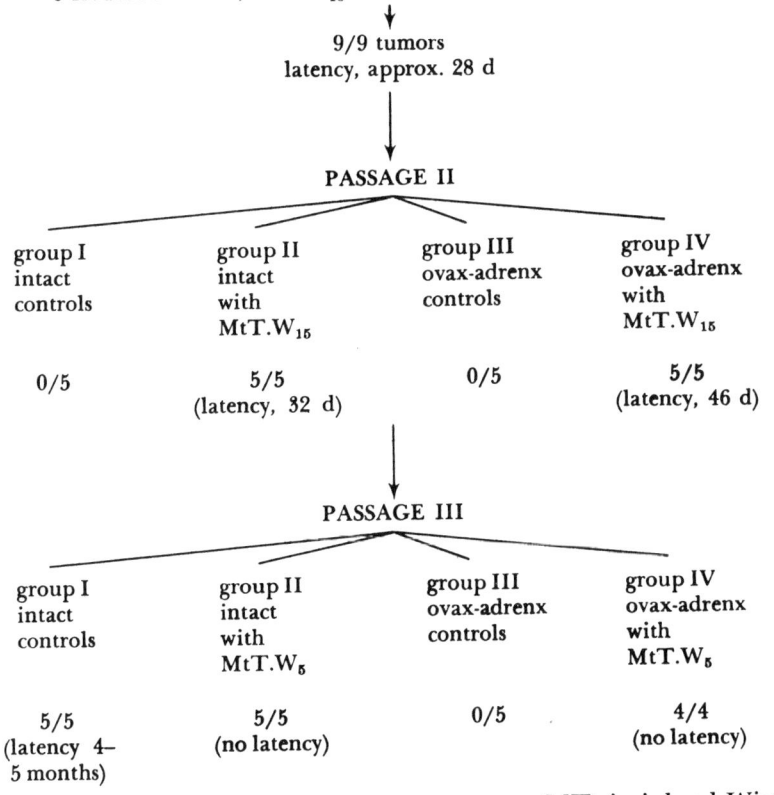

group I intact controls	group II intact with MtT.W$_{15}$	group III ovax-adrenx controls	group IV ovax-adrenx with MtT.W$_{15}$
0/5	5/5 (latency, 32 d)	0/5	5/5 (latency, 46 d)

↓
PASSAGE III

group I intact controls	group II intact with MtT.W$_5$	group III ovax-adrenx controls	group IV ovax-adrenx with MtT.W$_5$
5/5 (latency 4–5 months)	5/5 (no latency)	0/5	4/4 (no latency)

Fig. 1. Growth of transplanted mammary tumors (MT) in inbred Wistar-Furth rats with and without pituitary tumors (MtT.W$_{15}$ or MtT.W$_5$). (From D. Sinha, I. Weber, and J. Meites, unpublished)

from these two groups and two other groups (I and III) was grafted with MT (passage 2) derived from passage 1. The four groups were then treated as shown in figure 1. In the 5 intact control rats not transplanted with MtT.W_{15} (group I), no mammary tumor development was found, whereas all 5 rats with a MtT.W_{15} tumor (group II) developed mammary tumor (mean latency period was 32 days). None of the 5 ovariectomized-adrenalectomized controls (group III) showed mammary tumor growth, but all 5 ovariectomized-adrenalectomized rats with a MtT.W_{15} (group IV) developed palpable mammary tumors after a mean latency period of 46 days. All ovariectomy-adrenalectomies were performed a week or more before MT implantation.

In a third experiment (fig. 1), 10 rats (groups II and IV) were each grafted with a MtT.W_5 pituitary tumor which secretes large amounts of prolactin and growth hormone. At the end of 91 days, these rats and the rats of two control groups (I and II) were each implanted in the left inguinal region with mammary tumor tissue (passage 3). The MtT.W_5 tumors had reached approximately 1.7 cm in diameter at the time of MT transplantation. The transplanted mammary tumor in the control rats (groups I and III), initially palpable as a small nodule, disappeared shortly after transplantation. These tumors reappeared in all 5 intact control rats (group I), but not in the ovariectomized-adrenalectomized rats (group III), after a latency period of about 4 mo, although they never reached more than 1 cm in diameter. This suggests that the transplanted mammary tumor can grow in intact rats even in the absence of a pituitary tumor transplant, but that the latency period is prolonged and extent of MT growth is limited. In the rats of groups II and IV, with both MT and MtT.W_5 transplants, the MT began growing almost without any latency period. There appeared to be no significant difference in growth of this particular mammary tumor in the ovariectomized-adrenalectomized rats compared with that in the intact control rats, reflecting the primary dependency of this tumor on the anterior pituitary hormones from the MtT.W_5 rather than on steroid hormones. The nature of this mammary tumor shows very little difference from tumors induced by DMBA. DMBA-induced mammary tumors regress if ovariectomy is performed even in the presence of high blood levels of prolactin after median eminence lesions (6).

In a fourth experiment, 10 intact rats were implanted with an

MtT.W$_5$ and 58 days later were grafted with an MT (4th passage). The mammary tumor developed rapidly in all rats with almost no latency period. In 5 rats, the MtT.W$_5$ was removed 20 days after mammary tumor transplantation, and rapid regression of the mammary tumor was observed in all animals. The mammary tumor regressed to approximately 0.5 cm after MtT.W$_5$ removal and remained at that level for about 100 days, then grew slowly to a maximum size of about 1.0 cm in diameter. The mammary tumor in the 5 rats with MtT.W$_5$ continued to grow rapidly throughout the experimental period.

The results of the above four experiments show that transplanting a MtT.W$_{15}$ pituitary tumor, known to secrete large amounts of prolactin, growth hormone, and ACTH, can cause occasional induction of mammary tumors in intact Wistar-Furth rats. This is similar, therefore, to the development of mammary tumor in intact mice after transplantation of additional normal pituitaries (2). After passage to other rats of the original mammary tumor induced in the presence of MtT.W$_{15}$ in the present study, the mammary tumor grew rapidly only in the presence of the pituitary tumors, and regressed after the pituitary tumors were removed. In later passages they appeared to grow almost as quickly in the absence as in the presence of the ovaries and adrenals, indicating a primary dependence on the pituitary tumor hormones for maintenance of their growth. In the third experiment, when the mammary tumors were transplanted to rats with a palpable MtT.W$_5$ grafted 91 days earlier, there was no obvious latency period, presumably because large amounts of prolactin and growth hormone already were being secreted by the MtT.W$_5$.

The observation that some transplanted mammary tumors became palpable after a prolonged latency period of 4-5 mo in intact rats without an MtT transplant, or did not regress completely after MtT removal, suggests that the lower levels of hormones secreted by the in situ anterior pituitary of the host rats permitted minimal growth and maintenance of the mammary tumor. Since no tumors have been grafted in the hypophysectomized rats, we cannot be sure whether this tumor will grow in the absence of prolactin or other anterior pituitary hormones. Nonetheless, the present study emphasizes the important role of the anterior pituitary hormones for stimulation of growth of the transplantable mammary tumor in these rats.

Ability of Estrogen or Anterior Pituitary Hormones to Promote Mammary Carcinogenesis in Ovariectomized Rats Given 7, 12-Dimethylbenz(a)anthracene (DMBA)

In this experiment, we attempted to determine the relative importance of estrogen as compared with prolactin and growth hormone on carcinogen-induced mammary tumorigenesis. These results have been published previously (4) and will only be summarized here. Sprague-Dawley virgin female rats were randomly divided into six groups as indicated in table 1. When they reached 52 days of age, group I was sham operated (controls) and groups 2–6 were bilaterally ovariectomized. Seven days later, each rat was fed 20 mg of DMBA in 1 ml corn oil. Groups 1–5 were treated for 7 days before and 7 days after DMBA administration, as indicated in table 1. Group 6 was treated daily with gradually increasing doses of porcine growth hormone and ovine prolactin, beginning a day after ovariectomy and continuing for 75 days.

All 18 of the intact, sham-operated control rats (group 1) developed mammary tumors after a mean latency period of 68 days. None of the ovariectomized control rats injected with saline (group 2) showed mammary tumors. Ovariectomized rats injected with 1 or 10 μg estradiol for 14 days (groups 2 and 3) showed a mammary tumor incidence of 33% and 23% respectively. Ovariectomized rats injected with growth hormone (STH) and prolactin for 14 or 75 days (groups 5 and 6) showed a mammary tumor incidence of 44% and 66% respectively. All tumors were removed from these animals and found to be adenocarcinomas.

These results indicate that in ovariectomized rats given DMBA, either estrogen alone or prolactin and growth hormone permits development of mammary adenocarcinomas. Since no mammary tumors appeared in the ovariectomized controls, we can assume that the prolactin and growth hormone released from the in situ pituitary were insufficient to promote mammary carcinogenesis. Ovariectomy results in a significant decrease in secretion of anterior pituitary prolactin (12), and therefore the effects of ovariectomy can be attributed to a loss of ovarian hormones as well as to a decrease in anterior pituitary secretion. The ability of injections of prolactin and growth hormone to elicit mammary tumorigenesis in these ovariectomized rats suggests that estrogen action on the mammary gland is not a prerequisite for the action of DMBA. Inasmuch as the adrenals were

TABLE 1: EFFECTS OF HORMONE ADMINISTRATION ON MAMMARY TUMOR INDUCTION IN OVARIECTOMIZED RATS TREATED WITH DMBA

Group and Treatment[a]	Duration of Treatment (days)	Total No. of Rats	No. and % of Rats with Tumors	Average No. of Tumors per Tumor-bearing Rat	Range and Mean Latency Period (days)
1. Sham-operated controls, saline	14	18	18 (100)	3.9	52–110 (68)
2. Ovax-controls, saline	14	20	0 (0)	—	—
3. Ovax, 1 µg esd 1×daily	14	12	4 (33)	1.5	72–130 (104)
4. Ovax, 10 µg esd 1×daily	14	13	3 (23)	1.0	76–102 (89)
5. Ovax, 1 mg STH+1 mg prolactin 2×daily	14	9	4 (44)	1.8	114–210 (146)
6. Ovax, STH+prolactin[b] 1×daily	75	9	6 (66)	2.3	94–207 (122)

SOURCE: Talwalker, Meites, and Mizuno (4).

[a] Ovax = ovariectomized; STH = porcine growth hormone; esd = estradiol. DMBA was administered 7 days after ovariectomy.
[b] Dosages of STH and prolactin were increased every 15 days.

not removed from the ovariectomized rats in this experiment, we cannot conclude that all possible sources of ovarian hormones were removed. But it is clear that no mammary tumors were produced by DMBA in the absence of the ovaries, which suggests that any estrogen present in ovariectomized rats was too little to contribute to the mammary tumorigenesis in the presence of endogenous prolactin and growth hormone.

INHIBITION OF MAMMARY TUMOR GROWTH BY ESTROGEN: ITS RELATION TO PROLACTIN

That estrogens, particularly in large doses, can inhibit growth of mammary tumors in rats and human subjects appears to be well established. Indeed, it has been observed that the same doses of estrogen effective for inducing mammary tumors in ovariectomized rats can inhibit the growth of these tumors after they develop (3). It has been assumed that large doses of estrogens (and androgens) depress anterior pituitary secretion (13), and this in turn inhibits mammary tumor growth. I have always doubted this hypothesis, since no doses of estrogen actually were demonstrated to reduce anterior pituitary prolactin secretion in any species. On the contrary, even large doses of estrogen have been found to increase pituitary and blood prolactin levels (14), although small doses are more effective than large doses in this respect. I wished, therefore, to determine the relation of different doses of estrogen to induction and growth of mammary tumors in ovariectomized DMBA-treated rats and to measure their effects on serum prolactin concentration.

In this experiment, young Sprague-Dawley rats were ovariectomized at 45 days of age. Seven days later, all rats were given a single intravenous injection of 5 mg of DMBA. Beginning the next day, the rats were treated for 150 days as shown in table 2. The intact and ovariectomized controls (groups 1 and 2) were injected subcutaneously every other day with corn oil. Groups 3–5, all ovariectomized, were injected subcutaneously every other day with different doses of estradiol benzoate in corn oil.

Mammary tumors developed in all 18 control rats (group 1), but in none of the 10 ovariectomized control rats (groups 2). Of the ovariectomized rats given estradiol benzoate, the greatest development of mammary tumors (in 17 out of 19 rats) occurred in group 4, given 2 μg estradiol benzoate on alternate days. The percentage and number of spontaneously regressed tumors was greater in all

TABLE 2: EFFECTS OF GRADED DOSES OF ESTRADIOL BENZOATE (EB) ON MAMMARY TUMOR INDUCTION IN DMBA-TREATED, OVARIECTOMIZED RATS

Group and Treatment	No. of Rats	No. of Rats with Tumors	Average Latency Period (days)	% and No. of Completely Regressed Tumors[a]	Serum Prolactin Concentration (ng/ml)
1. Intact controls, no EB	18	18	59 ± 3	8 (11/143)	27.3 ± 2.6 (D)[b] 101.8 ± 23 (E)[c]
2. Ovax[d] controls, no EB	10	0	—	—	14.7 ± 2.4
3. Ovax, 0.2 µg EB	21	12	98 ± 10	19 (4/21)	20.8 ± 1.6
4. Ovax, 2.0 µg EB	19	17	73 ± 7	20 (16/79)	169.7 ± 23
5. Ovax, 20.0 µg EB	19	10	119 ± 7	39 (9/23)	177.0 ± 21

SOURCE: Nagasawa and Meites, unpublished.
NOTE: EB was injected every 2 days for 150 days.
[a] These are tumors that appeared first and later regressed spontaneously while rats were still on estrogen treatment.
[b] D = diestrous phase of cycle.
[c] E = estrous phase of cycle.
[d] Ovax = ovariectomized.

three groups given estradiol benzoate than in the intact controls (group 1). The greatest mammary tumor regression, 39%, occurred in group 5, which was given the highest dose of estradiol benzoate, 20 µg.

About 150 days after the experiment was begun, serum prolactin values in the intact controls (group 1) were 27.3 ng/ml serum in diestrous rats and 101.8 ng/ml in estrous rats. These animals continued to cycle normally, and the values reported here agree with previous reports from our laboratory on prolactin values in normal cycling rats (15). The ovariectomized controls (group 2) showed the lowest serum prolactin levels, and the 0.2 µg dose of estradiol benzoate (group 3) only slightly increased serum prolactin values. The highest serum prolactin levels were found in groups 4 and 5, which received the highest doses of estradiol benzoate. However, the tumor incidence in group 5 is markedly reduced in spite of the highest level of serum prolactin.

These results suggest that a dose of 2 µg estradiol benzoate injected every other day for 150 days to ovariectomized rats is very nearly optimal for producing mammary tumors in DMBA-treated rats, although the total number of tumors and average latency period were somewhat less than in the intact control rats. The incidence of tumor regression was greater in all the estradiol benzoate-injected rats than in the intact controls and was highest in the group given the largest dose (group 5). It is interesting that serum prolactin values were highest in the rats showing the greatest tumor regression (groups 4 and 5). It is apparent, therefore, that estradiol benzoate-induced mammary tumor regression in rats is associated with very high levels of serum prolactin and that mammary tumor regression cannot be explained on the basis of inhibition of pituitary prolactin secretion. Some other mechanism(s) must account for this phenomenon.

The two larger doses of estradiol benzoate inhibited body weight gains compared with the untreated intact controls, and this may account in part for the regression of the mammary tumors. However, the fact that a high percentage of mammary tumors developed in these rats suggests that the inhibitory effect on body growth was not the principal factor responsible for mammary tumor regression. Earlier work from our laboratory (16) suggests that although large doses of estrogen increase pituitary prolactin secretion, they render the mammary glands less susceptible to certain actions of prolactin. Thus large doses of estrogen, or combinations of estrogen and progesterone, stimulated mammary growth but prevented moderate doses of prolactin from initiating lactation in castrated rabbits. If estrogen administration was terminated, the same doses of prolactin initiated copious lactation. It appears possible, therefore, that large doses of estrogen alter the biochemical substrate of the parenchymal cells of the mammary gland so that prolactin can no longer exert a lactational effect. Large doses of estrogen may similarly inhibit the tumorigenic action of prolactin on the mammary gland in the presence of a carcinogen. Further work is necessary to discover the mechanism(s) by which large doses of estrogen inhibit these actions of prolactin on the mammary gland.

Acknowledgments

This research was aided by National Institutes of Health grants CA-10771 and AM-04784.

References

1. Noble, R. L., and Cutts, J. H. 1959. Mammary tumors of the rat: A review. *Cancer Res.* 19: 1125.
2. Muhlbock, O., and Boot, L. M. 1967. The mode of action of ovarian hormones in the induction of mammary cancer in mice. *Biochem. Pharm.* 16: 627.
3. Huggins, C.; Briziarelli, G.; and Sutton, H. 1959. Rapid induction of mammary carcinoma in the rat and the influence of hormones on the tumors. *J. Exp. Med.* 109: 25.
4. Talwalker, P. K.; Meites, J.; and Mizuno, H. 1964. Mammary tumor induction by estrogen or anterior pituitary hormones in ovariectomized rats given 7, 12-dimethyl-1, 2-benzanthracene. *Proc. Soc. Exp. Biol. Med.* 116: 531.
5. Clemens, J. A.; Welsch, C. W.; and Meites, J. 1968. Effects of hypothalamic lesions on incidence and growth of mammary tumors in carcinogen-treated rats. *Proc. Soc. Exp. Biol. Med.* 127: 969.
6. Welsch, C. W.; Clemens, J. A., and Meites, J. 1969. Effects of hypothalamic and amygdaloid lesions on development and growth of carcinogen-induced mammary tumors in the female rat. *Cancer Res.* 29: 1541.
7. Nagasawa, H., and Yanai, R. 1970. Effects of prolactin or growth hormone on growth of carcinogen-induced mammary tumor of adreno-ovariectomized rats. *Int. J. Cancer* 6: 488.
8. Welsch, C. W.; Jenkins, T. W.; and Meites, J. 1970. Increased incidence of mammary tumors in the female rat grafted with multiple pituitaries. *Cancer Res.* 30: 1024.
9. Welsch, C. W.; Clemens, J. A.; and Meites, J. 1968. Effects of multiple

pituitary homografts or progesterone on 7, 12-dimethylbenz(a)anthracene-induced mammary tumors in rats. *J. Nat. Cancer Inst.* 41: 465.
10. Welsch, C. W., and Meites, J. 1969. Effects of norethynodrel-mestranol combination (Enovid) on development and growth of carcinogen-induced mammary tumors in female rats. *Cancer* 23: 601.
11. Nagasawa, H.; Chen, C. L.; and Meites, J. 1969. Effects of estrogen implant in median eminence on serum and pituitary prolactin levels in the rat. *Proc. Soc. Exp. Biol. Med.* 132: 859.
12. Meites, J., and Nicoll, C. S. 1966. Adenohypophysis: Prolactin. *Ann. Rev. Physiol.* 28: 57.
13. Folley, S. J., and Malpress, F. H. 1948. Hormonal control of lactation. In *The Hormones,* ed. G. Pincus and K. V. Thimann, vol. I, chap. 16. New York: Academic Press.
14. Chen, C. L., and Meites, J. 1970. Effects of estrogen and progesterone on serum and pituitary prolactin levels in ovariectomized rats. *Endocrinology* 86: 503.
15. Amenomori, Y; Chen, C. L.; and Meites, J. 1970. Serum prolactin levels in rats during different reproductive states. *Endocrinology* 86: 506.
16. Meites, J. and Sgouris, J. 1953. Can the ovarian hormones inhibit the mammary response to prolactin? *Endocrinology* 53: 17.

Olof H. Pearson, A. Molina, T. P. Butler,
L. Llerena, and H. Nasr

Estrogens and Prolactin in Mammary Cancer   18

Mammary cancer is hormone-responsive in about one-third of the women with this disease. Ablation of the ovaries, adrenals, or pituitary gland can produce temporary tumor regression in some patients with metastatic disease. Pilot studies have shown that after an oophorectomy-induced remission, estrogen administration may reactivate tumor growth (1). After a hypophysectomy-induced remission, estrogens failed to reactivate the disease, suggesting that a pituitary factor was involved in the estrogenic stimulation of tumor growth (2). Because of the inherent difficulties of conducting such studies in humans, we sought an animal tumor model which might allow for more definitive studies of the endocrine factor, or factors, involved in maintaining mammary tumor growth (3).

Huggins and his coworkers (4) demonstrated that a single feeding of 7, 12-dimethylbenz(a)anthracene (DMBA) given to 50-day-old female Sprague-Dawley rats would produce breast cancer in 100% of the animals within 30 to 60 days. They also demonstrated that these cancers were hormone dependent. We have used this model system to study the endocrine factors involved in maintaining the growth of these tumors. Previous studies (5) showed that these cancers grow progressively in intact rats, and the animals die usually of inanition or infections. The tumors are adenocarcinomas which may invade local tissues but rarely, if ever, metastasize. Following oophorectomy and adrenalectomy or after hyphophysectomy, the tumors regress completely and the animals live for several months without recurrence of the tumors. After an oophorectomy and adrenalectomy-

The authors are affiliated with the Department of Medicine at Case Western Reserve University School of Medicine.

induced regression, estradiol benzoate in doses of 1 to 5 µg/day reactivates the growth of the tumors. When estradiol injections are discontinued, the tumors again regress. After a hypophysectomy-induced remission, estradiol benzoate injections failed to reactivate tumor growth even when cortisone and thyroxin injections were added to the estradiol. These results indicate that the pituitary plays a role in the estrogenic stimulation of rat mammary tumor growth, and they resemble the results obtained in women with hormone-responsive mammary cancer in the experiment referred to above. Further studies were undertaken in an attempt to define the pituitary factor involved in the growth of the rat mammary tumor.

Methods

The induction of mammary tumors in rats has previously been described (5). Bovine growth hormone used in these studies was prepared by the Armour Company. Ovine prolactin was supplied by the Endocrinology Study Section of the National Institute of Arthritis and Metabolic Diseases.

The radioimmunoassay of rat prolactin is done by a method similar to that recently reported by Niswender et al. (7). Rat prolactin (LTH) was prepared from organ culture incubates of rat pituitary gland using polyacrylamide gel electrophoresis. Purified rat prolactin (H96B) prepared by Ellis, Grindeland, and Nuenke (9) was used as the standard. Serum for prolactin assay was obtained from tail blood without anesthesia. Antiserum to purified rat prolactin was prepared in a rabbit and its specificity was tested by radioimmunoassay (10).

Results

Effects of Bovine Growth Hormone

Twelve rats with DMBA-induced mammary tumors underwent oophorectomy and adrenalectomy, which was followed by regression of the tumors to 0.25–0.50 cm^2. At this time bovine growth hormone 2 mg per day, was injected subcutaneously for periods of 7 to 41 days with an average treatment period of 35 days. There was no evidence that tumor growth was stimulated in any of these animals. Two animals received 4 mg of bovine growth hormone for an additional period of 43 to 52 days without evidence of stimulation of tumor growth.

Effects of Ovine Prolactin

Figure 1 shows the effects of ovine prolactin, 2 mg injected subcutaneously per day, on 16 rats whose mammary tumors had regressed after oophorectomy and adrenalectomy. Prolactin reactivated tumor growth and the tumors reached their original size in an average of 18 days. When the prolactin injections were discontinued, the tumors regressed to less than 0.3 cm^2 in an average of 14 days. Additional studies revealed that 0.5 mg of prolactin daily would reactivate tumor growth in about 75% of the animals.

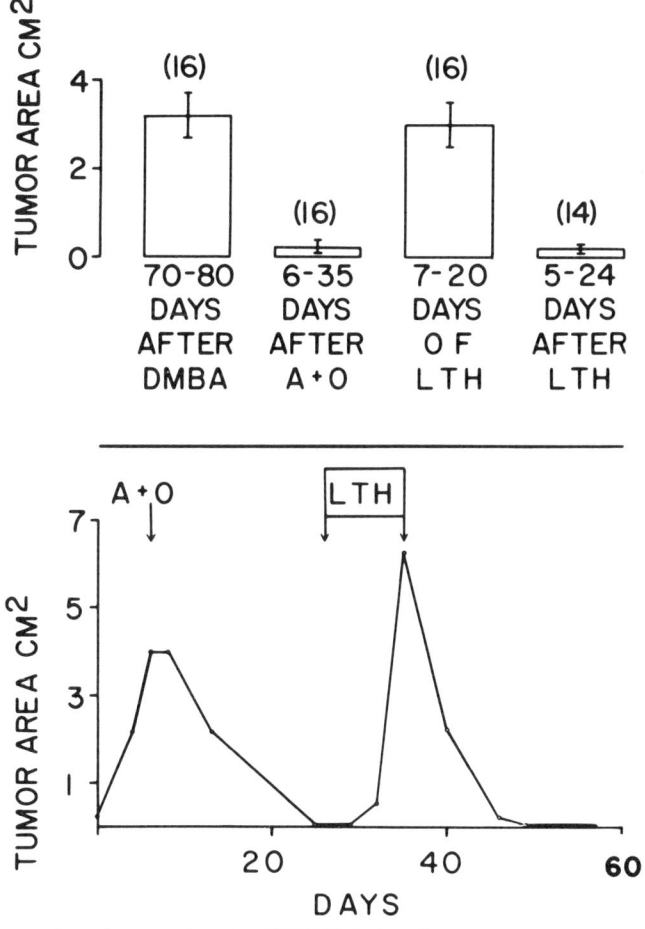

Fig. 1. Effects of ovine prolactin (LTH) injections on rat mammary tumor growth after oophorectomy and adrenalectomy $(A + O)$. The lower portion of the figure depicts the results in a single animal, and the upper part shows the mean tumor size and standard error of the mean in 16 rats.

Figure 2 presents the results of administering ovine prolactin, 1.5 mg per day subcutaneously, to 8 rats whose mammary tumors had regressed after hypophysectomy. Tumor growth was reactivated within 16 days after prolactin injections began. The tumors regressed promptly when prolactin was discontinued. Estradiol benzoate injections, 5 µg per day, were administered to 6 rats whose mammary

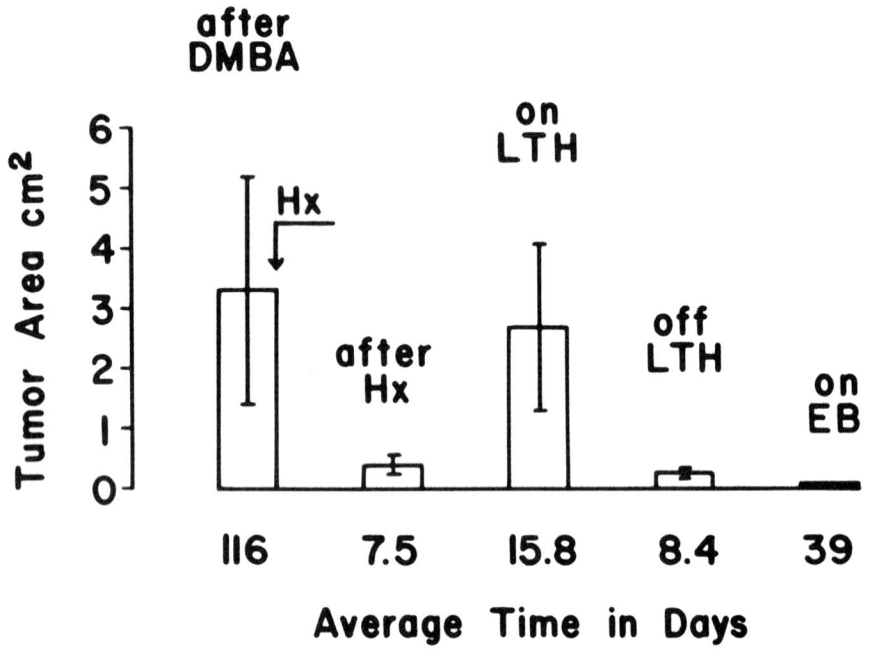

Fig. 2. Effects of ovine prolactin (*LTH*) and estradiol benzoate (*EB*) injections on rat mammary tumor growth after hypophysectomy (*Hx*). Mean tumor size and standard error of the mean in 8 rats are shown.

tumors had regressed after oophorectomy, adrenalectomy, and hypophysectomy. Prolactin reactivated tumor growth in all of these animals.

These results suggested that DMBA-induced rat mammary carcinoma is prolactin-dependent, and that the effects of estradiol on tumor growth might be mediated through effects on pituitary prolactin secretion.

Serum Prolactin Levels in the Rat

Radioimmunoassay of serum prolactin levels during the estrous cycle is shown in figure 4. A surge in prolactin secretion occurs on the

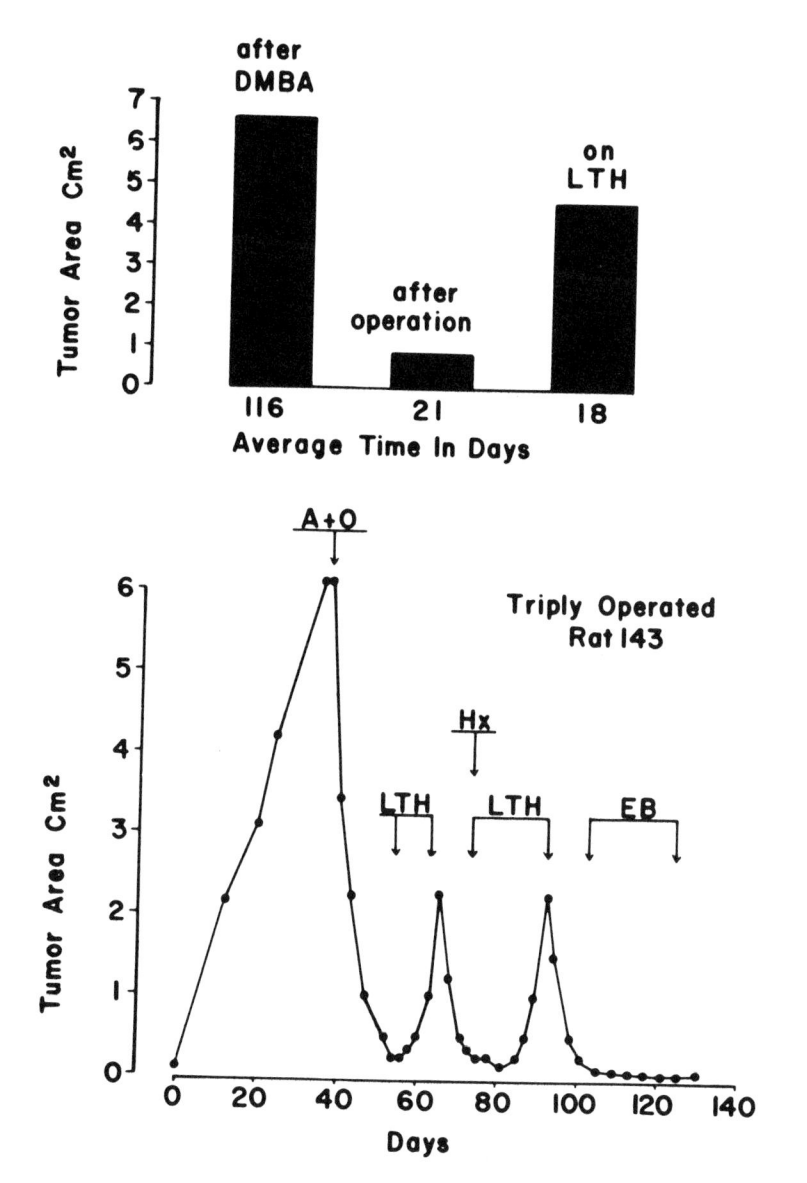

Fig. 3. Effects of ovine prolactin (*LTH*) injections on rat mammary tumor growth after oophorectomy, adrenalectomy, and hypophysectomy. The lower portion of the figure shows the results in a single animal, and the bars at the top depict the mean tumor size in 6 rats.

first day of estrus. Additional studies have shown that the rise in serum prolactin occurs on the evening of proestrus in rats with only one day of estrus (fig. 5). Similar observations have been reported by Kwa and Verhofstad (8) and Niswender et al. (7).

Figure 6 illustrates the effects of oophorectomy and adrenalectomy on serum prolactin levels. There is a prompt fall in serum prolactin

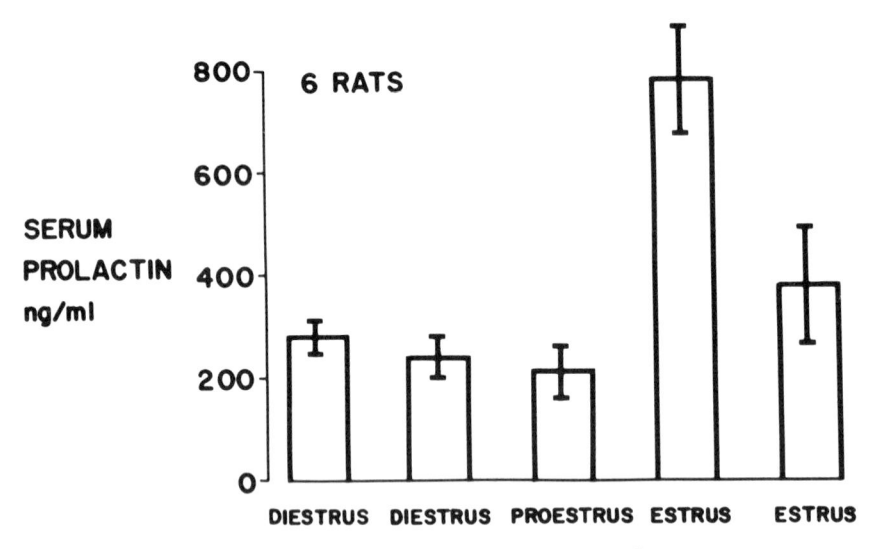

Fig. 4. Rat serum prolactin levels during estrous cycle

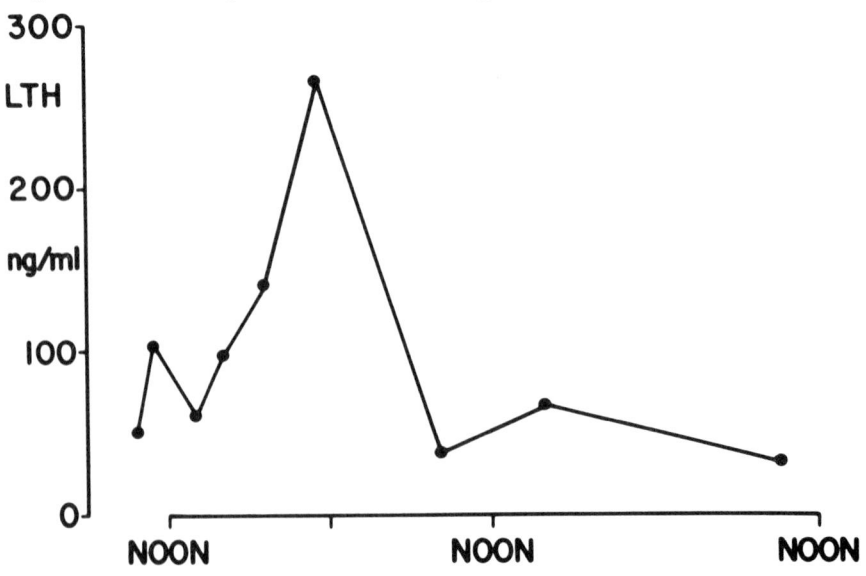

Fig. 5. Serum prolactin during estrous cycle

Estrogens and Prolactin in Mammary Cancer 293

levels, which remain low for at least one month. Daily measurements of serum prolactin in oophorectomized and adrenalectomized rats showed that there is no surge in prolactin secretion such as occurs during the estrous cycle. Figure 7 shows the effect of a single injection of estradiol benzoate on a castrated female rat. There is a prompt rise in serum prolactin levels. Figure 8 shows that administering

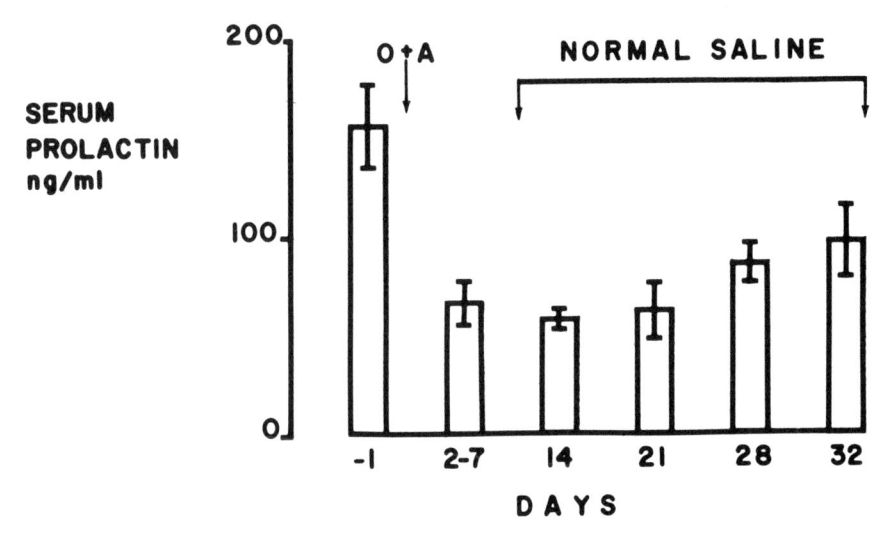

Fig. 6. Effects of oophorectomy and adrenalectomy on rat serum prolactin levels.

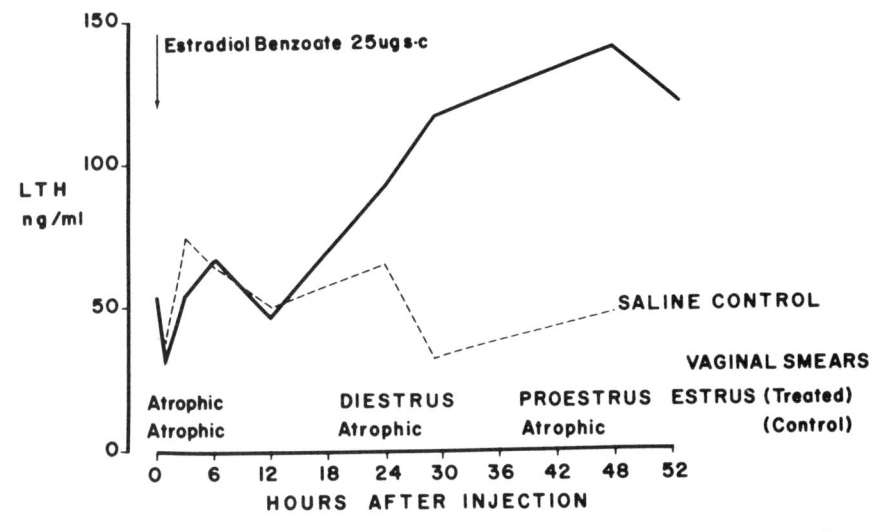

Fig. 7. Acute effects of estradiol benzoate on rat serum prolactin levels

5 μg of estradiol benzoate daily to male rats results in a prompt (within 6 hr) and sustained rise in serum prolactin levels. These data suggest that the surge in prolactin secretion at the time of estrus is probably controlled by circulating estrogen levels.

These observations are consistent with the concept that oophorectomy- and adrenalectomy-induced regression of rat mammary cancer is related to reduction in serum prolactin levels, and that estradiol-

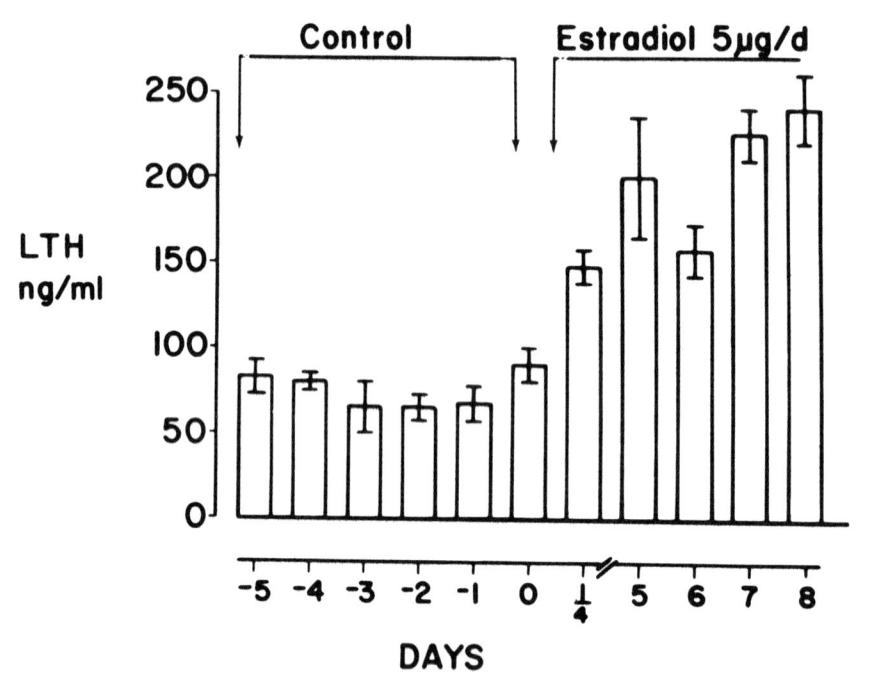

Fig. 8. Effects of estradiol benzoate on serum LTH levels in male rats

induced reactivation of mammary tumor growth is related to rising serum prolactin levels.

Effects of Perphenazine on Serum Prolactin Levels
and on Rat Mammary Tumor Growth

A number of workers have demonstrated that certain tranquilizing drugs, such as the phenothiazines, induce mammotrophic and lactogenic effects in animals and man (11). Ben-David (12) presented evidence that perphenazine treatment stimulates endogenous prolactin secretion in rats. Figure 9 shows the effects of a single injection of perphenazine (Trilafon) on each of two female rats. Serum prolactin levels rose markedly after 1 hr and returned toward control levels at 24 hr. Daily administration of perphenazine for 15 days also increased serum prolactin levels.

Perphenazine was administered to DMBA-fed rats to determine whether this drug would influence the development and rate of growth of mammary tumors. The results of one experiment are presented in figure 10. A group of rats who had been fed DMBA 2 mo previously and had not yet developed palpable tumors were injected with perphenazine and compared with a control group which received saline injections. Although tumors appeared in the treated

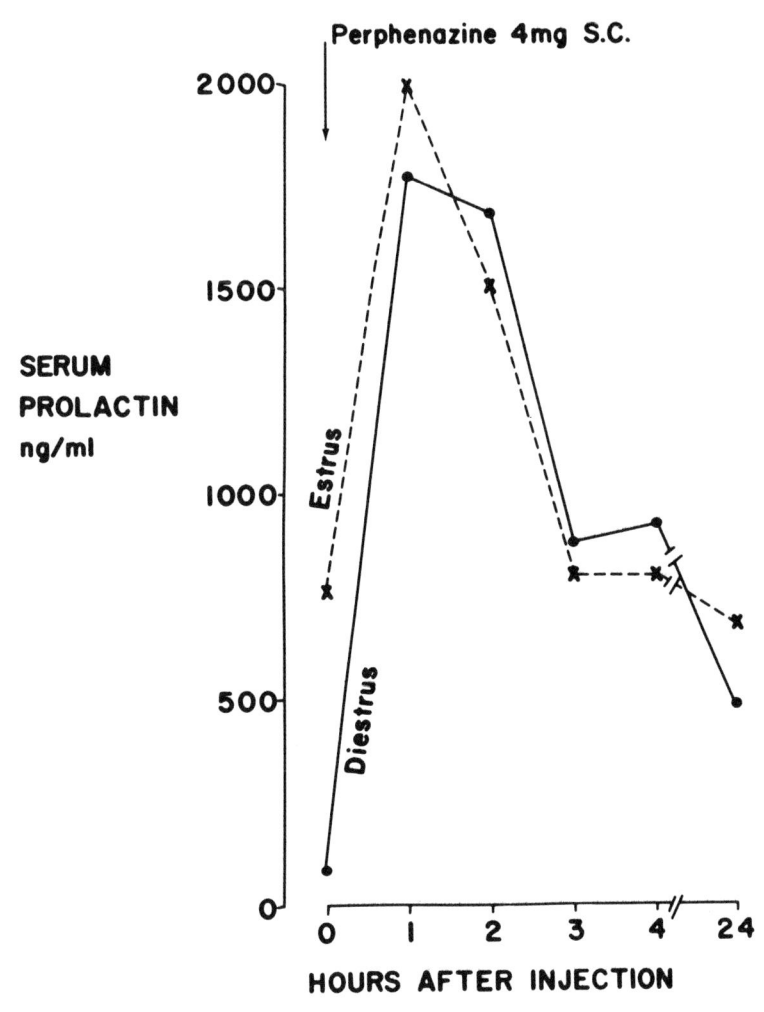

Fig. 9. Acute effects of perphenazine on rat serum prolactin levels

and control groups of animals at about the same time, the number and size of the tumors in the perphenazine-treated animals far exceeded those in the control animals. Histological examination of all the tumors in these animals revealed that they were mammary carcinomas. Serum prolactin levels were measured periodically and the mean

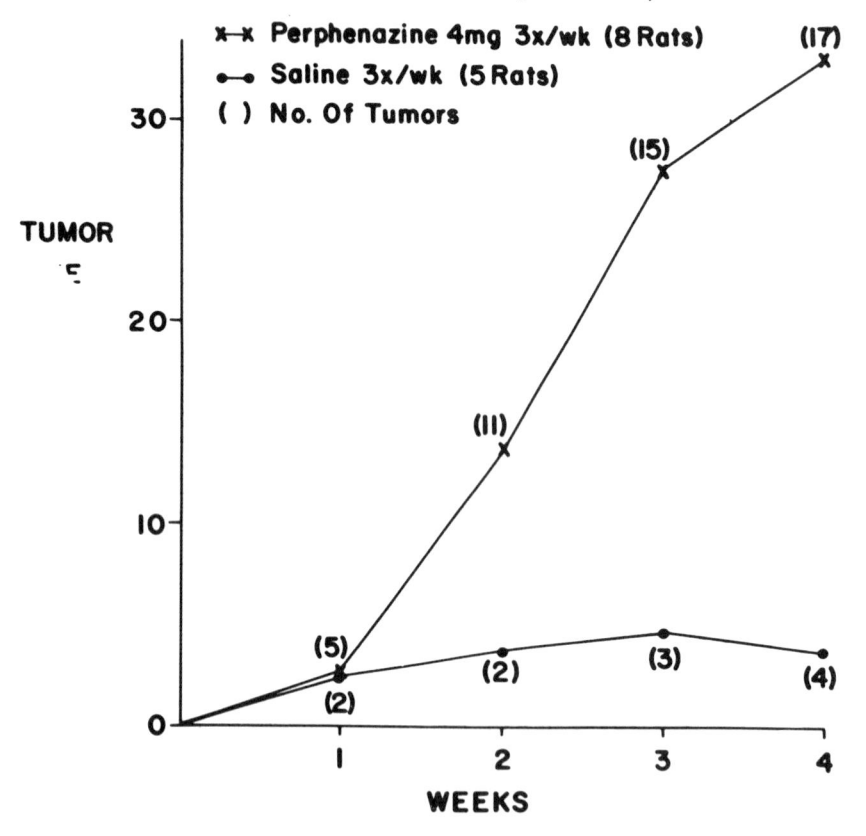

Fig. 10. Effect of perphenazine on growth of DMBA-induced rat mammary carcinoma.

values were invariably higher in perphenazine-treated animals than in the saline-injected controls.

Two additional experiments were carried out in which perphenazine injections were started immediately after the rats were fed DMBA. Nineteen animals received perphenazine injections and 17 received saline injections. After 5 mo, 70% of the saline-treated animals had mammary tumors, whereas all of the perphenazine-treated rats had mammary tumors. The number and size of the tumors in the perphenazine-treated group exceeded those in the control group by a factor of two. Thus, perphenazine stimulated the rate of growth of the mammary tumors.

Perphenazine was also given to DMBA-fed animals after oophorectomy and adrenalectomy. In this experiment, oophorectomy and adrenalectomy were performed 6 days after the rats were fed DMBA, and perphenazine injections were started 2 days postoperatively. Figure 11 shows that perphenazine stimulated the secretion of pro-

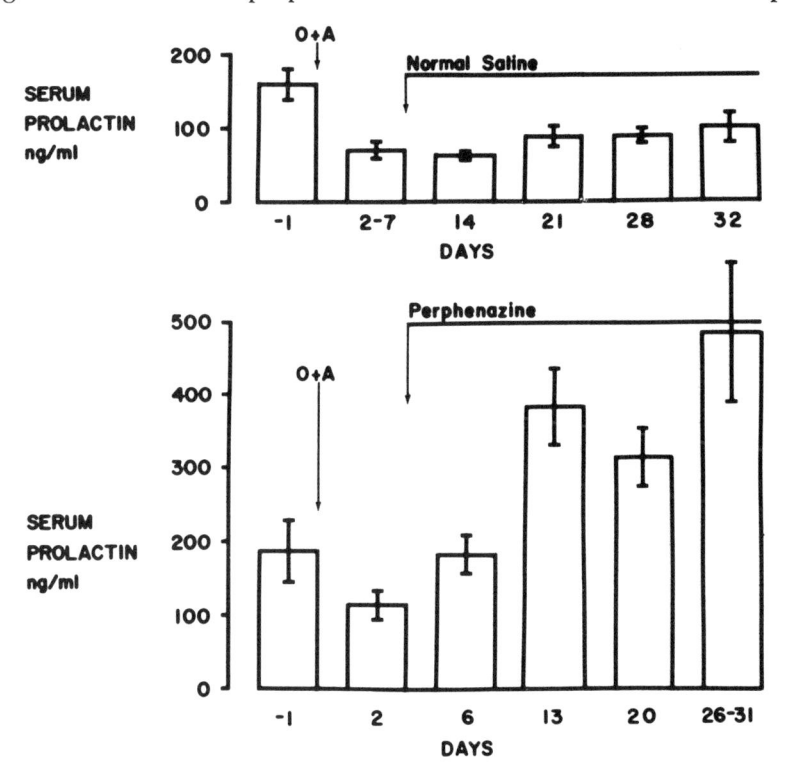

Fig. 11. Effects of oophorectomy and adrenalectomy and of perphenazine on rat serum prolactin levels.

lactin in these animals. After 5 mo of treatment with perphenazine, 1 mg daily, 7 out of 15 rats had a total of 15 tumors averaging 2.7 cm^2, whereas none of 11 control rats receiving saline injections developed palpable tumors.

Effects of Antiserum to Rat Prolactin on Rat Mammary Tumor Growth

The purpose of this study was to determine whether administering antiserum to purified rat prolactin could induce regression of rat mammary carcinoma. Unpublished observations in our laboratory indicated that antibodies to ovine prolactin failed to influence the growth of DMBA-induced rat mammary cancer. Antiserum to ovine prolactin also failed to block the prolactin activity of rat pituitary homogenates in the pigeon crop sac, and bioassay indicated species specificity of the prolactin. Thus, antiserum to purified rat prolactin was generated in rabbits for this study (6, 10). Ten rats with 20 growing DMBA-induced tumors received subcutaneous or intraperitoneal injections of antiserum twice daily for 36 days, and 9 control rats bearing 23 tumors received injections of normal rabbit

TABLE 1: EFFECT OF PROLACTIN ANTISERUM ON TUMOR GROWTH

Treatment	A Growing Tumors No.	(%)	B Stable Tumors No.	(%)	C Regressing Tumors No.	(%)
Normal rabbit serum 9 rats 23 tumors	13	(57)	7	(30)	3	(13)
Prolactin antiserum 10 rats 20 tumors	7	(35)	3	(15)	10	(50)

NOTE: $A + B + C, p < 0.05$; C vs. A, $p < 0.025$; $A + B$ vs. C, $p < 0.01$.

serum in the same manner. Table 1 shows the overall results in terms of growth and regression of the tumors; 50% of the antihormone-treated and 19% of the control tumors regressed. This difference is statistically significant. Figure 12 shows the size of the tumors before, during, and after treatment. Before the start of treatment, the two groups did not differ significantly, but after 36 days of injections there had been a fourfold increase in tumor area for the control rats, and the two groups differed significantly ($p < 0.01$). Further tumor growth in control rats could not be plotted because most of these rats died very shortly with large necrotic tumors. All tumors in the experimental group showed reactivation of growth after antiserum injections ceased, and all tumors decreased in size after oophorectomy.

In 5 of the 10 experimental rats, all tumors regressed during treatment. Variable tumor behavior was observed in 4 of the 10 rats, with some tumors regressing, some remaining stable, and some growing. One example is shown in figure 13. All tumors, including the 2 which had not responded to treatment, regressed dramatically after oophorectomy. In 1 of the 10 rats, both tumors continued to grow in spite of treatment. This rat unfortunately died immediately

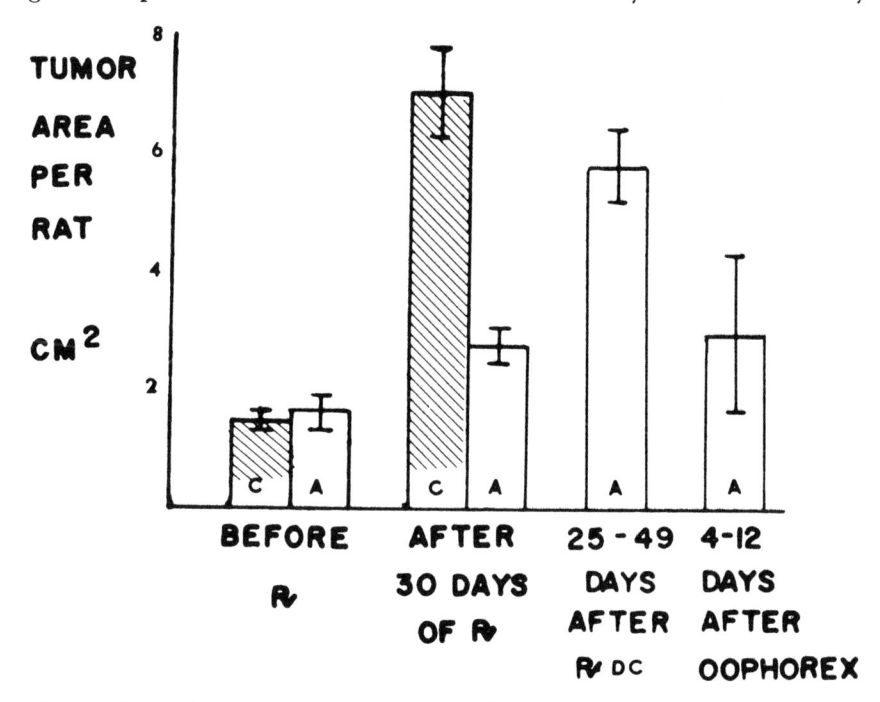

Fig. 12. Growth of tumors in control (C) and antihormone-treated (A) rats.

after oophorectomy, and therefore it could not be ascertained whether its tumors were hormone dependent.

Vaginal smears showed that all antihormone-treated rats continued to exhibit estrous cycle activity, though with somewhat less regularity than the controls. One experimental rat was in constant estrus for 2 wk, but no rat displayed prolonged or constant diestrus.

These results indicate that antihormones interfered with the growth of DMBA-induced rat mammary carcinoma, presumably by combining with and inactivating endogenous prolactin. Maintenance of estrus suggests that the tumor regression induced by prolactin antiserum was not due to a castration effect.

Effects of Estradiol Benzoate on Serum Prolactin Levels and Rat Mammary Tumor Growth

Figure 14 shows the effect on serum prolactin levels and tumor size of oophorectomy and adrenalectomy and subsequent administration of estradiol benzoate, 5 µg daily, to a group of 5 rats bearing DMBA-induced mammary tumors. After oophorectomy and adrenalectomy

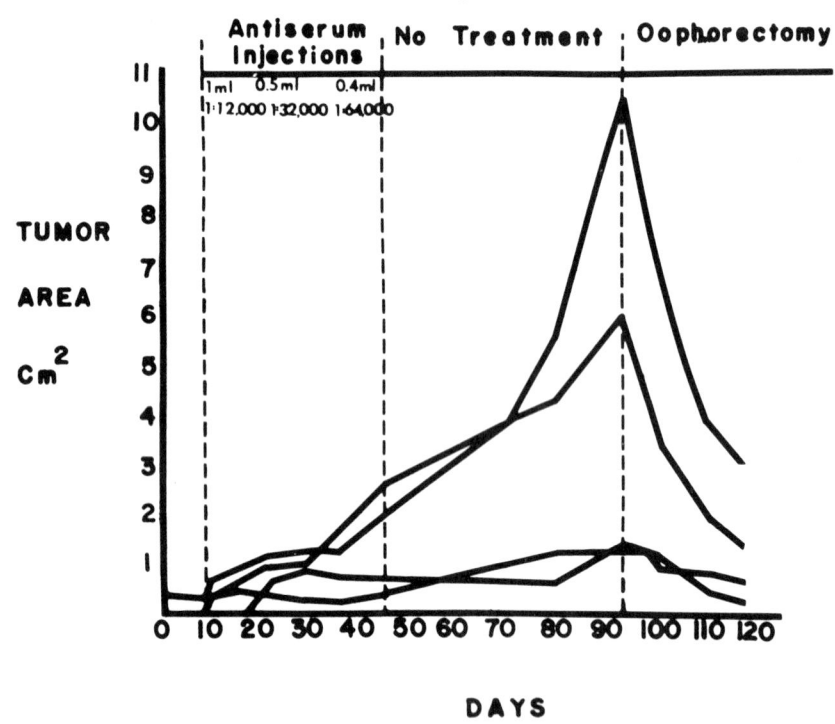

Fig. 13. Mixed response of tumor growth with prolactin antiserum

there was a significant fall in mean serum prolactin levels and in tumor size. After 11 to 29 days of estradiol administration there was a twofold increase in mean tumor area and a fivefold increase in serum prolactin levels; 5 to 15 days after estradiol was withdrawn, tumor area and serum prolactin levels had both declined. These findings are in accord with the concept that small doses of estradiol stimulate prolactin secretion, which in turn accelerates rat mammary tumor growth.

The well-known paradoxical effect of large doses of estrogen in women and in rats, which may induce tumor regression rather than stimulation, was investigated to determine whether large doses of estrogen suppress prolactin secretion. Figure 15 shows the effect on serum prolactin levels and tumor size of administering 500 μg of estradiol daily to 5 intact female rats bearing DMBA-induced

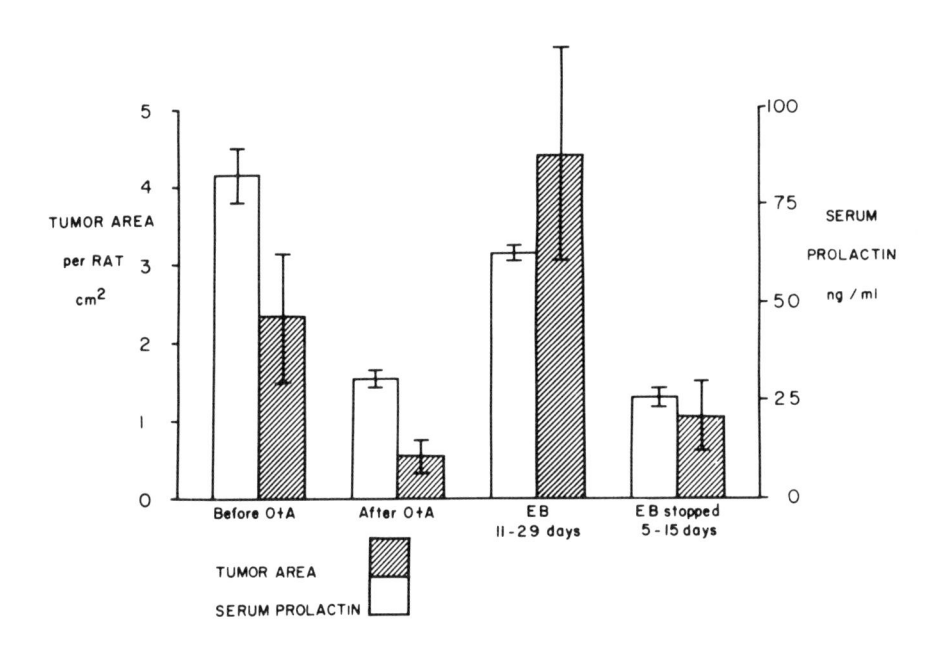

Fig. 14. Effect of $O + A$ and estradiol on mammary tumor growth and serum prolactin levels.

mammary tumors. It is apparent that tumor regression was associated with steadily increasing serum prolactin levels. Similar results were obtained in a group of animals which received 20 μg of estradiol benzoate daily. These results indicate that tumor regression induced by large doses of estradiol cannot be explained by suppression of prolactin secretion.

Preliminary studies suggest that large doses of estradiol may exert an antitumor effect by inhibiting the peripheral action of prolactin on mammary tumor growth. In this study oophorectomy was performed on a group of tumor-bearing rats. After partial regression of the tumors had occurred, perphenazine, 1 mg daily, was administered, which stimulated tumor growth and increased serum prolactin levels. While perphenazine injections were maintained, estradiol benzoate, 500 μg daily, was added to the regimen. This

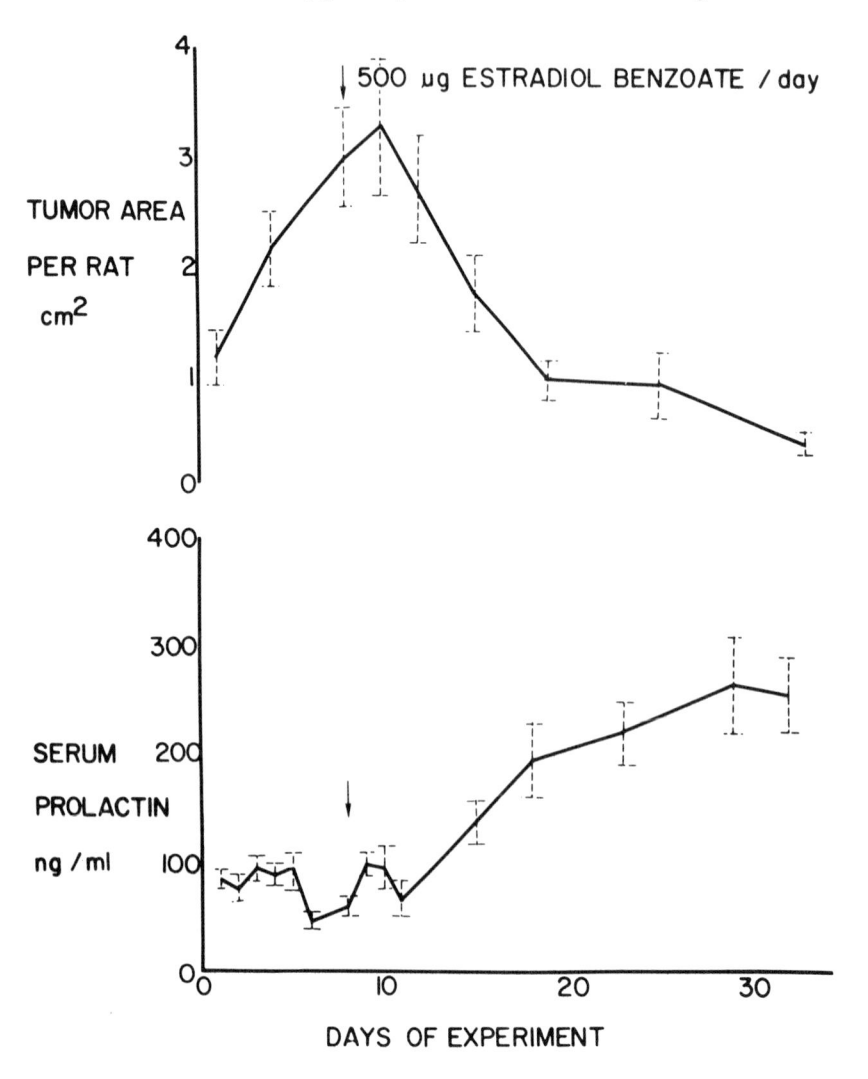

Fig. 15. Effects of estradiol on mammary tumor growth and serum prolactin levels.

resulted in regression of tumor size, suggesting that the estrogen was interfering with the action of prolactin.

DISCUSSION

The results presented appear to justify the conclusion that DMBA-induced rat mammary carcinoma is prolactin dependent, and that this hormone may be the only one of significance in maintaining the growth of this tumor. How does this model system apply to the problem of hormone-responsive breast cancer in man? Prolactin has not yet been isolated as a distinct hormone from normal human pituitaries. Purified human growth hormone preparations have been shown by bioassay to have prolactin activity, and this led to the postulate that these two hormonal activities might reside in the same peptide molecule in man. However, considerable indirect evidence suggests that prolactin is a separate hormone in man. Rimoin et al. (13) have demonstrated that growth-hormone-deficient midgets are capable of bearing children and nursing their infants. Serum growth hormone was undetectable during lactation in such an individual. Since it is believed that prolactin is essential for maintaining lactation, we presume that prolactin was being secreted. Peake et al. (14) have recently documented the presence of prolactin activity in a human pituitary tumor which was essentially devoid of growth hormone. Similar results were obtained by Nasr, Pensky, and Pearson (15). Tranquilizing drugs have been noted to induce lactation in women (11) and to produce gynecomastia in men (16). Isolating human prolactin and developing an immunoassay for it would facilitate further studies of this hormone in human breast cancer.

Knowledge of the endocrine factor, or factors, involved in the growth of human breast cancer would help significantly in managing this disease. Recent reports by Nissen-Meyer (17) and by Cole (18) indicate that castration at the time of mastectomy is more effective as a therapeutic procedure than when this therapy is reserved until metastases appear. This important observation suggests that if optimum endocrine control were introduced at the earliest phase of the disease, it would improve the management of breast cancer. If prolactin should turn out to be the important endocrine factor in human breast cancer, it is conceivable that appropriate medical control of the secretion of this hormone might even have prophylactic value.

Acknowledgments

The authors wish to acknowledge the expert technical assistance of Mr. Robert Sholl, Mr. Alan Pearson, and Mrs. Anita Clifford.

This investigation was supported by grant CA-05197-10 from the National Institutes of Health, United States Public Health Service, and by grant T46J from the American Cancer Society.

References

1. Pearson, O. H.; West, C. D.; Hollander, V.; and Treves, N. 1954. Evaluation of endocrine therapy for advanced breast cancer. *J.A.M.A.* 154: 234.
2. Pearson, O. H., and Ray, B. S. 1959. Results of hypophysectomy in the treatment of metastatic mammary carcinoma. *Cancer* 12: 85.
3. Pearson, O. H.; Llerena, O.; Llerena, L.; Molina, A.; and Butler, T. 1969. Prolactin-dependent rat mammary cancer: A model for man? *Trans. Ass. Amer. Physicians* 82: 225.
4. Huggins, C.; Grand, L. C.; and Brillante, F. P. 1961. Mammary cancer induced by a single feeding of polynuclear hydrocarbons and its suppression. *Nature (Lond.)* 189: 204.
5. Sterenthal, A.; Dominguez, J. M.; Weisman, C.; and Pearson, O. H. 1963. Pituitary role in the estrogen dependency of experimental mammary cancer. *Cancer Res.* 23: 281.
6. Llerena, L.; Molina, A.; and Pearson, O. H. 1969. Radioimmunoassay of rat prolactin. Annual Meeting of the Endocrine Society.
7. Niswender, . D.; Chen, C. L.; Midgley, A. R.; Meites, J.; and Ellis, S. 1969. Radioimmunoassay for rat prolactin. *Proc. Soc. Exp. Biol. Med.* 130: 793.
8. Kwa, H. G. and Verhofstad, F. 1967. Prolactin levels in the plasma of female rats. *J. Endocr.* 39: 455.
9. Ellis, S.; Grindeland, R. E.; and Nuenke, J. M. 1968. Isolation and characterization of prolactin from rat pituitary glands. *Excerpta Med.,* International Congress Series, No. 157, p. 77.
10. Butler, T. P., and Pearson, O. H. 1970. Regression of prolactin-dependent rat mammary carcinoma in response to antihormone treatment. *Proc. Amer. Ass. Cancer Res.* 11: 14.
11. Khazan, N.; Primo, C.; Damon, A.; Assael, M.; Sulman, F. G.; and Winnik, H. Z. 1962. The mammotrophic effects of tranquillizing drugs. *Arch. Int. Pharmacodyn.* 136: 291
12. Ben-David, M. 1968. Stimulation of endogenous secretion of prolactin (LTH) in adult Fisher rats by perphenazine treatment. *Excerpta Med.* International Congress Series, no. 157, p. 75.
13. Rimoin, D. L.; Merimee, T. J.; Rabinowitz, D.; Calvalli-Sforza, L. L.; and McKusick, V. A. 1968. Genetic aspects of growth hormone deficiency. In *Growth hormone,* ed. A. Pecile and E. E. Muller,

Excerpta Med. Foundation, International Congress Series, no. 158, p. 418.
14. Peake, G. T.; McKeel, D.; Jarett, L., and Daughaday, W. H. 1968. Prolactin in a pituitary tumor. *Proc. Central. Soc. Clin. Res.* 41: 76.
15. Nasr, H.; Pensky, J.; and Pearson, O. H. 1970. Prolactin content of a pituitary tumor in Forbes-Albright syndrome. *Annual Meeting of the Endocrine Society,* p. 129.
16. Margolis, I. B., and Gross, C. G. 1967. Gynecomastia during phenothiazine therapy. *J.A.M.A.* 199: 942.
17. Nissen-Meyer, R. 1968. Suppression of ovarian function in primary breast cancer. In *Prognostic factors in breast cancer,* ed. A. M. P. Forrest and P. B. Kunkler, p. 139. Edinburgh and London: E. & S. Livingstone.
18. Cole, M. P. 1968. Suppression of ovarian function in primary breast cancer. In *Prognostic factors in breast cancer,* ed. A. M. P. Forrest and P. B. Kunkler, p. 146. Edinburgh and London: E. & S. Livingstone.

Dilip Sinha and Thomas Dao

Estrogen and Induction of Mammary Cancer 19

Prolonged administration of an estrogen to an organism can induce tissue growth and neoplasia. This biological phenomenon is well known, but its mechanism is not understood. The effect of an estrogen on the target tissue can be either direct or indirect; for example, the capacity of an estrogen to induce a mammotrophic effect largely depends on the production of prolactin mediated by the anterior pituitary. It is not clear, however, whether the effect of an estrogen on the induction of a mammary tumor is similarly mediated by the pituitary gland or whether the estrogen exerts its effect by a local, direct action on the mammary epithelium.

In earlier studies by Jensen and Jacobson (1), tritiated estradiol of high specific activity, administered to ovariectomized rats, was retained and taken up by the target tissue, such as the uterus, vagina, and pituitary. This tissue appeared to contain a unique substance, the "receptor molecule," that has a striking affinity for estradiol. On the basis of ^{3}H-estrogen accumulation data, the mammary glands of rats, goats, and sheep have also been shown to be estrogen targets (2, 3). These studies demonstrate that estradiol interacts with a macromolecule species in the uterus, mammary gland, and so on. Whether this interaction is an essential step in hormone action is not known, but it certainly strongly indicates that an estrogen has a direct effect on the target tissues.

In any study concerned with the role of an estrogen in mammary tumorigenesis, we must define whether we are investigating the initi-

The authors are affiliated with the Department of Breast Surgery at the Roswell Park Memorial Institute of the New York State Department of Health at Buffalo.

ation or promotion phase of the process of carcinogenesis. The initiation phase, however brief it may be, is concerned with very early changes, whereas the promotion phase determines how rapidly a tumor appears and to what extent the growth rate is maintained. Thus Dao (4) previously reported the critical role of an estrogen in initiating the induction of mammary tumors by a chemical carcinogen. In that study it appeared that the presence of an estrogen is a sine qua non for the induction of mammary cancer. Although the results did not present conclusive evidence that estrogen can exert any effect in the absence of the pituitary gland, the data strongly suggest that estrogen acts directly on the mammary epithelium in conjunction with the effect on the carcinogenic stimulus of a polycyclic aromatic hydrocarbon. This chapter reports results from the first of a series of studies designed to define more precisely the role of an estrogen in chemical carcinogenesis in the mammary gland.

MATERIALS AND METHODS

The objective of our experiments was to elucidate how an estrogen and a chemical carcinogen interact in initiating neoplastic transformation of the mammary epithelium; particularly, we wished to determine whether estrogen exerts its effect directly on the mammary epithelium. If so, what is the role of the estrogen in this interaction?

We have developed a technique for inducing mammary tumors by direct application of minute quantities of a carcinogen, an estrogenic hormone, or both to individual mammary glands. In this study, the procedure was carried out as follows. A rat was lightly anesthetized with ether, and a small incision was made over the right inguinal region. The mammary gland was exposed, and a specified amount of diethylstilbestrol (DES), 7, 12-dimethylbenz(a)anthrancene (DMBA) or a combination of the two agents was "dusted" over the right inguinal mammary gland (fig. 1). The skin was then flipped back, and the wound was closed with Mitchell clips.

Since the amounts of DES and DMBA applied locally were very small, cholesterol powder was used as a vehicle. A suitable amount of DES or DMBA was weighed out and was uniformly mixed with an appropriate amount of cholesterol powder so that 2 mg of the final mixture contained the desired dose of DES or DMBA. In all control groups, each rat received 2 mg of cholesterol.

The rats were kept in a room with a controlled temperature (25° C ± 1). The lighting schedule was 14 hr of light and 10 hr of darkness, controlled by an automatic time switch. The animals were given laboratory food and water ad libitum.

The course of tumor development was determined by examining the animals at weekly intervals. We palpated each mammary gland and estimated tumor growth by caliper measurements of two diameters at right angles to each other for most tumors; but four diameters were measured for tumors of highly irregular shapes. Tumor sizes

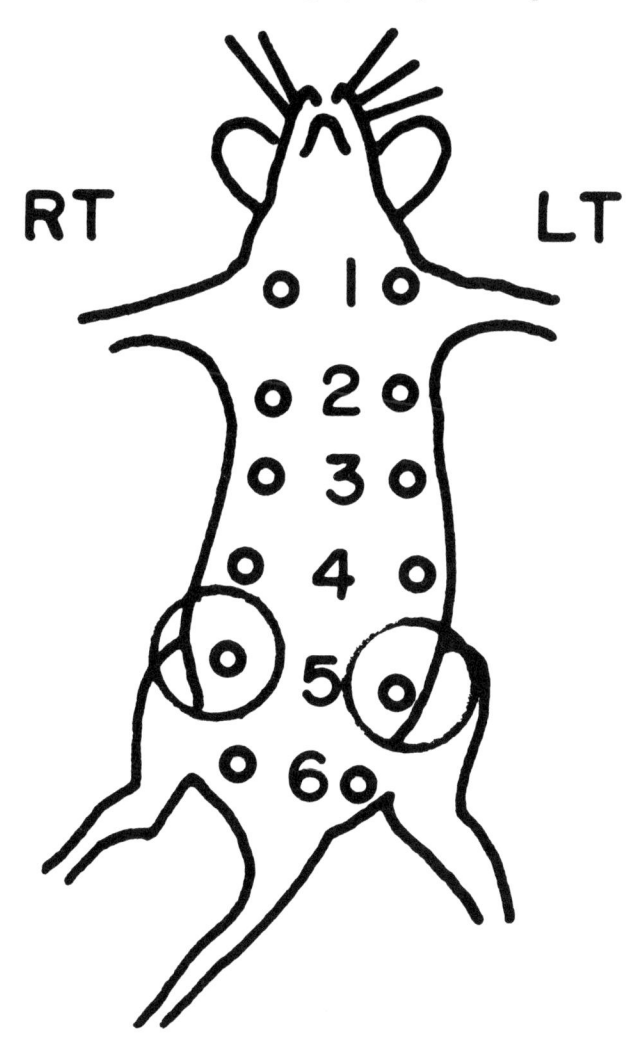

Fig. 1. Schematic diagram showing mammary glands of the rat. The right fifth mammary gland is used for local application of DMBA and DES. The left fifth gland serves as the control.

were calculated from the averages of the two or four diameters. At autopsy, tumors were fixed in small pieces in Bouin's fixative for histological examination.

All the mammary glands were checked for the presence of tumors during autopsy. Contralateral inguinal mammary glands were removed and fixed in Bouin's fixative for whole-mount preparation, as were treated glands that did not develop tumors. Only animals that developed adenocarcinoma of the mammary gland, confirmed by histological examination, were included in the data of this study. The pituitary, ovaries, uterine horns and adrenals were weighed, and sections were prepared for histological study.

RESULTS AND DISCUSSION

With the technique just described, tumors develop only in glands where the carcinogen has been applied. There was no tumor in any other gland in any of the 97 rats used. All the tumors were adenocarcinomas, with various degrees of acinar involvement.

The experimental groups were distributed according to the dose levels of DMBA and DES. The basic design of the experiments was to compare the effects of DMBA alone, DES alone, and DMBA and DES in combination on the induction of mammary cancer. Since we used cholesterol in weighing minute quantities of the hormones and the carcinogen, we included a control group treated with cholesterol alone. The dosages of DMBA used were 0.1, 0.5, and 1 mg, and those of DES were 50 and 100 μg. Each of these compounds, singly or in combination, was applied locally, once only, to the right inguinal mammary gland.

Table 1 summarizes the results, which show conclusively that an estrogen in combination with DMBA produces a significantly greater incidence of mammary cancer than does DMBA given alone. It appears that 1 mg of DMBA is an optimal dose for carcinogenesis when applied locally over the mammary gland. Adding DES to the carcinogen shortened the latent period for tumor appearance. When only 0.5 mg of DMBA was applied to the mammary gland, the tumor incidence was significantly reduced, to 42.8%, and the latent period of tumor appearance was markedly increased. Adding DES to 0.5 mg of DMBA produced a significant difference in mammary tumor induction. Whereas the mammary tumor incidence was 42.8% in rats receiving 0.5 mg of DMBA alone, it rose to 60% and 66.6% in groups in which rats were given 50 and 100 μg of DES, respectively, in addition to 0.5 mg of DMBA. These differences in tumor incidence are statistically significant. The latent period of tumor appearance was reduced from 83 to 65 days. If the dose of DMBA was further reduced to 0.1 mg, the tumor incidence decreased to only 14%. The tumor incidence was again markedly increased (to 42%), however, when 100 µg of DES was applied in combination with DMBA. Similarly, the latent period of tumor induction was greatly shortened. These results clearly demonstrate that DES and DMBA act in synergism to enhance tumor induction.

TABLE 1: EFFECT OF ESTROGEN ON MAMMARY TUMORIGENESIS BY 7, 12-DMBA

Treatment	No. of Rats	Rats with Tumors	Percentage	Average Latency Period (days)	Average Tumor Size (cm)
1 mg DMBA	12	11	91.6	65	1.2
1 mg DMBA+100 µg DES	12	12	100.0	54	2.5
1 mg DMBA+50 µg DES	14	12	86.6	50	2.2
0.5 mg DMBA	14	6	42.8	83	1.1
0.5 mg DMBA+100 µg DES	12	8	66.6[a]	65	2.0
0.5 mg DMBA+50 µg DES	5	3	60.0[b]	65	1.1
0.1 mg DMBA	7	1	14.0	112	0.7
0.1 mg DMBA+100 µg DES	7	3	42.0[c]	92	1.4

NOTE: All p values were calculated by Student's t-test.
[a] $p < 0.01$ (from 0.5 mg DMBA). [c] $p < 0.1$ (from 0.1 mg DMBA).
[b] $p < 0.01$ (from 0.5 mg DMBA).

The enhancement of carcinogenesis by DES was not limited to shortening the latency period and inducing more tumors. Tumor growth was much faster in the estrogen-treated groups. Figure 2 illustrates the growth rate and development of the tumors in two experiments. It demonstrates that whenever DES was added to DMBA, tumors appeared much earlier, the rate of growth was much faster, and the sizes of the tumors were always greater.

There was also a definite pattern in how the tumors appeared in different groups (fig. 3). About 40% of the rats in a group treated with 1 mg of DMBA in combination with 100 µg of DES had tumors by 42 days after treatment, whereas only 10% of the animals receiving 1 mg of DMBA alone developed tumors. By 65 days, all the animals treated with both DES and DMBA had tumors; but in the group receiving DMBA alone, tumors continued to appear until 80 days after treatment. In the rats where the dose of the carcinogen was smaller (0.5 mg), tumors appeared at a later date, but the general pattern was the same; that is, tumors appeared much sooner whenever estrogen was given in addition to DMBA. Although tumors always appeared in the

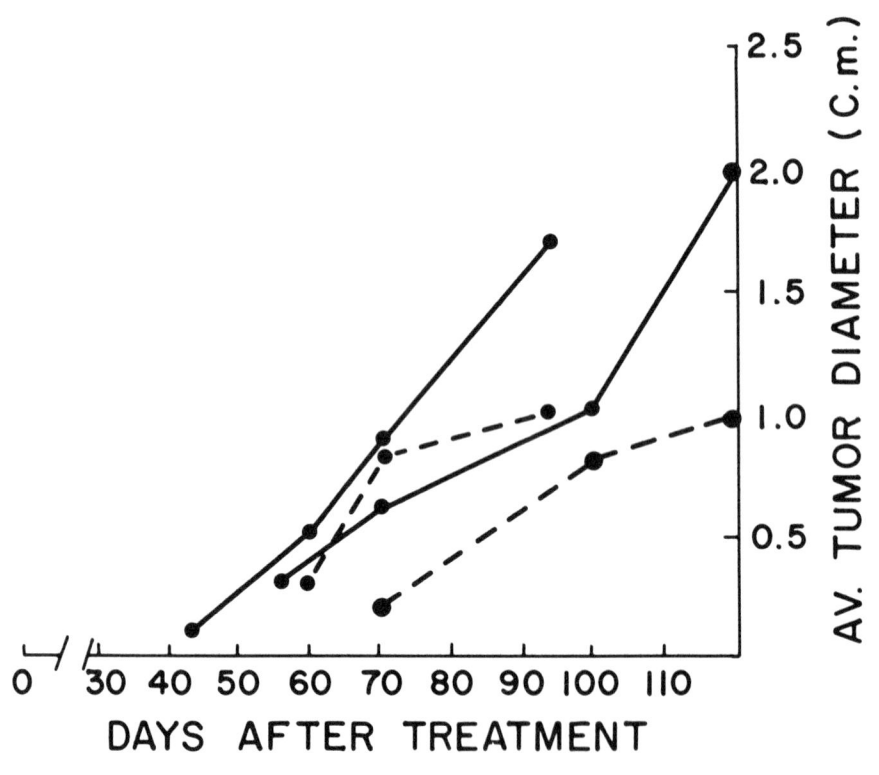

Fig. 2. Effect of DES in combination with DMBA on growth rate of mammary tumors. ●----------●, DMBA alone. DMBA. ●——————●, DES +

particular gland where the carcinogen had been applied, the number of tumors in the gland varied, depending on the treatment. In most cases there was only one tumor in the gland; but in many instances multiple tumors developed. It appears that the number of tumors increased only when the dose of the carcinogen was increased (fig. 4).

The weights of the uterine horns, ovaries, adrenals, and pituitaries in these animals at the end of the study are shown in table 2. None of the endocrine organs exhibited any significant difference in weight

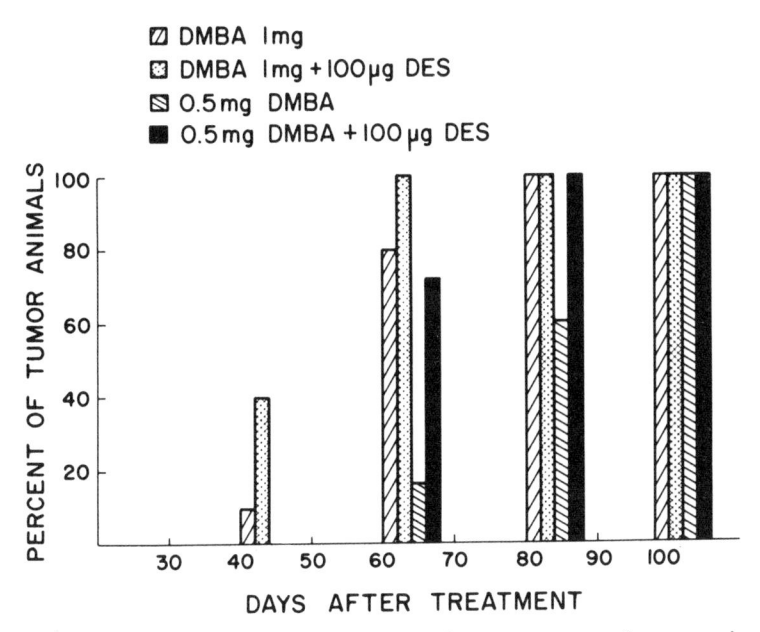

Fig. 3. Histogram showing the pattern of appearance of tumor in different treatment groups. Percent tumor animal is the percentage of the tumor-bearing animal of a particular group.

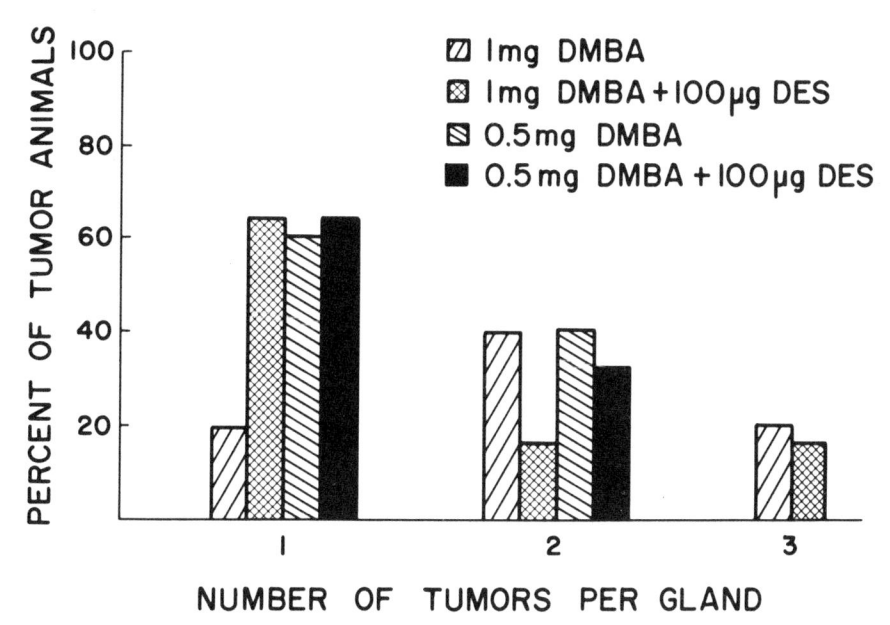

Fig. 4. Relationship between the dose of carcinogen and number of tumors per gland. Note that only in the high-dose groups a certain percentage of the tumor-bearing rats had more than two tumors per gland.

between groups receiving DMBA alone and in combination with DES. Histological examinations of these tissues revealed no discernible morphological differences among these groups. These results suggest that local application of small amounts of an estrogen caused no systemic changes in endocrine functions.

In all control groups in which rats were given 100 or 300 µg of DES only, without DMBA, no mammary tumor was ever observed during the experimental period of 6 mo.

TABLE 2: EFFECT OF DIETHYLSTILBESTROL AND 7, 12-DMBA ON ORGAN WEIGHTS

Treatment	No. of Rats	Ovary	Uterine Horn	Anterior Pituitary
100 µg DES	9	45.00±3.5	193.00±3.5	14.5 ±0.9
1 mg DMBA	12	34.24±2.1	182.50±2.4	13.85±0.7
1 mg DMBA+100 µg DES	12	38.63±1.1	202.06±5.2	13.03±0.9
1 mg DMBA+50 µg DES	14	35.88±1.5	169.91±3.3	14.48±1.1
500 µg DMBA	14	35.00±3.2	182.17±5.2	15.68±0.8
500 µg DMBA+100 µg DES	12	36.32±0.9	183.34±4.3	14.82±0.7
500 µg DMBA+50 µg DES	5	40.72±2.3	196.72±5.1	13.40±0.7
Control	9	41.25±2.1	195.00±6.3	14.20±0.9

Perhaps the most important and interesting observation in this study is the demonstration that an estrogen acts in synergism with a chemical carcinogen in inducing mammary cancer in rats. In some way, the estrogen apparently enhances or facilitates the interaction between the carcinogenic agent and the mammary epithelial cells in initiating carcinogenesis. It appears that this action of the estrogen is localized in the mammary gland, since there is no evidence to suggest a systemic effect as a result of local application of minute quantities of an estrogen.

In our laboratory we (5, 6) have demonstrated that DMBA affects the synthesis of macromolecules in the mammary gland. Although the data from these studies showed that DMBA caused significant inhibition of both DNA and RNA synthesis in the mammary gland, only the effect of DMBA on RNA synthesis was found to be estrogen dependent. The alteration in RNA synthesis represents an early biochemical change in the mammary gland as a result of DMBA treatment, but how it is related to carcinogenesis remains to be elucidated. Even so, the fact that these changes (inhibitory effect on RNA synthesis) can be nullified by the absence of an estrogen suggests that estrogen plays an important role in the interaction between a chemical carcinogen and the macromolecules of the target tissue.

Bresciani (7) and Banerjee and Walker (8) have also shown that control of both initiation and duration of DNA synthesis in mouse mammary glands is influenced by ovarian hormones. Increased stimulation by both endogenous and exogenous estrogens can augment the initiation and decrease the duration of the S phase of the cell cycle. Furthermore, it has been demonstrated that an estrogenic hormone has a definite role during the S phase of the mitotic cycle in hormone-induced precancerous hyperplastic alveolar nodules in mice (9). Probably in the same way in our experiments, the minute amount of an estrogen might have changed the rate of cell proliferation in the mammary gland, thus enhancing the interaction between the chemical carcinogen and the mammary epithelial cells and hence the induction of tumors.

The role of pituitary hormones, prolactin in particular, during the early phase of mammary carcinogenesis cannot be entirely disregarded. Although it is possible that the sensitive response of the pituitary to exogenous estrogen stimulation may cause increased prolactin secretion, it is too small to elicit any morphological changes in the target tissues. There is no conclusive evidence that levels of serum prolactin are correlated with mammary tumorigenesis. We have demonstrated that a single pituitary graft placed in the mammary gland can induce mammary gland growth and lactation, but no systemic effect was observed, since the contralateral mammary gland was not stimulated (10). In addition, tumors failed to develop in these locally stimulated mammary glands (11). Serum prolactin levels are now being measured in these estrogen-treated rats. The lack of any evidence to demonstrate excess prolactin secretion as a result of estrogen treatment in our experiments leads us to believe that in the presence of "normal" amounts of prolactin in an intact animal, an estrogen, in conjunction with a chemical carcinogen, acts directly on the mammary gland to induce carcinogenesis.

Acknowledgments

This investigation was supported by grant CA-04632-11 from the National Cancer Institute, National Institutes of Health.

References

1. Jensen, E. V., and Jacobson, H. I. 1960. Fate of steroid estrogens in target tissues. In *Biological activities of steroids in relation to cancer,* ed. G. Pincus and E. P. Vollmer, p. 161. New York: Academic Press.
2. Glascock, R. F., and Hoekstra, W. G. 1959. Selective accumulation of tritium-labeled hexestrol by the reproduction organs of immature female goats and sheep. *Biochem. J.* 72: 673.
3. Sander, S. 1968. The uptake of 17β-estradiol in breast tissue of female rats. *Acta Endocr.* 58: 49.
4. Dao, T. L. 1962. The role of ovarian hormones in initiating the induction of mammary cancer in rats by polynuclear hydrocarbons. *Cancer Res.* 22: 937.
5. Libby, P. R., and Dao, T. L. 1966. Rat mammary gland RNA: Incorporation of C^{14}-formate and effect of hormones and 7, 12-dimethylbenz(a)anthracene. *Science* 153: 303.
6. Tominaga, T.; Libby, P. R.; and Dao, T. L. 1970. An early effect of 7, 12-dimethylbenz(a)anthracene on rat mammary gland DNA synthesis. *Cancer Res.* 30: 118.
7. Bresciani, F. 1965. Effect of ovarian hormones on duration of DNA synthesis in cells of the C_3H mouse mammary gland. *Exp. Cell Res.* 38: 13.
8. Banerjee, M. R., and Walker, R. J. 1967. Variable duration of DNA synthesis in mammary gland cells during pregnancy and lactation of C_3H/He mouse. *J. Cell Physiol.* 69: 133.
9. Banerjee, M. R. 1969. Hormonal control of DNA synthesis: Altered responsiveness of hyperplastic alveolar nodules of mouse mammary gland. *J. Nat. Inst.* 42: 227.
10. Dao, T. L. 1962. Mammary carcinogenesis by 3-methylcholanthrene. IV. Effect of pituitary homograft on mammary-gland growth and tumorigenesis. *J. Nat. Cancer Inst.* 29: 107.
11. Dao, T. L., and Gawlak, D. 1963. Mammotrophic effect of a pituitary homograft in rats. *Endocrinology* 72: 884.

Clifford W. Welsch

Effect of Brain Lesions on Mammary Tumorigenesis 20

INTRODUCTION

It has been known for many years that the central nervous system (CNS) plays an influential role in tumorigenesis. Several clinical studies have correlated a medical history of psychological stress with increased incidence of breast cancer (1), cervical cancer (20), leukemia (8), and other types of neoplasms (13). Laboratory investigations, using experimental animals, have substantiated these clinical observations. Lacassagne and Duplan (12) were among the first to demonstrate that tranquilizers such as reserpine hasten the development of mammary tumors in mice, an observation recently confirmed in rats by Welsch and Meites (23).

Recent studies in our laboratories have sought to determine which specific sites in the CNS significantly influence mammary tumorigenesis in rats. The results reported here demonstrate that disrupting the median eminence–arcuate nucleus area of the hypothalamus in female rats by electrolytic lesions causes a significant increase in growth of carcinogen-induced mammary tumors, incidence of spontaneous mammary tumors, and secretion of pituitary prolactin.

MATERIALS AND METHODS

Placement of Lesions

The electrodes were prepared from size 1 steel insect pins, insulated with four coatings of epoxylite and oven baked after each coating at 140° C for 3 hr. The electrodes used for median eminence lesions

The author is affiliated with the Department of Anatomy at Michigan State University.

were ground flat at the tip to produce lesions which extend horizontally and not vertically. The median eminence lesions were produced bilaterally by passing a direct current of 2–3 ma through the electrodes for 7–10 sec. The median eminence area was located with the aid of a Stoelting stereotaxic instrument and de Groot's (3) atlas of the rat brain. Properly placed lesions in the median eminence resulted in total destruction of the median eminence, and nearly complete destruction of the arcuate nucleus, but in little or no damage to the pituitary stalk (fig. 1). When the rats were killed,

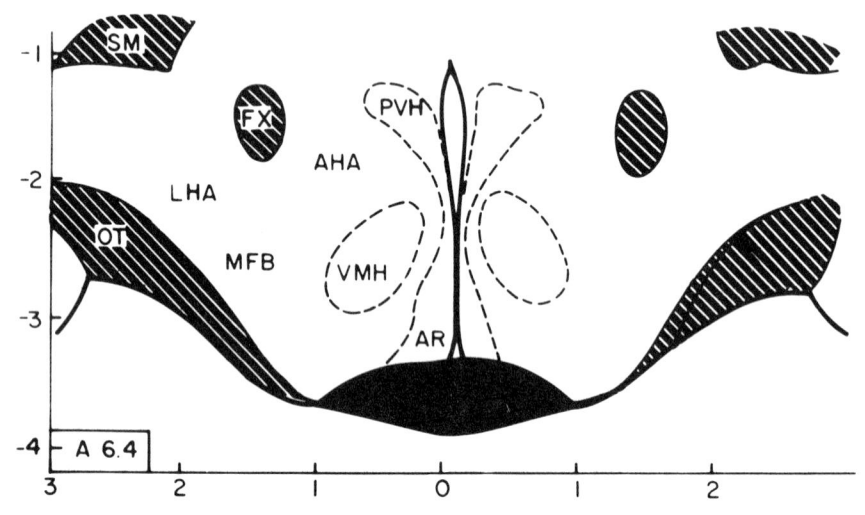

Fig. 1. Diagrammatic cross-section of rat brain Solid black area represents the approximate region of the median eminence lesion.

if any doubt existed regarding the site of the lesion, that rat was not included in computing the data. Sham lesions were placed in rats by making bilateral lesions on the skull at the midline (bregma).

Effect of Median Eminence Lesions on Growth of Carcinogen-induced Rat Mammary Tumors

One hundred twenty-seven female Sprague-Dawley rats, 55 days of age, were given single intravenous injections of a lipid emulsion containing 5 mg of 7, 12-dimethylbenz(a)anthracene (DMBA). Seventy to 90 days after carcinogen treatment, when all rats had at least one palpable mammary tumor, they were divided into groups and treated as follows: (*a*) intact controls, sham-operated; (*b*) intact, with lesions placed in the median eminence; (*c*) ovariectomized controls, sham-operated; and (d) ovariectomized, with lesions placed in the median eminence. Median eminence lesions were made in intact rats on the day of estrus or the first day of diestrus. At 0, 10, and 25 days after the lesions were placed, all rats were examined for number of palpable mammary tumors. All tumors 1 cm or larger were measured with a vernier caliper at the largest diameter.

Twenty-five days after the lesions were placed, the rats were killed. Statistical analysis within each group was prepared according to the mean increase or decrease in the number of palpable mammary tumors and in the tumor diameter (mm) at 0–10 and 0–25 days after lesion placement. The significance of differences between means was calculated by Student's t-test.

Effect of Median Eminence Lesions on Development of Spontaneous Rat Mammary Tumors

Forty-four 10-mo-old multiparous female Sprague-Dawley rats were divided into two groups and treated as follows: (a) intact controls, sham-operated; and (b) intact, with lesions placed in the median eminence. At the time lesions were placed, all rats were free of palpable mammary tumors. Twenty-five weeks after lesions were placed all rats were killed. Blood was withdrawn and assayed for prolactin by the radioimmunoassay method of Niswender et al. (17). Mammary tumors were excised for histological evaluation. The significance of differences between number of rats with mammary tumors and total number of mammary tumors in each group was determined by chi-square analysis.

Effect of Median Eminence Lesions on Pituitary Prolactin Secretion

Twenty-four 3-mo-old nulliparous female Sprague-Dawley rats were divided into two groups and treated as follows: (a) intact controls, sham-operated; and (b) intact, with lesions placed in the median eminence. Blood was withdrawn by cardiac puncture 0, ½, 1, 2, and 4 hr after lesions were placed for prolactin analysis.

One hundred seventy-five 4-mo-old, nulliparous female Sprague-Dawley rats were divided into groups and treated as follows: (a) intact controls, sham-operated; (b) intact, with lesions placed in the median eminence; (c) ovariectomized controls, sham-operated; and (d) ovariectomized, with lesions placed in the median eminence. Median eminence lesions were made in intact rats on the day of estrus or the first day of diestrus. Ten or 25 days after placement of the lesions, the rats were killed and blood was withdrawn for prolactin analysis.

Thirty-three 3-mo-old nulliparous female Sprague-Dawley rats were given lesions in the median eminence and subsequently divided into four groups; 2, 3, 4, and 5 months after lesions were placed, the rats were killed and blood was withdrawn for prolactin analysis. The significance of differences between mean blood prolactin levels was calculated by analysis of variance.

RESULTS

Effects of Median Eminence Lesions on Growth of
Carcinogen-induced Rat Mammary Tumors

Intact rats bearing mammary tumors responded 10 and 25 days after lesions were placed in the median eminence with 130% and 200% increases respectively in number of palpable mammary tumors per rat, in contrast to an increase of only 23% and 27% respectively in the intact controls (table 1). In addition, a slight but significant increase in mean tumor diameter was observed at 10 days, but not at 25 days, after lesions were placed in these rats (fig. 2).

Rats that had lesions placed in the median eminence and that were ovariectomized immediately thereafter responded 10 days later with a 25% *increase* and 25 days later with a 35% *decrease* in number of palpable mammary tumors per rat, in contrast to 40% and 58% decreases at 10 and 25 days respectively in the ovariectomized controls (table 2). In addition, a significant increase in the mean tumor diameter was seen at 10 days, followed by a marked decrease in tumor diameter 25 days after the lesions were placed (fig. 2). By contrast, when ovariectomy preceded the median eminence lesions by 10 days, no significant effect of the lesions on the number of mammary tumors per rat or mean tumor diameter was observed (table 2, fig. 2).

Effect of Median Eminence Lesions on Development
of Spontaneous Rat Mammary Tumors

Mature mammary-tumor-free female rats, when given lesions in the median eminence, responded 25 wk later with a significant increase in incidence of mammary tumors (table 3). Twelve of 23 rats (52%) developed a total of 20 mammary tumors in the group with lesions in the median eminence, in contrast to 4 of 21 rats (19%) which developed a total of 4 mammary tumors in the sham-lesioned controls.

TABLE 1: EFFECT OF MEDIAN EMINENCE LESIONS ON MAMMMARY TUMOR GROWTH IN INTACT FEMALE RATS TREATED WITH 7, 12-DIMETHYLBENZ(a)ANTHRACENE (DMBA)

| | | | Average Number of Palpable Mammary Tumors ||||||
Group	Treatment[a]	No. of Rats	At Time of Lesion	10 Days after Lesion	% Change	25 Days after Lesion	% Change
I	Intact+sham lesion	22	3.0 ± 0.3[b]	3.7 ± 0.4[c]	+23%	3.8 ± 0.4[d]	+27%
II	Intact+median-eminence lesion	20	2.6 ± 0.4	6.2 ± 0.8[e]	+138%	7.8 ± 0.9[f]	+200%

[a] DMBA was administered at 55 days of age. Bilateral lesions were made 70–90 days after DMBA treatment.
[b] Standard error of the mean.
c/e, d/f = $p < 0.001$.

Histological examination of the mammary tumors revealed an adenomatous type of tumor in the rats with lesions in the median eminence (fig. 3), in contrast to a relatively fibrous type of tumor, containing considerably fewer glandular elements, in the sham-lesioned controls (fig. 4). Fifteen of the 20 mammary tumors in the median eminence-lesioned group were highly differentiated glandular

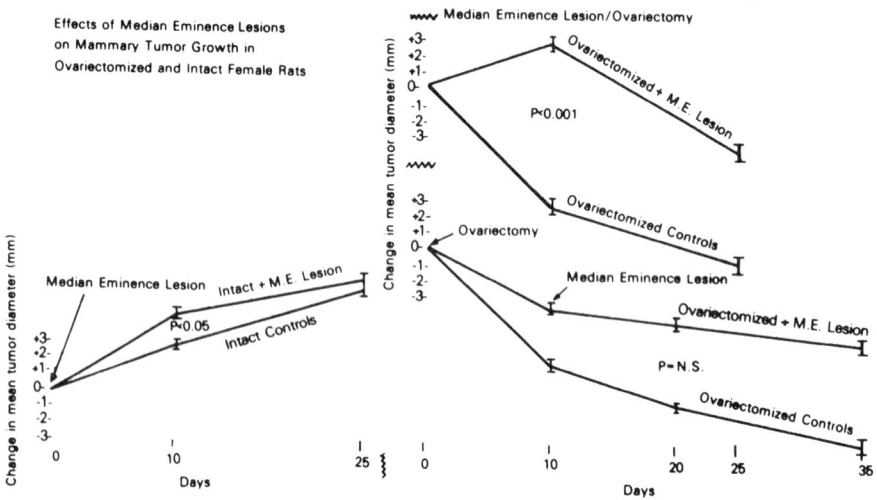

Fig. 2. Changes in mean diameter of carcinogen-induced mammary tumors 10 and 25 days after lesion was placed. *Bottom left,* intact rats with lesions in the median eminence (*ME*) and intact controls. *Top right,* ovariectomized rats with lesions in the ME and ovariectomized controls. Bottom right, ovariectomized rats with lesions placed in the ME 10 days later and ovariectomized controls. N.S. = not significantly different.

neoplasms, 4 were glandular neoplasms containing an abundance of connective tissue, and 1 was entirely a fibrous tumor. Carcinomatous tumors were not observed in animals of either group. The majority of the mammary tumors in the rats with lesions in the median eminence were quite large, over 4 cm in diameter. No evidence of metastases or invasiveness of tumors was observed in either group.

Effect of Median Eminence Lesions on Pituitary Prolactin Secretion

Intact female rats with lesions in the median eminence responded, 30 min after the lesion, with approximately a tenfold increase (59.5 mμg/ml → 583.3 mμg/ml) in serum prolactin levels (fig. 5). Serum

TABLE 2: EFFECT OF MEDIAN EMINENCE LESIONS ON MAMMARY TUMOR GROWTH IN OVARIECTOMIZED RATS TREATED WITH 7, 12-DIMETHYLBENZ(a)ANTHRACENE (DMBA)

Group	Treatment[a]	No. of Rats	At Time of Lesion	10 Days after Lesion	% Change	25 Days after Lesion	% Change
I	Ox+sham lesion	24	4.0±0.4[b]	2.4±0.3[c]	−40%	1.7±0.2	−58%
II	Ox+ME lesion	21	4.3±0.6	5.4±0.6[d]	+25%	2.8±0.4	−35%
III	Ox —10 days→ sham lesion	24	2.4±0.3	2.0±0.3	−16%	1.5±0.2	−25%
IV	Ox —10 days→ ME lesion	16	3.9±0.4	3.5±0.4	−10%	3.4±0.4	−13%

Average Number of Palpable Mammary Tumors

NOTE: ME = median eminence lesion; OX = ovariectomized.

[a] DMBA was administered at 55 days of age. Bilateral lesions were placed in the median eminence area of the hypothalamus approximately 80 days after DMBA treatment.

[b] Standard error of the mean.

c/d = $p < 0.001$.

prolactin levels remained significantly increased for at least 6 mo after the lesion (table 3, fig. 6).

Ovariectomized rats with lesions in the median eminence also responded with a significant increase in serum prolactin levels 10 days after the lesion (table 4). If ovariectomy preceded the lesion by 10 or 25 days, a considerably higher level of serum prolactin (248.6 mμg/ml and 286.4 mμg/ml) was observed, in contrast to those rats lesioned and ovariectomized during the same day (102.7 mμg/ml) or to intact lesioned rats (82.3 mμg/ml).

TABLE 3: EFFECTS OF MEDIAN EMINENCE LESIONS ON DEVELOPMENT OF SPONTANEOUS MAMMARY TUMORS AND SERUM PROLACTIN LEVELS IN FEMALE RATS

Group	Treatment[a]	No. of Rats	Serum Prolactin Levels (mμg/ml)	No. and % of Rats with Tumors	Total No. of Tumors
I	Controls, sham lesion	21	50.9 ± 9.6[b]	4 (19%)[b]	4[b]
II	Median eminence lesions	23	179.8 ± 23.9[c]	12 (52%)[c]	20[c]

[a] All rats were killed 25 wk after placing of median eminence or sham lesion. Serum prolactin levels are represented as the mean value ± standard error.

[b]/[c] = $p < 0.001$.

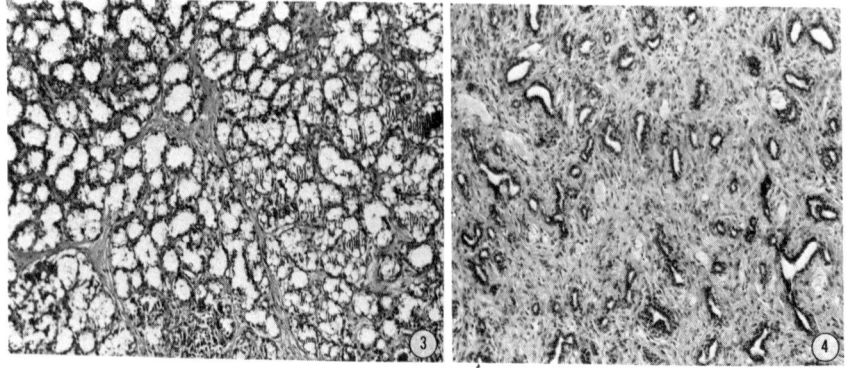

Figs. 3–4. Representative histological sections of spontaneous mammary tumors from (3) median eminence-lesioned rat and (4) sham-lesioned control rat. × 200.

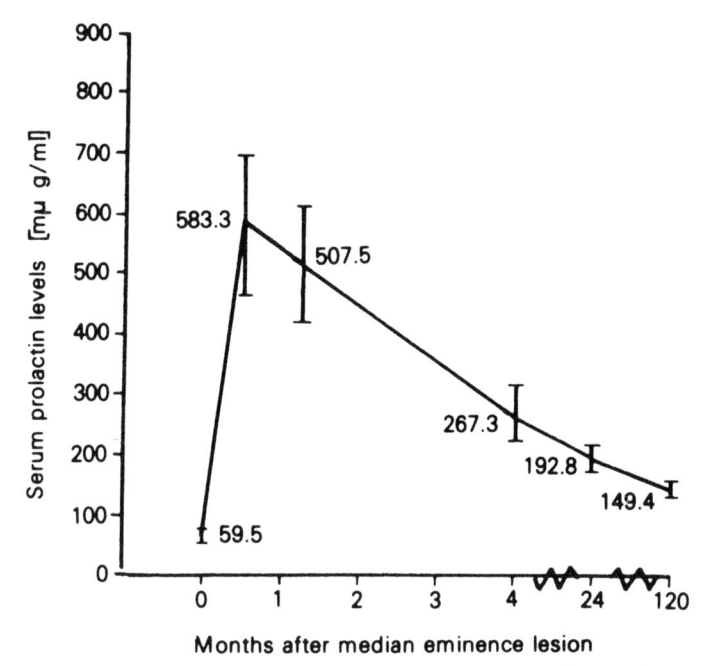

Fig. 5. Effect of median eminence lesions on serum prolactin levels in female rats 1/2, 1, 4, 24, and 120 hr after placing of lesions.

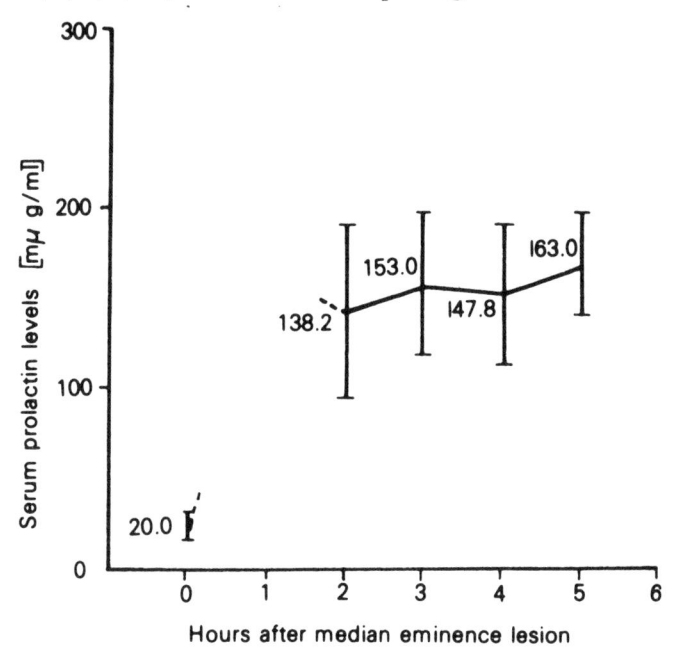

Fig. 6. Effect of median eminence lesions on serum prolactin levels in female rats 2, 3, 4, and 5 mo after placing of lesions.

Discussion

Bilateral electrolytic lesions placed in the median eminence–arcuate nucleus area of the hypothalamus of female rats result in increased growth of carcinogen-induced mammary tumors, increased incidence of spontaneous mammary tumors, and increased serum prolactin levels. These results support our hypothesis that certain neoplasms, particularly those which are hormone responsive, may be related etiologically to specific anomalies in the CNS. The probability that

TABLE 4: EFFECT OF MEDIAN EMINENCE LESIONS ON BLOOD PROLACTIN LEVELS IN INTACT AND OVARIECTOMIZED FEMALE RATS

Group	Treatment[a]	No. of Rats	Serum Prolactin Levels (mμg/ml)
I	Intact+sham lesion	20	20.0± 1.5[b]
II	Intact+ME lesion	24	82.3±18.6[c]
III	Ox+sham lesion	15	18.2± 2.9[d]
IV	Ox+ME lesion	20	102.7±15.2[e]
V	Ox (10 days) sham lesion	10	19.0± 2.8[f]
VI	Ox (10 days) ME lesion	22	248.6±29.3[g]
VII	Ox (25 days) ME lesion	21	286.4±40.0[h]

NOTE: ME = median eminence lesions; OX = ovariectomized.

[a] All rats were killed 10 days after placing of the lesion. Serum prolactin levels are represented as the mean ± standard error.

b/c, d/e, f/g + h = $p < 0.05$.

prolactin is important in murine mammary tumorigenesis is further supported by these studies.

It has been proposed that many tumors may develop as a consequence of hormonal imbalances. The concept that the CNS may influence the endocrine system was suggested as early as 1904 (5). Only in the past few years have we been able to say, with a reasonable degree of confidence, that the endocrine system is not independent of, but to a significant degree controlled by, the CNS. Numerous experiments have demonstrated that there are separate hypothalamic neural control mechanisms for each of the anterior pituitary hormones (14). Proof that the link between the hypothalamus and the anterior pituitary was neurovascular came with the extraction of the agents affecting pituitary secretion from hypothalamic tissue (14).

Six factors (neurohormones) have been extracted from the mammalian hypothalamus: corticotrophin-releasing factor (CRF), thyrotrophin-releasing factor (TRF), growth hormone-releasing factor (GHRF), follicle-stimulating hormone-releasing factor (FSHRF), luteinizing hormone-releasing factor (LRF), and prolactin inhibitory factor (PIF). Prolactin appears to be controlled by an inhibitory neurohormone (15). The neurohormones are believed to be secreted by the nerve fibers which end on the capillary loops in the median eminence, from which the hypothalamic-hypophyseal portal vessels arise (6).

Electrolytic lesions placed in the median eminence act, at least in part, by disrupting the hypothalamic-hypophyseal portal system, thus preventing the neurohormones from reaching the anterior pituitary gland. The subsequent effect would be decreased secretion of all anterior pituitary hormones except prolactin, which is increased. The marked increase in serum prolactin levels as a consequence of median eminence lesions, as observed in this study, is in accord with this principle.

The stimulatory effects of the median eminence lesion on carcinogen-induced mammary tumor growth provide substantial evidence that prolactin may be the principal *pituitary* hormone in promoting growth of this tumor. Such results suggest that other pituitary hormones may not be essential for growth of this tumor. The possibility cannot be excluded, however, that median eminence lesions may also contribute to the growth of mammary tumors by depressing the secretion of other anterior pituitary hormones such as ACTH. It has been reported that removing the adrenals of rats bearing DMBA-induced mammary tumors enhances growth of the tumors (9). Other studies, however, have indicated that adrenalectomy does not significantly influence the incidence of carcinogen-induced rat mammary tumors (19).

The absence of continued growth of mammary tumors observed in ovariectomized rats 25 days after median eminence lesions were placed and the lack of effect in rats ovariectomized 10 days before the lesions were placed is most interesting, in view of the observations that serum prolactin levels are markedly increased during the latter experimental conditions. One can postulate that ovarian hormones are essential for sensitizing mammary tumors to the stimulatory effects of prolactin; that growth hormone elicits a synergistic response with prolactin in stimulating growth of mammary tumors; or both. The first postulate is supported by in vitro studies in our laboratory which demonstrate that prolactin is not capable of promoting DNA synthesis of DMBA-induced mammary tumors obtained from ovariectomized rats, but is very active in stimulating DNA synthesis of mammary tumors obtained from intact female rats (24). On the other hand, other studies have indicated that pituitary hormones alone can stimulate growth of carcinogen-induced rat mammary tumors in vivo. Kim and Furth (10) reported that in rats with mammary tumor regression after ovariectomy, grafts of pituitary tumors which secreted prolactin, GH, and ACTH caused resumption of tumor growth. Since these rats were not adrenalectomized, one cannot exclude the possibility that adrenal steroids synergized with the pituitary hormones in promoting tumor growth. More recently, Pearson et al. (18) demonstrated that administering prolactin to DMBA-treated rats manifesting mammary tumor regression as a result of adrenalectomy, ovariectomy, and hypophysectomy (triply operated) caused resumption of tumor growth. However, the concept that ovarian hormones can synergize with prolactin is supported by our observation of an initial increase and subsequent decrease in mammary tumor growth in rats given lesions in the median eminence and ovariectomized simultaneously. Presumably, residual circulating ovarian hormones were available in sufficient quantities within approximately 10 days after the combined surgical treatment. The lack of effect of lesions in the median eminence on mammary tumor growth of rats ovariectomized 10 days before the lesioning is in accord with this concept.

The role of growth hormone in promoting mammary tumor growth is less comprehensible. Pearson et al. (18) failed to demonstrate any significant effect of bovine growth hormone on mammary tumor growth in DMBA-treated rats. On the other hand, Talwalker, Meites, and Mizuno (21) reported enhanced mammary tumor development in DMBA-treated, ovariectomized rats injected with growth hormone and prolactin, and Young (25) demonstrated a significant incidence of 3-methylcholanthrene-induced mammary tumors in hypophysectomized female rats treated with ovarian hormones and bovine growth hormone.

The significant increase in incidence of *spontaneous* mammary tumors in mature female rats with lesions in the median eminence provides evidence that a hormonal imbalance, consisting of an increased secretion of prolactin and decreased secretion of all other anterior pituitary hormones favors the development of mammary tumors in the rat. There is little doubt that ovarian hormones participated in this process, but their degree of involvement remains to be determined. It is unlikely that an increase in mammary tumor incidence takes place in rats with median eminence lesions in the absence of ovaries. Marked mammary stimulation is observed in these rats *only* initially, whereas marked mammary atrophy typically occurs 3 to 4 wk after lesions are placed (22).

Hypothalamic-hypophyseal activity is also influenced and perhaps, at least in part, controlled by a variety of extrahypothalamic afferent neural pathways arising principally from the limbic system and the reticular formation. Although very little is known about the nature of this influence, small electrolytic lesions placed in these neural structures result in marked changes in endocrine activity (2, 4, 7, 26). That extrahypothalamic areas significantly influence tumor growth was recently reported by Welsch, Clemens, and Meites (22). We observed regression of carcinogen-induced mammary tumors in rats given lesions in the amygdaloid complex, a component of the limbic system.

To my knowledge there are only two other published reports pertaining to the direct manipulation of the CNS and its effect upon tumorigenesis (11, 16). Montemurro and Toy (16) recently reported in an abstract that electrolytic lesions in various areas of the hypothalamus of mice decreased the latency period of spontaneous mammary tumor appearance. They concluded that hypothalamic damage stimulated mammary tumorigenesis by producing a hormonal imbalance, involving an elevated secretion of pituitary prolactin. Klaiber et al. (11) recently confirmed our report (22) that median eminence-hypothalamic lesions markedly influence development and growth of carcinogen-induced rat mammary tumors. This experimental approach to understanding the development and growth of tumors, particularly those which are markedly hormone responsive, will require extensive investigation to obtain essential and reliable data; our knowledge in this area is almost nil and the problem is vastly complex. It is therefore important to initiate studies of this nature, since investigations involving the brain are well behind those of other anatomical regions, although the brain has long been considered the most crucial to the function of the organism.

Acknowledgments

I wish to express appreciation to E. E. Cassell, D. J. Dickinson, and M. D. Squiers, graduate students in the Department of Anatomy, for their interest and efforts in this research. Appreciation is also extended to Drs. C. L. Chen, J. A. Clemens, and H. Nagasawa for their collaboration in these studies and to Dr. J. Meites for his continuous interest and collaboration. A portion of this research was completed while I was a special research fellow of the National Cancer Institute (U.S.A.) in the laboratory of Dr. J. Meites.

This investigation was supported in part by National Science Foundation research grant GB-17034 and the American Cancer Society, Michigan Division.

References

1. Bacon, C. L.; Rennecker, R.; and Cutler, M. 1952. A psychosomatic survey of cancer of the breast. *Psychosom. Med.* 14: 453–60.
2. Critchlow, B. V. 1958. Blockade of ovulation in the rat by mesencephalic lesions. *Endocrinology* 63: 596–610.
3. Groot, J. de. 1958. The rat hypothalamus in stereotaxic coordinates. *J. Comp. Neurol.* 113: 389–400.
4. Elwers, M., and Critchlow, B. V. 1961. Precocious ovarian stimulation following interruption of stria-terminalis. *Amer. J. Physiol.* 201: 281–84.
5. Erdheim, J. 1904. Über Hypophysenganggeschwulste und Hirnocholesteatone. *Sitzber Akad. Wiss. Wien, Math-Nat. Kl.*, abst. III, 113, pp. 537–726.
6. Ganong, W. F. 1966. Neuroendocrine integrating mechanisms. In *Neuroendocrinology*, ed. L. Martini and W. F. Ganong, pp. 1–13. New York: Academic Press.
7. Green, J. D.; Clemente, C. D.; and Groot, J. de. 1957. Rhinencephalic lesions and behavior in cats. *J. Comp. Neurol.* 108: 505–36.
8. Greene, W. A., Jr.; Young, L.; and Swisher, S. N. 1956. Psychological factors and reticuloendothelial disease. II. Observations on a group of women with lymphomas and leukemias. *Psychom. Med.* 18: 284–303.
9. Kim, U. 1965. Pituitary function and hormonal therapy of experimental breast cancer. *Cancer Res.* 25: 1146–61.
10. Kim, U., and Furth, J. 1960 Relation of mammary tumors to mammotropes. II. Hormone responsiveness of 3-methylcholanthrene induced mammary carcinomas. *Proc. Soc. Exp. Biol. Med.* 103: 643–45.
11. Klaiber, M. S.; Gruenstein, M.; Meranze, D. R.; and Shimkin, M. B. 1969. Influence of hypothalamic lesions on the induction and growth of mammary cancers in Sprague-Dawley rats receiving 7, 12-dimethylbenzanthracene. *Cancer Res.* 29: 999–1001.

12. Lacassagne, A., and Duplan, J. F. 1959. Le mécanisme de la cancérisation de la mamelle chez la souris, considéré d'après les résultats d'expériences au moyen de la réserpine. *C. R. Acad. Sci.* 249: 810–12.
13. Le Sham, L. 1959. Psychological states as factors in the development of malignant disease: A critical review. *J. Nat. Cancer Inst.* 22: 1–13.
14. McCann, S. M., and Dhariwal, A. P. S. 1966. Hypothalamic releasing factors and the neurovascular link between the brain and the anterior pituitary. In *Neuroendocrinology,* ed. L. Martini and W. F. Ganong, pp. 261–96. New York: Academic Press.
15. Meites, J. 1966. Control of mammary growth and lactation. In *Neuroendocrinology,* ed. L. Martini and W. F. Ganong, pp. 669–707. New York: Academic Press.
16. Montemurro, D. G., and Toy, Y. C. 1968. Effect of hypothalamic lesions on the genesis of spontaneous mammary gland tumors in mice. *Excerpta Med.* 157: 136.
17. Niswender, G. D.; Chen, C. L.; Midgley, A. R.; Meites, J.; and Ellis, S. 1969. Radioimmunoassay for rat prolactin. *Proc. Soc. Exp. Biol. Med.* 130: 793–97.
18. Pearson, O. H.; Llerena, O.; Llerena, L.; Molina, A.; and Butler, T. 1969. Prolactin-dependent rat mammary cancer: A model for man? *Trans. Ass. Amer. Physicians* 82: 225–38.
19. Shay, H.; Harris, C.; and Gruenstein, M. 1960. Further studies in prevention of experimental induced breast cancer in the rat: Some endocrine aspects. *Acta Un. Int. Cancr.* 16: 225–32.
20. Stephenson, J. H., and Grace, W. J. 1954. Life stress and cancer of the cervix. *Psychosom. Med.* 16: 287–94.
21. Talwalker, P. K.; Meites, J.; and Mizuno, H. 1964. Mammary tumor induction by estrogen or anterior pituitary hormones in ovariectomized rats given 7, 12-dimethylbenzanthracene. *Proc. Soc. Exp. Biol. Med.* 116: 531–43.
22. Welsch, C. W.; Clemens, J. A.; and Meites, J. 1959. Effects of hypothalamic and amygdaloid lesions on development and growth of carcinogen-induced mammary tumors in the female rat. *Cancer Res.* 29: 1541–49.
23. Welsch, C. W., and Meites, J. 1968. Effects of reserpine on development of carcinogen-induced mammary tumors in rats. *Twenty-Fourth Intern. Congr. Physiol. Sci.* 6:466. Washington, D.C.
24. Welsch, C. W., and Rivera, E. 1970. The differential effects of prolactin and estrogen on growth of dimethylbenzanthracene (DMBA)-induced rat mammary tumors *in vitro. Tenth Int. Cancer Congr.,* Houston, Texas.
25. Young, S. 1961. Induction of mammary carcinoma in hypophysectomized rats treated with 3-methylcholanthrene, estradiol-17β, progesterone and growth hormone. *Nature (Lond.)* 190: 356–57.
26. Zouhar, R. L., and Groot, J. de. 1963. Effects of limbic brain lesions on aspects of reproduction in female rats. *Anat. Rec.* 145: 358.

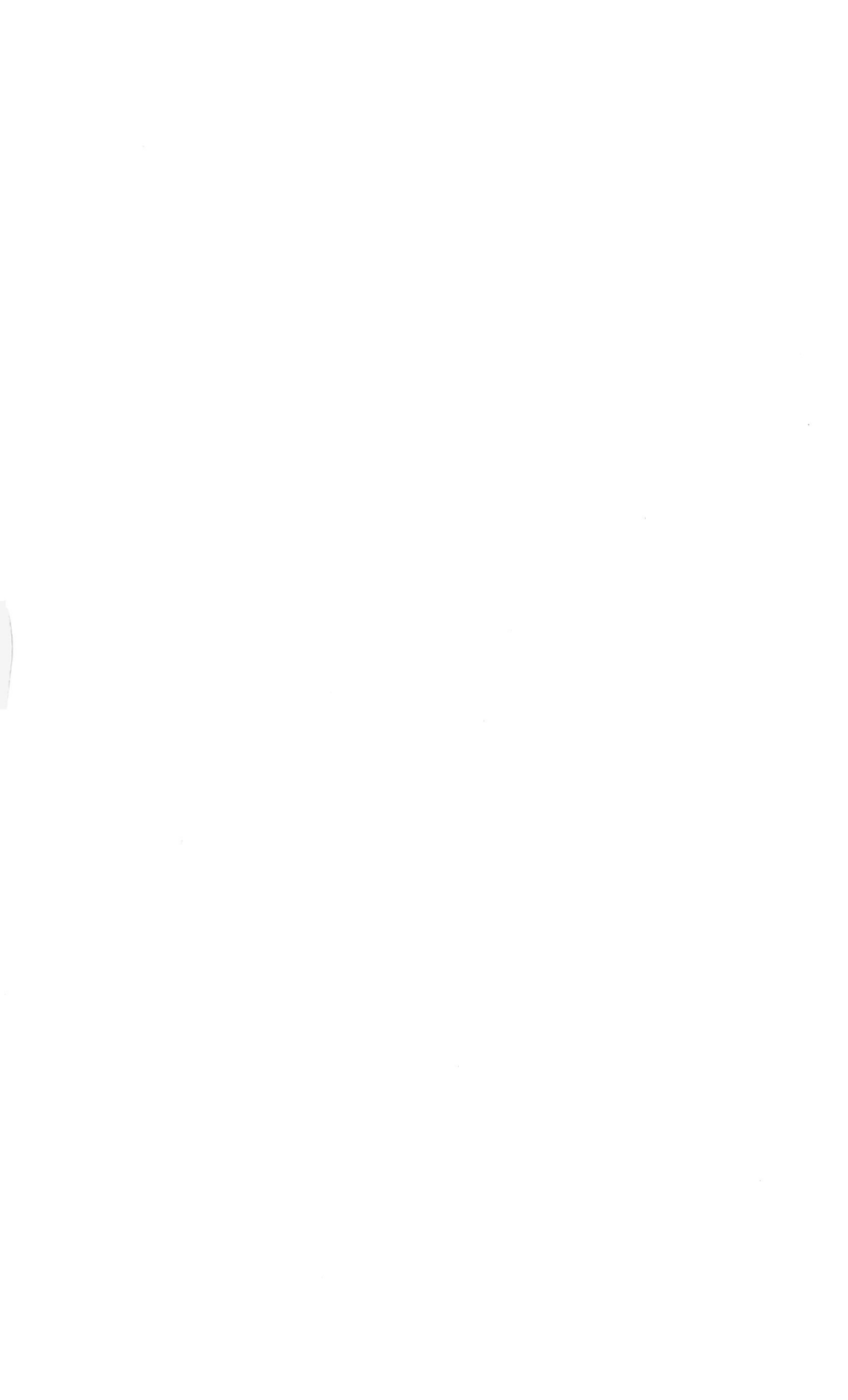

Charles B. Huggins, Hisao Oka, and George Fareed

Induction of Mammary Cancer in Rats of Long and Evans Strain   21

Two tissues of the rat are foremost among cells of living mammals in their susceptibility to the induction of cancer by polycyclic aromatic hydrocarbons. The neoplasms rapidly become evident. These immensely vulnerable target cells of a rat are the mammary acini and hemopoietic stem cells. Mammary carcinoma (8) and leukemia can be evoked by a flash exposure of the cells to aromatics, achieved by intravenous injection of lipid emulsions of powerful carcinogenic hydrocarbons. The propensity of these two classes of rat cells to undergo malignant disease is exceeded only by stem-cell fibroblasts of chickens inoculated in vivo with a single type of virus, Rous Sarcoma Virus I (17).

This paper is concerned with (*a*) the growth of rats of Long and Evans strain (L-E) in early life; (*b*) the induction of mammary cancers by pulse-doses (intravenous injection) of homogenized 7, 8, 12-TMBA[1] and (*c*) enzyme characteristics of these tumors. It was found that L-E rats are advantageous for studies where prolonged observation of the animals is desirable.

Long and Evans (12) described a strain of rats which arose from descendants of a cross, made in 1915, between albino females and a wild gray male caught in Berkeley, California. It is a vigorous stock. Mammary cancer was not observed in L-E rats injected for prolonged periods with pituitary growth hormone (15) in Evans's

---

The authors are affiliated with the Ben May Laboratory for Cancer Research at the University of Chicago.

[1] Abbreviations: 7, 12-DMBA = 7, 12-dimethylbenz(a)anthracene; 7, 8, 12-TMBA = 7, 8, 12-trimethylbenz(a)anthracene; NAD-nicotinamide adenine dinucleotide; ± = standard deviation of the mean.

laboratory. Spontaneous leukemia was detected in one rat among 6,000 female rats, maintained as breeding stock in our colony until age 6 mo, whereas spontaneous mammary cancer has not been observed.

Two polycyclic aromatic hydrocarbons are more efficient than all others in eliciting cancer in rat and mouse. In a remarkable paper, Bachmann and Chemerda (1) reported the synthesis of these intensely carcinogenic compounds, 7, 12-DMBA and 7, 8, 12-TMBA. Both compounds evoke cancer (2) when applied to the skin or when injected in muscle of rat or mouse. Lipid emulsions of these compounds are sterile and stable; intravenous injection of such homogenates of 7, 12-DMBA or 7, 8, 12-TMBA is simple and constitutes an effective technique for rapidly eliciting cancer in every rat or mouse. The dose of these compounds causing death of half of the rats in 21 days has been determined (5): LD_{50} for 7, 12-DMBA is 60 mg/kg; LD_{50} for 7, 8, 12-TMBA is 125 mg/kg.

Mammary cancer can also be elicited by feeding these compounds dissolved in vegetable oil. A single feeding (7) of 7, 12-DMBA, 20 mg, induced multiple cancers of the mammary gland rapidly in all Sprague-Dawley (S-D) female rats, whereas under identical conditions rats of the Long and Evans strain (18) had a low incidence (16%) of mammary cancer, with a delayed induction time and few tumors.

A single pulse-dose of 7, 12-DMBA, 13 mg/kg, was given to young adult female rats of two strains and the incidence (18) of mammary cancer was S-D strain, 100%; L-E strain, 9%. But when multiple pulse-doses of 7, 12-DMBA (18) or 7, 8, 12-TMBA (9) were given to rats of L-E strain the incidence of mammary cancer was 100% and myriads of mammary cancers emerged in all of these animals.

In male rats of S-D strain (6) a single pulse-dose of 7, 12-DMBA elicited a few mammary and sebaceous gland tumors, but leukemia was not observed. Multiple pulse-doses enhanced the yield of these tumors and leukemia (73%); many S-D rats (36%) in this series died early with pneumonitis and aplastic anemia.

The first biochemical characterization (16) of hormone-dependent mammary cancer utilized hydrocarbon-induced carcinoma of the mammary glands of S-D rats. Malic dehydrogenase had the greatest activity in normal mammary glands of pregnant and lactating rats; lactic dehydrogenase occupied the first rank in mammary cancer.

METHODS

Biological

The experimental animals were not inbred; they were male and female rats of Long and Evans and Sprague-Dawley strains. Our colony of L-E rats has been maintained by breeding at random inter se for more than 11 years; S-D rats were purchased from a dealer. The animals were housed in metal cages in air-conditioned rooms at 25° C ± 2, fed a commercial ration (Rockland Mouse/Rat Diet, Teklad, Inc., Monmouth, Illinois) and given water ad libitum; 3 times each week the animals were weighed. Every day the vaginal smear of each female was examined using a Pasteur pipette and saline.

Lipid emulsions of 7, 12-DMBA or 7, 8, 12-TMBA were injected in a caudal vein; the first injection is denoted day 0. The experiments were terminated when the tumors were in an advanced stage or on day 135.

Tissue sections were stained with hematoxylin and eosin. Alkaline phosphatase was exhibited histochemically by the method of Gomori (4).

Biochemical

Mammary glands and cancers were excised rapidly, weighed and homogenized in an ice-cold solution of 0.15 N NaCl containing 0.003 M $NaHCO_3$; 100–200 mg of tissue was homogenized in 5 ml of the buffered saline. The chilled homogenates were centrifuged at 11,000 g in a refrigerated centrifuge. Enzyme assays were performed on the supernatant fluids.

Lactic Dehydrogenase (LDH). The reaction mixture contained 0.083 M Tris, pH 7.4; 0.003 M sodium pyruvate; 0.0001 M NADH.
Malic Dehydrogenase (MDH). The reaction mixture contained 0.083 M Tris, pH 7.4; 0.001 M sodium oxalacetate; 0.0001 M NADH.

Three ml samples of reaction mixture were placed in silica cuvettes of 1 cm light path and 0.02 ml of homogenate was added to start the reaction. The initial rate of oxidation of NADH at 25° C was measured for 1 min in a spectrophotometer; the optimal enzyme concentration yielded an absorbance change of 0.015–0.025 OD units/mg/min at 340 mμ.

One unit of LDH or MDH is defined as that activity which oxidizes 1 μmole of DPNH/min/g of tissue under the stated conditions.

Alkaline phosphatase. Alkaline phosphatase was determined by a method (10) described previously. One unit of alkaline phosphatase liberates 1 μmole of *p*-nitrophenol/0.5 hr/g of tissue at 38° C.

Protein Determination.

The concentration of protein was determined by the method of Lowry et al. (13). Specific activity is defined as units/mg protein/min.

Electrophoresis of LDH Isozymes

LDH isozymes were separated by electrophoresis on a cellulose acetate slide in a mixture (1:1) of 0.2 M Tris, pH 8.3, and 0.075 M sodium barbital, pH 8.6. The relative migration and concentration of isozymes was measured in an electrophoresis densitometer. The isozymes are designated $H_4(LDH_1)$, $H_3M(LDH_2)$, $H_2M_2(LDH_3)$, $HM_3(LDH_4)$, and $M_4(LDH_5)$.

RESULTS

Rate of Body Growth: Onset of Puberty in L-E Rats

The growth of groups of male and of female L-E rats was identical in the age period 25–50 days (fig. 1); after 50 days the females grew more slowly than the males.

Compared with companion rats of S-D strain, L-E females had smaller initial body mass at age 25 days and slower rate of body growth thereafter (fig. 2); the vaginal plate opened later and the first estrus was delayed (table 1).

The interval between the first and second estrus was determined: in L-E rats it was 7.4 ± 3.6 days; in S-D rats 6 ± 1.5 days. After

TABLE 1: ONSET OF PUBERTY IN RATS OF LONG-EVANS AND SPRAGUE-DAWLEY STRAINS

	Day of Vaginal Opening		Day of First Estrus	
Strain	Range	Mean	Range	Mean
L-E	33–63	44.3 ± 9	33–63	50 ± 6.5
S-D	30–39	32.9 ± 3	30–39	34.5 ± 2.8

NOTE: There were 20 rats in each group.

the second estrus, periodicity was regular and identical for both strains (4.1 ± 0.2 days) for the 30 ensuing periods.

Induction of Neoplasms with Pulse-doses of 7, 8, 12-TMBA

Members of a group of 15 S-D females were given 3 pulse-doses of 7, 8, 12-TMBA, 35 mg/kg, at biweekly intervals starting at age 50 days; 12 of these animals (80%) succumbed from aplastic anemia and pneumonitis before day 31, whereas 15 uninjected control sisters survived free from disease.

L-E rats injected with a set of leukemogenic pulse-doses of 7, 8, 12-TMBA are more resistant to intercurrent illness than are S-D females. Forty-five rats of L-E strain, males and females, were

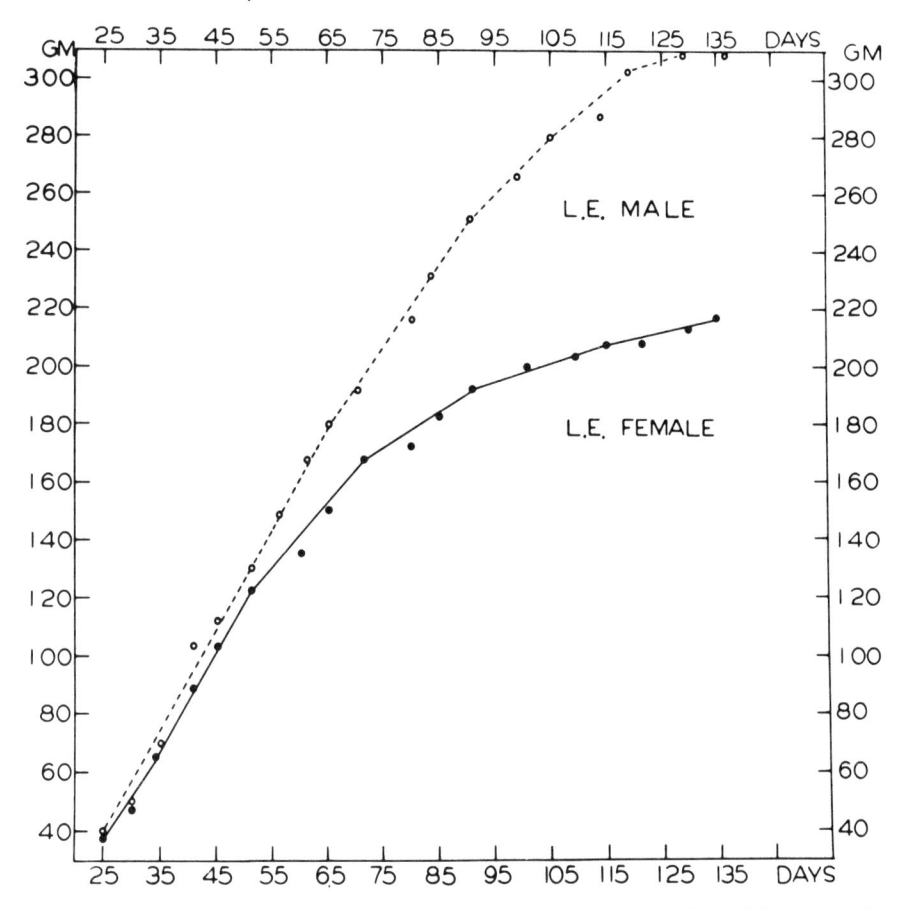

Fig. 1. Curves of body weight of normal males and females of Long and Evans strain of rats.

injected with 5 pulse-doses of 7, 8, 12-TMBA, 30 mg/kg, at intervals of 14 days beginning at age 50 days. There were 6 deaths (13%) before day 60: aplastic anemia, 4 rats; pneumonitis, 2 rats. Within 4.5 mo (table 2) 20 effective males developed the following neoplasms: leukemia, 11 rats (55%); mammary cancer, 0. The accompanying group of 19 virgin females developed the following tumors: leukemia, 10 rats (53%), mammary cancer, 15 rats (79%) (table 2).

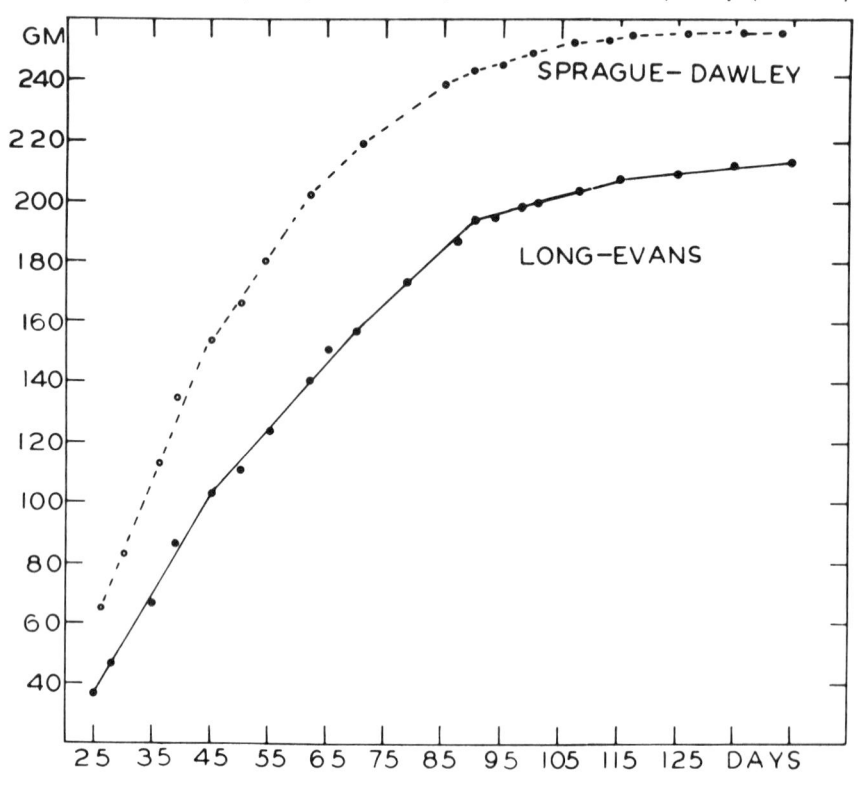

Fig. 2. Curves of body weight of normal females of Long and Evans and Sprague-Dawley strains.

In the group of female rats, mammary cancer was detected in 68.1 ± 17 days (table 2); at autopsy 64 mammary cancers were found in 15 rats and the neoplasms infiltrated the adjacent muscle and skin.

Enzymes in Hyperplastic Mammary Glands and in Mammary Cancers

When expressed as units/g of tissue, the activities of LDH and MDH in mammary cancer exceeded those in the normal hyperplastic glands or in pregnancy and lactation (table 3). To eliminate the contribution of fat to the gross weight of tissue, which would influence enzyme concentration of the normal mammary glands, all activities were calculated, in addition, in terms of units/mg protein/min, and this is denoted specific activity.

In normal mammary gland, enzyme activities in lactation exceeded

TABLE 2: MAMMARY CANCER AND LEUKEMIA EVOKED IN YOUNG ADULT LONG AND EVANS RATS BY A SET OF PULSE-DOSES OF 7, 8, 12-TMBA

Sex	No. Rats	Early Deaths[a]	Mammary Cancer Detected No. Rats	Range (days)	Mean (days)	Leukemia Detected No. Rats	Range (days)	Mean (days)
M	23	3	0	—	—	11	44–134	65.3 ± 25
F	22	3	15	41–93	68.1 ± 17	10	56–98	80.8 ± 16

NOTE: The animals received 5 pulse-doses of 7, 8, 12-TMBA, 30 mg/kg, at biweekly intervals starting at age 50 days; the experiment was terminated on day 135.

[a] Early deaths occurred before day 60.

TABLE 3: ALKALINE PHOSPHATASE AND LACTIC AND MALIC DEHYDROGENASES IN HYPERPLASTIC MAMMARY GLANDS AND MAMMARY CANCER

	Alkaline Phosphatase	LDH	MDH	LDH/MDH[a]
Pregnancy, day 8				
Units/g	15.3 ± 5.0	13.6 ± 2.3	37.9 ± 15.6	0.36
Units/mg protein	0.52 ± 0.11	0.48 ± 0.12	1.32 ± 0.54	
Pregnancy, day 13				
Units/g	25.5 ± 10.4	16.4 ± 3.3	44.2 ± 11.2	0.37
Units/mg protein	0.92 ± 0.26	0.61 ± 0.12	1.66 ± 0.39	
Lactation, day 6				
Units/g	51.5 ± 13.9	67.7 ± 11.7	163.5 ± 15.1	0.41
Units/mg protein	0.58 ± 0.14	0.77 ± 0.14	1.87 ± 0.25	
Mammary cancer				
Units/g	14.3 ± 7.6	192.7 ± 36.8	137.8 ± 36.9	1.41
Units/mg protein	0.21 ± 0.11	2.12 ± 0.43	1.63 ± 0.52	

NOTE: The rats were females of L-E strain. There were 8 rats in each group. Tumors were induced by pulse-doses of 7, 8, 12-TMBA. The results are expressed in units/g of tissue, wet weight, and as specific activity. Means with standard deviation ± are given.

[a] LDH/MDH is the ratio of LDH to MDH.

those in pregnancy; the ratio LDH/MDH was ~0.4. An important difference between normal mammary hyperplasias and cancers was the absolute and relative increase in concentration of LDH and the reversal in malignant disease of the ratio LDH/MDH (~1.4). These results agree with those of Rees and Huggins (16) for mammary tissues of S-D rats.

The content of alkaline phosphatase (table 3) was less in mammary cancer than in the normal hyperplastic states. These enzyme results

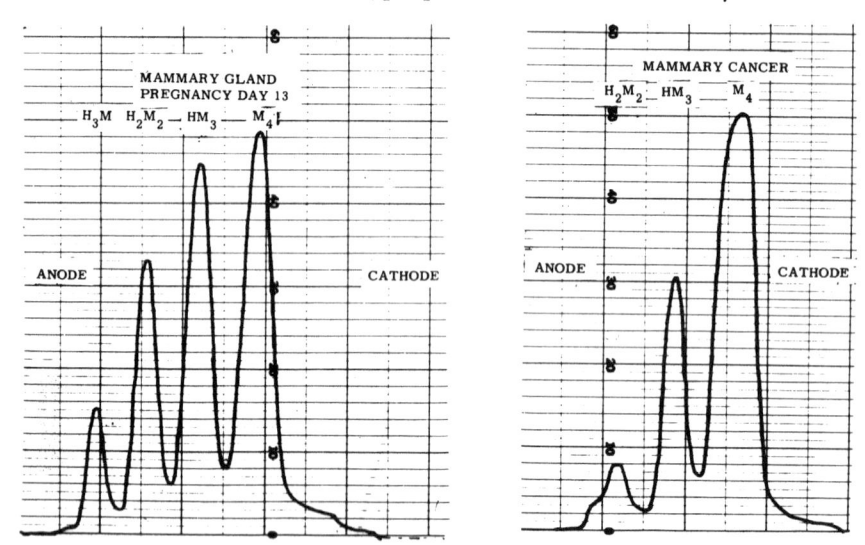

Fig. 3. Densitometer tracings of bands formed by isozymes of lactic dehydrogenase from mammary gland of pregnancy, day 13, and mammary cancer of Long and Evans strain female. Equivalent amounts of enzyme-protein were subjected to electrophoresis at 100 volts for 33 min at 4° C. Movement in the electrophoresis is along the horizontal axis.

are consonant with histochemical observations which showed alkaline phosphatase to be located principally in myoepithelial cells surrounding the mammary acini. In the mammary cancers there is a moderate reduction of the myoepithelial component.

Isozymes of Mammary Tissue

In all normal states of proliferation the pattern of isozymes in mammary gland was similar to that of skeletal muscle (fig. 3); in mammary cancer, the most striking finding was an absolute increase in isozymes of skeletal muscle type with no detection of H_4 or H_3M isozymes.

Discussion

There is a profound difference between two strains (S-D; L-E) of rats in their susceptibility to mammary cancer which is reflected in the incidence of spontaneous mammary cancer and in the development of cancer of the mammary gland after pulse-doses of homogenized 7, 12-DMBA and 7, 8, 12-TMBA. In addition, there is a difference in the rate at which the strains reach sexual maturity.

Sprague-Dawley female rats had the following characteristics: (*a*) the incidence of spontaneous mammary cancer was 1.2%; (*b*) a single pulse-dose of 7, 8, 12-TMBA (35 mg/kg) elicited mammary cancer in every animal, and the neoplasms were evident in 42 ± 11 days; (*c*) multiple biweekly pulse-doses of 7, 8, 12-TMBA, 35 mg/kg, resulted in a high mortality before day 31 because of susceptibility to epidemics of pneumonitis; and (*d*) the rats exhibited rapid growth in early life and early sexual maturity.

Long and Evans female rats had the following characteristics: (*a*) spontaneous mammary cancer has not been observed in our large colony; (*b*) a single pulse-dose of 7, 8, 12-TMBA evoked mammary cancer in 0–10% of the animals; (*c*) multiple pulse-doses of 7, 8, 12-TMBA elicited mammary cancer in high yield and the neoplasms were evident in 68.1 ± 17 days; (*d*) the rats were very resistant to epidemics of pneumonitis; and (*e*) they exhibited slower increment of body mass and later sexual maturity.

In this experiment, L-E males had a 55% incidence of induced leukemia, whereas mammary cancer was not observed.

The mammary cancers of L-E females resembled those of S-D females in their biochemical characteristics. The increase in concentration of LDH and reversal of the ratio LDH/MDH are striking characteristics of cancer of the breast in both strains. In an earlier study, Meister (14) found that the level of LDH in tumors of rodents is frequently higher than in the corresponding tissues of origin. In accord with previously reported results (3), a pronounced shift toward the most cationic, slow moving LDH isozymes was observed in mammary cancer.

Conclusion

The Long and Evans strain of rats is highly advantageous for studies of leukemia or mammary cancer in experiments where prolonged observation of the animals is desirable. It is highly resistant to pneumonitis and to the toxicity of a carcinogenic set of pulse-doses of 7, 8, 12-trimethylbenz(a)anthracene, and mammary cancer or leukemia or both neoplasms together can be induced rapidly and in high yield by very simple methods.

The enzymes of mammary cancer of L-E rats are characterized by decrease of alkaline phosphatase, increase of lactic dehydrogenase, and reversal of the ratio LDH/MDH. The increased LDH isozymes are principally of the most cationic, slow moving type similar to those of skeletal muscle.

Acknowledgments

We thank John Pataki of the Ben May Laboratory for Cancer Research, University of Chicago, for the synthesis of 7, 8, 12-TMBA, and Paul E. Schurr, of the Upjohn Company, Kalamazoo, Michigan, for lipid emulsion.

This work was supported by grants from the American Cancer Society and the Jane Coffin Childs Memorial Fund for Medical Research, and by grant CA-11603 from the United States Public Health Service, National Institutes of Health.

References

1. Bachmann, W. E., and Chemerda, J. M. 1938. The synthesis of 9, 10-dimethyl-1, 2-benzanthracene, 9, 10-diethyl-1, 2,-benzanthracene and 5, 9, 10-trimethyl-1, 2-benzanthracene. *J. Amer. Chem. Soc.* 60: 1023–26.
2. Bachmann, W. E.; Kennaway, E. L.; and Kennaway, N. M. 1938. The rapid production of tumours by two new hydrocarbons. *Yale J. Biol. Med.* 11: 97–102.
3. Goldman, R. D.; Kaplan, N. O.; and Hall, T. C. 1964. Lactic dehydrogenase in human neoplastic tissues. *Cancer Res.* 24: 389–99.
4. Gomori, G. 1952. *Microscopic histochemistry: Principles and practice.* Chicago: University of Chicago Press.
5. Huggins, C. B.; Ford, E.; and Jensen, E. V. 1965. Carcinogenic aromatic hydrocarbons: Special vulnerability of rats. *Science* 147: 1153–54.
6. Huggins, C. B., and Grand, L. 1966. Neoplasms evoked in male Sprague-Dawley rats by pulse-doses of 7, 12-dimethylbenz(a)anthracene. *Cancer Res.* 26: 2255–58.
7. Huggins, C.; Grand, L. C.; and Brillantes, F. P. 1961. Mammary cancer induced by a single feeding of polynuclear hydrocarbons and its suppression. *Nature (Lond.)* 189: 204–7.
8. Huggins, C.; Grand, L.; and Fukunishi, R. 1964. Aromatic influences

on the yields of mammary cancers following administration of 7, 12-dimethylbenz(a)anthracene. *Proc. Nat. Acad. Sci. USA* 51: 737–42.
9. Huggins, C.; Grand, L.; and Oka, H. 1970. Hundred day leukemia: Preferential induction in rat by pulse-doses of 7, 8, 12-trimethylbenz(a)anthracene. *J. Exp. Med.* 131: 321–30.
10. Huggins, C., and Morii, S. 1961. Selective adrenal necrosis and apoplexy induced by 7, 12-dimethylbenz(a)anthracene. *J. Exp. Med.* 114: 741–60.
11. Huggins, C. B., and Sugiyama, T. 1966. Induction of leukemia in rat by pulse-doses of 7,12-dimethylbenz(a)anthracene. *Proc. Nat. Acad. Sci. USA* 55: 74–81.
12. Long, J. A., and Evans, H. McL. 1922. The oestrous cycle in the rat and its associated phenomena. *Memoirs of the University of California* 6.
13 Lowry, O. H.; Rosebrough, N. J.; Farr, A. L.; and Randall, R. J. 1951. Protein measurement with the folin reagent. *J. Biol. Chem.* 193: 265–75.
14. Meister, A. 1950. Lactic dehydrogenase activity of certain tumors and normal tissues. *J. Nat. Cancer Inst.* 10: 1263–71.
15. Moon, H. D.; Simpson, M. E.; Li, C. H.; and Evans, H. McL. 1950. Neoplasms in rats treated with pituitary growth hormone. III. Reproductive organs. *Cancer Res.* 10: 549–56.
16. Rees, E. D., and Huggins, C. 1960. Steroid influences on respiration, glycolysis and levels of pyridine nucleotide-linked dehydrogenases of experimental mammary cancers. *Cancer Res.* 20: 963–71.
17. Rous, P. 1911. A sarcoma of the fowl transmissible by an agent separable from the tumor cells. *J. Exp. Med.* 13: 397–411.
18. Sydnor, K. L.; Butenandt, O.; Brillantes, F. P.; and Huggins, C. 1962. Race-strain factor related to hydrocarbon-induced mammary cancer in rats. *J. Nat. Cancer. Inst.* 29: 805–14.

Kenneth DeOme, *Chairman*

Discussion: Part III 22

DR. MUHLBOCK: We have studied the hormonal aspects of mammary tumorigenesis in the mouse. We implanted a hypophysis at a site far from the hypothalamus in the female mouse. This is a very good induction method for mammary tumors without viral involvement. There is no inhibitory effect from the hypothalamus, so prolactin is produced continuously. Since mammary tumor induction is successful only if estrogenic hormones are present, it does not work in a male animal, in which no excessive prolactin production occurs. This system can be used to investigate the effect of estrogenic hormones or other steroid hormones on the development of mammary tumors in the presence of a hypophyseal graft in the male mouse. Results in table 1 show that mammary tumor did not develop in gonadectomized male F1-hybrid mice with a hypophyseal graft in the kidney capsule. If large doses of estrone were given continuously in drinking water, no mammary tumors developed. If we gave the same doses intermittently, that is, if we continued this dose for 5 days and stopped for 5 days, 65% of the animals developed mammary tumors. If a low dose of estrone was given, 55% of these animals developed mammary tumors. This means that prolactin is produced only with certain doses of estrogenic hormone; higher doses of estrogen inhibit prolactin release, hence tumors developed. In the mouse progesterone certainly plays an important role; in the same system it can induce mammary tumors in 29% of the animals. If progesterone is combined with a low dose of estrone, 100% of the animals develop a mammary tumor.

DR. MEITES: My comment is related to some of the apparent contradictions in the talk I presented, and to that of Dr. Welsch. Dr.

The chairman is affiliated with the Cancer Research Genetics Laboratory at the University of California at Berkeley.

Welsch produced median eminence lesions in ovariectomized rats that already had DMBA-induced tumors. Stimulation of tumor growth occurred only during the first 10 days after the lesions were placed, and this was followed by regression of the mammary tumors. I should point out that median eminence lesions increase prolactin secretion but decrease secretion of all the other hormones, including growth hormone. This is also true of the pituitaries that Dr. Muhlbock transplanted in the mouse, which also

TABLE 1: MAMMARY TUMORS IN CASTRATED (C57BL × CBA) F1 MALE MICE WITH HYPOPHYSEAL ISOGRAFTS

Treatments	No. of Animals	With Tumor %	With Tumor Average Age (days)	Without Tumor Average Age at Death (days)
No treatment	36	0	—	587
Estrogen, 2 mg/l drinking water daily	37	0	—	439
Estrogen, 2 mg/l drinking water at 5-day intervals	31	65	488	504
Estrogen, 0.25 mg/l drinking water daily	35	40	466	477
Progesterone, 2 mg pellets subcutaneously, 3 times	12	25	577	553
Estrogen, 0.25 mg/l drinking water daily + progesterone	42	100	271	—

produce prolactin but very little growth hormone. Only in the presence of prolactin and growth hormone were we able to maintain mammary tumor growth in ovariectomized-adrenalectomized rats. I find most interesting the work reported by Dr. Sinha and Dr. Dao demonstrating tumor induction by local application of estrogen and DMBA to the mammary gland of the rat, and the synergism they observed of estrogen with DMBA on mammary tumor induction. Dr. Sinha made the point that he obtained local mammary tumor growth by adding estrogen directly to the mammary gland without increasing prolactin secretion. However, we cannot rule out the possibility that prolactin was increased. There are

Discussion

indications in the literature that when estrogen is applied locally to the mammary gland it increases development of the blood vessels and also increases the circulation. So even though there is no systemic increase in blood levels of prolactin, there might still be a local increase of prolactin in the mammary gland as a result of increased blood supply to this tissue.

DR. NANDI: Is it possible that the pituitary tumors Dr. Meites is using are capable of producing steroid hormone? If they are indeed producing a small quantity of steroid hormone, they can act synergistically in tumorigenesis. Therefore, until one proves that these tumors are not producing steroid hormones, one cannot say that prolactin or prolactin and growth hormones are the main hormones responsible for the tumorigenesis of the mammary gland. Also, are there any ectopic adrenal or ovarian tissues in these animals? If there are ectopic tissues, they could be producing small amounts of steroid hormones.

DR. MEITES: I am unaware of any evidence that pituitary tumors can produce estrogens, although I am not certain that anyone has looked for them. In reference to the ectopic tissues, our experience with adrenalectomized inbred Fisher rats suggests that these animals do not have ectopic adrenal tissues, since they do not survive without saline solution.

DR. NANDI: Even if the pituitary tumor, like the mammotropic tumors, can induce mammary tumor in the oophorectomized and adrenalectomized rats, it does not necessarily mean that in normal intact females prolactin is the only hormone involved in mammary tumorigenesis.

DR. MEITES: We have recently determined the effects of DMBA, methylcholanthrene, and benzopyrene on serum levels of prolactin (Nagasawa and Meites, unpublished) and found no effect whatsoever, which indicates that these carcinogens do not act on the mammary gland by increasing prolactin secretion. I should mention that we induced the original mammary tumors with a pituitary tumor ($MtT.W_{15}$) not in ovariectomized-adrenalectomized rats but in intact rats. We transplanted the mammary tumors to adrenalectomized-ovariectomized rats, and they were dependent only on pituitary hormones for their growth.

DR. ROSEN: Since most of the polypeptide hormones exert their actions on target tissues by altering the levels of the cyclic AMP in tissue, I wonder if Dr. Welsch has any evidence that in these tumors there is a difference in the metabolism of cyclic AMP. Also, you indicate that if you give growth hormone to these ovariectomized rats with median eminence lesion, the tumor will continue to grow. But in fact, you get a tumor regression.

DR. WELSCH: Dr. Meites mentioned that failure of mammary tumor growth in ovariectomized rats with median eminence lesions may be due, at least in part, to a lack of growth hormone. It is possible that if growth hormone was administered to these rats tumor growth would accelerate or at least continue. In Dr. Meites's experiments both growth hormone and prolactin were administered concurrently. However, I seem to recall an experiment from the laboratory of Dr. Nandi which demonstrates in vitro that prolactin alone can induce lobuloalveolar growth of the rat mammary gland. Dr. Meites has shown that growth hormone can enhance the prolactin effect. Dr. Nandi raised the question whether prolactin and growth hormone alone can induce mammary tumors. I cannot think of any experiment or experimental model in which one can be absolutely certain of an absence of steroid hormones. After the ovaries and adrenals are removed, steroid hormones are still found in the circulation under certain conditions. Thus, it seems that other tissues certainly have the potential and capacity to produce them. It is therefore impossible to design experiments in vivo to show conclusively the pituitary hormones alone can produce mammary tumors in the absence of steroid hormones.

DR. DAO: Dr. Welsch's suggestion that steroid hormones were being produced in these animals after both ovaries and adrenals were removed needs some clarification. There is evidence that breast cancer tissue has the capacity to convert precursors to physiologically active hormones; similar data are not available for normal mammary gland tissue. There has been no report to indicate that the normal mammary gland may be a site where transformation of the steroid precursors into physiologically active hormones can take place. I would agree that if tumors were present in the rats it would be possible for the tumor to perform the conversion. In tumorigenesis of the mammary gland it is rather doubtful that prolactin alone, in conjunction with a chemical carcinogen, can induce mammary tumors in the ovariectomized rats. In spite of Dr. Welsch's and Dr. Meites's insistence that prolactin is the "key" pituitary hormone in rat mammary carcinogenesis, their evidence is not sufficient for such a conclusion. In fact, Dr. Welsch's own data clearly show the opposite results. In his ovariectomized-lesioned animals, he clearly shows that in the absence of ovaries the very elevated level of prolactin is inconsequential to mammary tumorigenesis. Instead of stimulating tumor growth in the presence of high prolactin levels in ovariectomized-lesioned rats, the tumors regress, whether the lesions are placed before or after ovariectomies. These data in my opinion represent more evidence supporting the concept of Nandi and others who suggest that there is synergism between estrogen and prolactin. Particularly pertinent to this possibility is Dr. Welsch's demonstration that there was an initial rise of tumor size followed by regression in the group of rats in which ovariectomy was done immediately after median eminence lesions were placed. The initial growth activity might be due to circulating estrogen. The tumors subsequently regressed in spite of the presence of high-level circulating prolactin. These confusing but rather interesting studies must be further elucidated. I think that the male rats are ideal models for this experiment.

DR. DE OME: In the rodent system one has to consider that neoplastic transformation occurs at two levels: at the level of nodule formation and at the level of tumor formation. For this reason it is important that we consider the persistence of the chemical carcinogens used. We are inclined to think that these agents persist for only a short time, but recent experiments by Dr. Medina in our laboratory suggest that the effect of treatment with chemical carcinogens may persist for some time in a mammary gland cell population. For example, when a nodule outgrowth line was treated with one of these agents and then serially transplanted into untreated hosts, the tumor incidence was high in the first and second transplant generation, decreased in the third generation, and was not significantly different from the untreated control in the fourth transplant generation. The persistence of the effect of the carcinogen in these experiments suggests that we should be cautious in our estimates of the persistence of the active carcinogenic agent.

DR. TURKINGTON: A number of investigators have commented on the hypertrophy of the gastrointestinal tract and the growth of the host after mammotrophic pituitary tumor transplants. I wonder whether the nutritional factor in prolactin's effect plays some role in maintaining growth in the transplanted or DMBA-induced tumors.

DR. MEITES: There is good evidence that food intake can influence mammary development. A reduction in food intake has a profound effect on pituitary hormone secretion, resulting in a decreased secretion of anterior pituitary hormones, including prolactin. In the rat pituitary tumors, which secrete large amounts of GH and prolactin, the animals actually eat more, and they certainly grow more. It is quite possible, therefore, that the growth effect exerted by the pituitary tumor on the mammary gland is partly due to increased food intake.

DR. DE OME: Although the direct effect of nutritional deficiency on the endocrine organs occasionally can be demonstrated, one is still faced with the possibility that the level of metabolism and of protein synthesis in the whole animal is also reduced. It is very difficult to determine whether such a deficiency has a direct effect upon tumorigenesis or simply depresses the whole metabolic level of the animal.

DR. PEARSON: The DMBA tumor in the rat is extremely sensitive to starvation, and if the animals lose weight during an experiment tumor regression may be due to a starvation effect.

DR. SINGH: Decreased dietary protein reduces thyroxine secretion rate. Dr. Meites's laboratory and Dr. Turner's laboratory have demonstrated that thyroxine plays an important role in the secretion of prolactin in vivo and in vitro. Thyroxine increases prolactin secretion. An increase in prolactin secretion may significantly enhance mammary tumorigenesis. Decreased dietary protein reduces TSR, and therefore reduction in prolactin secretion which will affect tumorigenesis. On the whole, nutritional deficiency has an indirect effect upon tumorigenesis by affecting endocrine glands. Estrogen induces secretion of prolactin in vivo and in vitro. In ovariectomized rats, both TSR secretion and prolactin secretion are decreased. Since thyroxine increases the prolactin secretion to the same level obtained by estrogen, is it possible that thyroxine-stimulated prolactin secretion can induce tumor growth? Have you done any experiments studying the combined effect of thyroidectomy, oophorectomy, thyroxine and estrogen, and so on?

DR. MEITES: You are quite correct in stating that thyroidectomy decreases prolactin secretion and that administering thyroxine increases prolactin secretion, as we have shown recently. We haven't studied the combined effect of thyroidectomy and ovariectomy, or of thyroxine and estrogen. This would be interesting.

DR. O'MALLEY: It seems to me that we are asking a lot to understand the sophistication and paradoxes of tumor generation. In my own mind I think about it simply as a disorder of cell regulation. One can alter the genome in certain species by putting a carcinogen on it. This damage can be expressed in various manners. A mutation can be forced during future replications. A viral remnant could be activated. Rapid cell growth and transcription could allow expression of any existing defect. An example of this might be breast tumors and prolactin and estrogen; the hormones simply promote expression of existing defects but are not the basic cause of the malignancy. At this time, we know very little about the regulation of a cell, such as transcription and the link between RNA synthesis

Discussion

and protein synthesis, and DNA cycle and replication of the cell. The more we know about the regulation of the normal cell, the more we know about disorders in cell regulation, of which cancer may be our most important example.

DR. BRENNAN: It has been reported that there is better frequency and duration of remission following oophorectomy in women with metastatic breast cancer if the treatment is supplemented with thyroid extract afterward. At least it is clear that the dosage of thyroxine used in clinical medicine does not compensate for a prolactin shutdown as a result of oophorectomy and restore tumor growth in oophorectomized patients.

DR. SARFATY: Relating to the pharmacological doses of steroids and response, I wish to ask whether in Dr. Pearson's systems any steroids other than large doses of estradiol influence circulating prolactin.

DR. PEARSON: We studied the effects of progesterone in large doses and they suppress prolactin levels without influencing tumor growth. The tumors continued to grow, but we do not know whether they grow faster or slower than without progesterone since we did not have a control group in this experiment. Testosterone had little influence on prolactin levels and yet some tumors shrank while others grew. I have already mentioned that large doses of estrogen raise the serum prolactin levels, and yet tumors shrink. Our preliminary experiment suggests that large doses of estradiol may block the peripheral action of prolactin. In these experiments rats bearing DMBA-induced tumors were oophorectomized to induce tumorigenesis. After the tumors had partially regressed, perphenazine was administered, 1 mg daily subcutaneously, which brought reactivation of tumor growth. At this point perphenazine injections were continued and estradiol benzoate injections, 500 μg daily, were started. This resulted in prompt regression of the tumors. Although our serum prolactin data have not been completed, the results of this experiment suggest that estradiol interfered with the stimulating effects of perphenazine which causes an increase in prolactin secretion. I do not know how specific the effect of perphenazine on prolactin secretion is. We have not measured its effect on growth hormone, FSH, and LH secretion.

DR. MEITES: We have done experiments with chloropromazine, which is similar to promazine. Chloropromazine appears to act similarly to a median eminence lesion; that is, it increases prolactin secretion but decreases secretion of all other anterior pituitary hormones. It should also be mentioned that stimulating mammary growth by hormones before administering a carcinogen inhibits mammary carcinogenesis. In other words, if we induce a median eminence lesion or transplant a pituitary, either of which increases mammary growth, it appears to make the mammary gland refractory to the action of a carcinogen. On the other hand, the same treatment given after the mammary tumor is already present increases the tumor's growth.

DR. DAO: An overstimulated mammary gland is refractory to the action of the carcinogen. We first reported that mammary gland in pregnant rats was completely refractory to chemical carcinogenesis (*J. Nat. Cancer Inst.* 25: 991, 1960). However, if we give carcinogen first and then mate the rats, the subsequent pregnancy will accelerate the tumor development.

Dr. Welsch's and Dr. Meites's experiments are almost identical to the observation we made many years ago. Dr. Huggins also reported that injecting estradiol and progesterone, before DMBA administration, could inhibit tumor induction. All these experiments have a common denominator—a hyperfunctional mammary gland. It appears that cells undergoing active division and proliferation are resistant to carcinogenesis. We must also consider the possibility that carcinogen and steroid hormones may be competing for receptor sites.

DR. HILF: I think we should keep in mind that what we have been talking about may be specific for the DMBA-induced tumor. In the transplantable rat tumor we have studied, the R3230AC mammary carcinoma of the Fischer rat, whatever manipulations we employ to increase the level of prolactin, such as injecting ovine prolactin daily, or implanting a mammotrophic tumor which secretes prolactin, or injecting a phenothiazine compound (fluphenazine) which increases the secretion of endogenous prolactin, all cause a decrease in tumor growth, not an increase. Now, whether the DMBA-induced tumor is a true model of breast cancer or just one particular model, or whether the R3230AC transplantable tumor is also a valid model, has not been resolved. I do think it is important that we keep in mind that one can get different effects with various hormones depending on the system studied, and until we know which system is the best experimental model, we are not able to translate these effects in terms of human breast cancer.

DR. DE OME: The tumor biologist must remember that two histologically similar tumors of a single tissue type derived from one animal may be quite different in other characteristics. For example, differences in antigenicity are regularly encountered under these conditions.

Discussion

Furthermore, the population of cells composing a given tumor is not homogeneous. For example, part of the cell population in a mammary gland tumor may show considerable secreting activity, whereas the remainder of the cell population shows little evidence of hormone responsiveness.

Faced with problems of this magnitude, we can generalize only after many tumors have been tested.

Kenneth DeOme, *Chairman*

Summary: Part III 23

The occurrence of receptor proteins in certain tissues of the body suggests two important lines of investigation. First, the receptor proteins may provide a mechanism by which target cells trap hormones and convey them into the nucleus. If this hypothesis is correct, it may be possible to investigate at the molecular level the action of specific hormones within cells. Second, the presence or absence of specific receptors in lesions of the target tissues could provide evidence concerning the hormonal requirements of the lesions. For mammary tumors, information of this kind would have great clinical significance. It is too early to assess the importance of receptor proteins in either case, but we must be cautious about our interpretations, especially with mammary tumors.

The attempt to demonstrate a relationship between receptor proteins and hormone dependence of tumors assumes that we can objectively measure hormone dependence. In the mouse and rat, the organ culture technique is an acceptable method of assessment. This method, however, has not been tested adequately with human material. If we are to find meaningful relationships between receptor proteins for specific hormones and hormone dependence of mammary tumors, it is not enough to define dependence in general terms such as ovary-dependent or adrenal-dependent. We must define dependence in terms of specific hormones and we must develop suitable test methods.

For man and for the dog we need precise information concerning the hormonal requirements for the development of normal mammary gland tissues. A considerable body of data is available for the mouse and the rat. In the last two species, both in vivo and in vitro methods

The chairman is affiliated with the Cancer Research Genetics Laboratory at the University of California at Berkeley.

can be employed. In the first two species only in vitro methods seem appropriate and suitable test material is not readily available. Nonetheless, this task must be undertaken. Knowledge concerning the hormone dependence of tumor cell population has only limited meaning without reasonably precise information about the hormonal requirements of normal tissue.

Our experience with experimental animals has taught us that the growth, development, and function of mammary gland tissues depend upon the interaction of these tissues with many hormones. The importance of an individual hormone has been emphasized from time to time, but the fact remains that no single hormone is sufficient when administered at a physiologic level. The deviation from normal hormone requirements found in abnormal tissue must be measured in terms of requirements for a variety of hormones rather than the requirements for a single hormone.

Samples of mammary tissues represent mixtures of epithelial and stromal elements. Mammary tumors of man, the dog, and the rat vary greatly in this regard. Some tumors contain a preponderance of epithelial elements and others contain mostly stromal elements. Samples of normal mammary tissues taken at various stages of development also are variable in this regard. Measurements made on tissue samples must be interpreted with great care unless the relative amounts of epithelial and stromal elements in the samples are known. Attempts to concentrate epithelial or stromal elements in cell suspensions isolated from tissue samples have been successful in the mouse, and these methods should be extended to other species.

There is a large body of knowledge concerning the development of malignant tumors in the mouse and in the rat. In these two species most of the malignant tumors appear to arise from preexisting hyperplastic lesions. It is important to realize that the first demonstrable effect of an oncogenic agent on the mammary tissues of these two species is the formation of preneoplastic lesions. These lesions contain cell populations that are altered from normal. Comparing normal and malignant mammary gland tissues may reveal differences, but many of these differences may have arisen when the preneoplastic lesions appeared. Enumerating tumors is not an adequate measure of an oncogenic event. A knowledge of the states of receptor proteins in malignant tumors is desirable, but this knowledge is incomplete without equivalent information concerning the tissues from which the tumors arose. Attempts to extend the rodent model to man and to the dog are in progress, but it is too early to predict the results. Nonetheless, one must be cautious in interpreting data.

Participants

DR. JOHN ADAMS
University of New South Wales
Sidney, Australia

DR. LEONARD BEUVING
Wistar Institute
Philadelphia

DR. MICHAEL BRENNAN
Detroit Cancer Institute
Detroit

DR. SAMUEL BROOKS
Detroit Cancer Institute
Detroit

DR. THOMAS DAO
Roswell Park Memorial Institute
Buffalo

DR. KENNETH DE OME
University of California
Berkeley

PROF. A. P. M. FORREST
University of Edinburgh
Edinburgh, Scotland

DR. NEVILLE GLEAVE
National Welsh Medical School
Cardiff, Wales

DR. KEITH GRIFFITHS
National Welsh Medical School
Cardiff, Wales

DR. RUSSELL HILF
University of Rochester
Rochester

DR. JEROME HORWITZ
Detroit Cancer Institute
Detroit

PROF. CHARLES B. HUGGINS
University of Chicago
Chicago

DR. RIGOBERTO IGLESIAS
Instituto de Medicina Experimental
Santiago, Chile

DR. ELWOOD JENSEN
University of Chicago
Chicago

DR. STANLEY KORENMAN
University of Iowa
Iowa City

DR. PAUL LIBBY
Roswell Park Memorial Institute
Buffalo

DR. MORTIMER LIPSETT
National Institutes of Health
Bethesda

DR. RUTHANN MASARACCHIA
Roswell Park Memorial Institute
Buffalo

DR. WILLIAM MC GUIRE
University of Texas Medical School
San Antonio

DR. JOSEPH MEITES
Michigan State University
East Lansing

DR. CHARLES MORREAL
Roswell Park Memorial Institute
Buffalo

PROF. O. MUHLBOCK
Het Nederlands Kanderinstituut
Amsterdam, The Netherlands

DR. SATYABRATA NANDI
University of California
Berkeley

DR. BERT O'MALLEY
Vanderbilt University
Nashville

DR. OLOF PEARSON
Western Reserve University
Cleveland

DR. FRED ROSEN
Roswell Park Memorial Institute
Buffalo

DR. GORDON SARFATY
Cancer Institute
Victoria, Australia

DR. D. V. SINGH
Detroit Cancer Institute
Detroit

DR. DILIP SINHA
Roswell Park Memorial Institute
Buffalo

PROF. OLAV TORGERSEN
Institutt for Patologisk Anatomi
Oslo, Norway

DR. ROGER TURKINGTON
University of Wisconsin
Madison

DR. CLIFFORD WELSCH
Michigan State University
East Lansing

DR. GUY WILLIAMS-ASHMAN
University of Chicago
Chicago

Author Index

Adams, J., 116, 144, 151, 153, 158, 178, 223, 238–42, 246, 247, 249, 251, 252
Allfrey, V. G., 74, 85, 87, 97
Ames, B. N., 205
Attramadal, A., 26

Bachmann, W. E., 334
Baird, D., 146
Barker, K. L., 85
Baulieu, E. E., 26, 153, 176
Bekhor, I., 97
Ben-David, M., 294
Bern, H. A., 257, 260
Beuving, L., 257, 264, 266
Bonner, J., 69, 86, 97, 108
Brennan, M., 112, 113, 237, 241, 251
Bresciani, F., 26, 47, 117
Breuer, H., 221
Britten, R. J., 19
Brooks, S., 110, 240, 243, 244
Brown, J. B., 144
Bruchovsky, N., 157
Bulbrook, R. D., 142, 151, 158
Busch, H., 108
Bustin, M., 69

Cameron, E. H. D., 237
Chalkley, R., 69
Chang, E., 144
Charransol, G., 223
Chemerda, J. M., 334
Cleland, W. W., 207
Clemens, J. A., 329
Cole, M. P., 303
Cole, R. D., 69
Cowan, D. M., 157
Creange, J. E., 221

Dahm, K., 221
Dahmus, M. E., 86
Dao, T. L., 32, 33, 114, 117, 132, 144, 153, 163, 164, 223, 238, 239, 240, 247, 253, 263, 264, 307, 308, 346, 348, 352
Davidson, E. H., 19
DeGroot, J., 318
Delang, R. J., 69
DeOme, K., 109, 241, 349, 352
Dilley, W. G., 116
Dixon, G. H., 74
Dorfman, R. I., 135
Dunker, A. K., 213
Duplan, J. F., 317

Ekins, R. P., 61
Elias, J. J., 261
Engel, L. L., 164
Evans, H. McL., 333

Feher, T., 169
Fishman,, J., 222
Folca, P. J., 34

Forchielli, E., 135
Forrest, A., 117
Furth, J., 276, 328

Glascock, R. F., 34
Gleave, E. N., 158
Gomori, G., 334
Gorski, J., 26, 85, 103
Griffith, K., 107, 237–40, 247, 251

Hamilton, T. H., 85, 96
Hedrick, J. L., 211
Hilf, R., 352
Huang, R. C., 97
Huggins, C., 102, 153, 257, 287, 333, 340, 352

Ichii, S., 135
Inman, D. R., 157
Irvine, W. T., 14

Jacobson, H. I., 59, 307
Jensen, E., 59, 85, 89, 101, 102, 104, 106, 107, 109, 110, 112, 115, 117, 120, 218, 227, 238, 239, 243, 248, 251, 252, 253, 276, 307
Jensen, V., 141
Jones, D., 132
Jungmann, R. A., 252

Kim, U., 328
King, R. J. B., 153, 157

359

Index

Klaiber, M. S., 329
Kleinsmith, J. J., 71, 74
Korenman, S., 15, 26, 102, 104, 106, 111, 114, 117, 120, 237, 239, 243, 247, 251
Kung, G. M., 97
Kwa, H. G., 292

Lacassagne, A., 317
Langan, T. A., 71, 72, 74, 96, 97, 121
Lasnitzki, I., 153
Leiberman, S., 221
Lewin, S., 97, 109
Libby, P. R., 109, 121, 223, 242
Ling, V., 74
Lipsett, M., 104, 112, 237, 238, 243, 246, 247, 249, 251
Lockwood, D. H., 122
Lonergan, P., 164
Long, J. A., 333

Macartney, J. C., 243
MacDonald, P. C., 239
McGuire, W., 15, 103, 251
Mainzer, K., 153
Mans, R. J., 13
Marmorston, J., 136
Martin, R. G., 205
Marushige, K., 74
Masarcchia, R., 244
Means, A. R., 85, 96
Medina, D., 349
Meister, A., 341
Meites, J., 102, 112, 115, 116, 117, 275, 277, 281, 283, 317, 328, 329, 345, 346, 348, 349, 350, 351
Menon, K. M. J., 135
Mills, E. S., 114
Mirsky, A. E., 74, 75, 85, 87, 97
Mitchell, F. L., 127
Miyazaki, M., 221
Mizuno, H., 281, 328
Montemurro, D. G., 329
Morreal, C., 132, 163, 164, 247

Muhlbock, O., 345
Murawec, T., 223

Nagasawa, H., 283
Nandi, S., 114–17, 260, 346, 348
Nasr, H., 303
Nirenberg, M. W., 12, 13
Nissen-Meyer, R., 303
Niswender, G. D., 292, 319
Novelli, G. D., 13

Oertel, G. W., 145, 238
Ogawa, Y., 96
O'Malley, B., 15, 86, 107, 120, 121, 122, 350
Ord, M. G., 71
Osborn, M., 208

Panyim, S., 69
Peake, G. T., 303
Pearson, O. H., 109, 113, 249, 252, 253, 303, 328, 349, 351
Pegg, A. E., 122
Pensky, J., 303
Pogo, B. G. T., 85, 87, 97
Pradhan, D. S., 75
Puca, G. A., 74, 117

Riggs, T. R., 244
Rimoin, D. L., 303
Ris, H., 108
Rivera, E., 261
Robel, P., 153
Roberts, S., 223
Rosen, F., 347
Rueckert, R. R., 213
Ryan, K. J., 126, 127, 164

Sarfaty, G., 112, 351
Schertz, G. L., 47
Schubert, K., 176
Shackleton, C. H. L., 127
Sherod, D., 78
Singh, D. V., 114, 349
Sinha, D., 276, 277, 307, 346
Smith, A. J., 211
Smith, E. L., 70

Smith, I. N., 223
Smith, O. W., 126, 127, 164
Sreenivasan, A., 75
Stedman, E., 96
Stevely, W. S., 72
Stocken, L. A., 71, 72
Strominger, J. L., 243
Stumpf, N. E. 76
Sutherland, E., 121
Sweat, M. L., 239
Sylven, B., 172
Szego, C. M., 221, 239

Takaku, F., 97
Talwalker, P. K., 281, 328
Thomas, P. Z., 243
Toft, D., 85
Topper, Y., 114
Torgerson, O., 106, 240, 241, 252
Touchstone, J. C., 223
Toy, Y. C., 329
Treiber, L., 145, 238
Turkington, R., 96, 108, 109, 111, 113, 114, 116, 121, 349

Varela, R. M., 132
Verhofstad, F., 292

Walker, L. M., 244
Warren, J. C., 85
Weber, I., 276, 277
Weber, K., 208
Welsch, C., 317, 329, 345, 347–49, 352
West, C. D., 163
Williams-Ashman, H. G., 101, 109, 122, 238, 242, 243
Wilson, J. D., 157
Wissler, R. W., 32, 33
Wong, M. S. F., 153
Wood, S., 32, 33
Wotiz, H. H., 26, 223

Yoshizawa, I., 221
Young, S., 328

Zahier, W., 207

Subject Index

Acetate, conversion of, 136, 137
Acetate kinase, 93
Aceto-CoA kinase, 86
Acetyl-CoA, 93, 87
Acetylation of histone
  Effect of aldactone on, 94
  Effect of estradiol on, 87, 88, 95
  Effect of photohemagglutinin on, 85, 87
ACTH, 142, 145, 174, 202, 279, 327, 328
  in bronchogenic carcinoma, 145, 174
Actinomycin D, 24
Adenohypophysis. *See* Pituitary, anterior
Adenosine-3'-phosphate-5'-phosphosulfate (PAPS), 195, 196, 202–4, 207, 216, 242, 245
Adenyl cyclase, 74, 96
Adenylsulfate kinase, 195, 197
  and synthesis of steroid sulfate, 197
Adrenalectomy, 33, 34, 52, 53, 55, 117, 139, 144–46, 163, 176, 178, 182, 186, 189, 190, 191, 193, 194, 248, 252, 261, 262, 275, 278, 281, 284, 287, 288, 290, 291, 293, 297, 300, 319, 324, 326, 328
  and serum prolactin, 293, 297, 300
Adrenal gland, 268, 280, 287, 312
  bovine, 202
  DHEA sulfate, 151
  estrogen, 112, 239
  human, 213, 214
Alanine, 210
Aldactone, 94, 95
Aldosterone, 86, 93, 94
  prolactin synergism, 114

Amino acid
  analysis, 206, 207, 216
  composition, 210, 215, 216
  histone, 109
  sequence of histone, 70
Androgen, 55, 65, 112, 113, 145, 263, 282
Androst-5-ene-3β, 17β-diol-16-one, 168
Androst-5-ene-3β, 16α, 17β-triol (α-triol), 129, 130, 132, 139, 141, 142, 153, 163, 168, 172
  in postmenopausal women, 139, 141, 142
  in premenopausal women, 141
5α-Androstane-3α, 17β-diol, 156, 157, 169, 177, 178
  formation in prostate, 157
5α-Androstane-3, 17-dione, 169, 177, 178
Androstenedione, 127, 128, 135, 151, 153, 154, 157, 169, 176–78, 252
  perfusion of breast tumor with, 155
Androsterone, 169, 170, 177, 178
Antibody, 107
Antiestrogen. *See* Antiuterotrophic compounds
Antigen, 106, 107
Antiserum, to prolactin, 297–300
Antiuterotrophic compounds
  cis-clomiphene, 24, 63
  ethamoxytriphetol, 24
  nafoxidine, 24, 31, 32, 36, 89, 90
  Parke-Davis CI-628, 27, 34–36, 43, 44, 47, 63
Arcuate nucleus, 317, 318, 326
Arginine, 210

361

Aromatase, 145, 164, 178
  system in breast cancer, 132, 145, 163, 247
Aspartic acid, 210
Association constant, 60, 248
Avidin, 4

Binding protein, 102
Binding sites, 64, 106, 114
Breast, 3, 60, 76, 86, 90, 110–12, 114, 116, 117, 146, 176, 184, 185, 262, 263, 269, 285, 307–9, 314, 334, 338, 339, 351, 352, 355, 356
  cancer, 33, 34, 36, 37, 39, 43, 44, 47, 60, 62, 65, 112, 129, 138, 144–46, 151, 153–55, 157, 158, 163, 164, 169, 172, 173, 176, 182, 189, 191–93, 252, 253, 257, 259, 264, 268, 269, 271, 276, 277, 278, 281, 283, 287, 290, 294, 295, 299, 303, 317, 333, 334, 337, 338
    ascites cells, 70
    enzymes in
      alkaline phosphatase, 339, 340
      isozymes, 340, 341
      lactic dehydrogenase (LDH), 339, 340
      malic dehydrogenase (MDH), 339, 340
    growth of, 277, 278, 279, 288, 302, 303, 318, 321, 327, 328
    induction of, 270, 276, 280, 282, 283, 287, 288, 307, 308, 310, 314
    spontaneous, 319, 341
    transplanted, 259, 277, 278, 279
  enzymes in
    alkaline phosphatase, 336, 339, 340, 342
    isozymes, 340
    lactic dehydrogenase (LDH), 335, 339, 340, 342
    malic dehydrogenase (MDH), 335, 339, 340, 342
  fat pad, 258, 259, 261, 262, 263
  growth of, 257, 270, 275
  tumor, 31, 110, 111, 113, 114, 117, 127, 318–20, 322–29, 356
  tumorigenesis, 257, 260, 262, 275, 270, 311
Bronchogenic carcinoma, 145, 174

s-Carboxymethylcysteine, 206, 210
Casein, 77, 144
Cells
  chronic lymphocytic leukemia, 79
  endothelial, 7, 109
  epithelial, 109, 114, 241, 356
  eukaryotic, 96, 97
  goblet, 7
  hepatoma, 79
  mammalian, 70
  mammary carcinoma, 79
  mucosal, 4
  oviductal, 14
  proliferation of, 113, 114
  stromal, 109, 241, 356
  tubular gland, 4, 5
  uterine, 4
Cervical cancer, 317
p-Chloromercuribenzoate, 202, 210
Chloropromazine, 351
Cholesterol, 127, 133, 137, 169, 178, 237, 252
  cleaving enzyme, 248
  metabolism in breast cancer, 134, 168, 177
  sulfate, 129, 181
Cholesteryl sulfate, 129
Chorionic gonadotrophin, 112, 145
Chromatin, 12, 30, 74, 89, 107, 108
  DNA template activity, 85
  histone component of, 73
  liver, 86
  oviduct, 86
Cis-clomiphene, 24, 63
Corticosteroid, 113, 116, 117
Corticosterone, 182
Corticotrophin. See ACTH
Cortisol, 63, 75, 76, 86, 94, 201, 261
  binding globulin, 64
  9α-fluro, 94
  and liver chromatin, 86
Cortisone, 140, 163
Cushing's syndrome, 174
Cyclic AMP, 74, 75, 96, 346, 347
  activation of histone kinase, 73, 74
Cycloheximide, 5, 93
Cysteic acid, 206
Cysteine, 204, 206, 210, 218
Cystine, 204
Cytodifferentiation, 4, 8, 12, 13

Index

Cytosol, 26–29, 30–32, 35, 39, 44, 64, 102, 103, 111, 247
   sedimentation pattern in breast cancer, 42–45, 47, 49, 50
   tumor, 32, 35, 44, 45, 47, 48, 50, 51, 62, 64
   uterine, 28, 29

Deconjugation of DHEA sulfate, 153
Dehydroepiandrosterone. *See* DHEA
Dehydroepiandrosterone sulfate. *See* DHEA sulfate
Dehydrogenase
   alcohol, 205, 209
   in breast cancer, 164
   17β-estradiol, 221, 226-28, 234
   hydroxy steroid, 238
   3β-hydroxy-Δ^5 steroid isomerase, 144
   lactic, 334, 335, 338–40, 342
   malic, 334, 338–40, 342
   17β-ol, 164, 176, 178, 226
Deoxycorticosterone. *See* DOC
DES. *See* Diethylstilbestrol
Desmolase, 132, 134, 135, 142
   activity in breast cancer, 132, 135, 136, 178
DHEA, 128, 139, 151, 153, 154, 158, 163–65, 168–72, 176, 178, 182, 185, 197, 202, 204, 213, 217, 237, 240
   conversion in liver tissue, 171
   conversion in placenta, 129
   16α-hydroxy, 129, 139, 140, 153, 168, 176, 247
   metabolism in breast cancer, 127, 130, 132, 133, 168, 177
   urinary level of, 140
DHEA sulfate, 126, 129, 151, 153, 154, 164, 165, 168, 176, 178, 181, 184, 190, 192, 194, 196, 198, 201, 202, 221, 237
   estrogenic activity of, 145
   fetal adrenal, 240
   infusion of, 139, 143, 144
   metabolism in breast cancer, 131, 154, 168, 177
   perfusion of breast cancer with, 155
   plasma level, 159
Diaphragm, 24
Diethylstilbestrol, 6, 8, 10, 12, 14–16, 244, 245, 247, 308, 310–12, 314
   effect on ornithine decarboxylase, 5
   metabolism of, in liver, 244, 245

Differentiation, 15–17
   estrogen-induced, 12, 18
   estrogen-mediated, 4, 7, 12, 14, 15, 18
   lobuloalveolar, 116, 261, 262
   mammary epithelial cell, 79
   mechanism of, 3
   morphologic, 5, 7
   oviduct, 14
5αDihydrotestosterone, 63–65, 153, 154, 156, 157, 248
7, 12-Dimethylbenz(a)anthracene. *See* DMBA
Dimethylstilbestrol, 63
Dissociation constant, 106
DMBA, 103–5, 110–13, 262–64, 269, 278, 280, 282, 287, 290, 295, 308–12, 314, 315, 318, 321, 323, 327, 328, 334, 335, 341, 346
DNA, 72, 115, 269, 314, 315, 328, 350
   coiling of, 72
   cycle, 350
   synthesis
      in DMBA-induced mammary tumor, 328
      in insulin-stimulated mammary epithelial cells, 73
      in phytohemagglutinin-stimulated lymphocytes, 73
      polyamines, 6
      putrescine, 6
      in regenerating liver, 73
      stimulation by polyamines, 6
      transcription by RNA polymerase, 73
DNase, 103
DNA polymerase, 72, 76
DNA-RNA competition, 14, 79
DOC, 94, 181, 183, 261

Elements
   epithelial, 109, 114, 241, 356
   stromal, 109, 241, 356
Embryogenesis, of uterus, 4
Endometrial cancer, 117
Endometrium, 109
Endoplasmic reticulum, 114
Enzymes in mammary gland and cancer, 338–40
Epiestriol, 63, 166, 172, 247
17-Epiestriol, 247

Equilibrium, association-dissociation, 201
Erythro MEA, 63
Estradiol, 5, 23, 29, 31, 36, 37, 38, 39, 44, 47, 52, 87, 90, 91, 111, 163, 164, 166, 167, 168, 170, 171, 173–78, 182, 183, 185, 197, 204, 225–28, 232, 233, 247, 282, 283, 284, 301, 307
 benzoate,
  and tumor growth, 228, 283, 284, 290, 300–302
  and serum prolactin, 293–94, 300, 302
 -3, 17β-disulfate, 222, 225
 -17α-ethynyl, 23, 24
 -11β-hydroxy, 144, 163
 -6α-hydroxy, 17β sulfate, 222
 and mammary gland histone acetokinase, 90, 92
 metabolism of, in breast cancer, 136
 -3-methyl ether, 204
 ornithine decarboxylase, 5
 RNA polymerase, 86
 sulfate, 186, 192, 194, 196, 198, 199, 232
 -3-sulfate, 221, 223, 225, 227
 -17β sulfate, 222
 and uterine nuclear RNA, 85
17β-Estradiol. See Estradiol
17β-Estradiol-estrone oxidoreductase, 243
Estriol, 23, 63, 114, 126, 128, 132, 136, 139, 144, 163, 164, 165, 168, 171, 176, 178, 182, 204, 207, 246, 247
 -2-hydroxy, 165, 177
 urinary, 136
Estrogen, 144, 221, 229, 233, 251, 260–63, 268–71, 275, 280, 282, 284, 285, 307, 308, 311, 313, 314, 315, 346
 action, 3, 4, 59, 86, 101
 binding of, 23, 24, 26, 35, 52, 54, 64, 101, 102, 110, 114, 254, 276
  in mammary gland, 62
  in mammary tumor, 31, 35, 60
  in premenopausal women, 111, 114
  and response to therapy, 52–55
 conjugation in plasma, 224
 control of
  oviductal transcription, 11
  oviductal translation, 7
 effect on gene activation, 16
 effect on gene transcription, 12
 fate, of, 223
 hepatic metabolism of, 222
 and histone acetylation, 85, 86
 inhibitors of (see also Antiuterotrophic compounds)
  dimethylstilbestrol, 63
  Erythro MEA, 63
 -2-methoxy, 222
 nuclear site of action, 4
 in oophorectomized, adrenalectomized patients, 144
 on ornithine decarboxylase induction, 5
 oviduct protein synthesis, 7, 8
 physical shape of, 107
 plasma, 224, 227, 228, 239
 in postmenopausal women, 239
 receptors, 20, 23, 27, 31–34, 40, 54, 64, 101, 103, 110, 111, 112, 114, 117, 233, 234, 251, 254, 355
  in DMBA-induced tumor, 103, 110, 111
  in human breast cancer, 33
  in mammary gland, 110, 112
  in target tissue, 34
 synthesis of ribosome, 8, 9
 tetroxy, 168, 177
 uptake
  by breast cancer, 36–40, 47, 60
  by hormone-dependent tissue, 24
  by hormone-dependent tumors, 31
  by mammary gland, 31, 60
  by pituitary, 26
  by uterus, 26, 31, 39, 89, 226–28
  by vagina, 26, 31
 on uterotrophic activity, 59, 145
Estrogen sulfotransferase
 amino acid composition of, 210, 215
 isolation of, 205
 isozymes of, 207, 208, 212, 213
 property of,, 202, 209
 in sulfation of estrogen, 204
Estrone, 53, 63, 144, 163, 164, 166–68, 171, 173, 175–78, 204, 205, 216, 224, 226, 227, 229, 232, 247, 345
 16α-hydroxy, 165, 166, 167, 172, 173, 176, 177

Index

11β-hydroxy, 144, 163
metabolism in breast cancer, 172, 177
2-methoxy, 174, 175, 177, 223
sulfate in plasma, 204, 216, 221–25, 227, 229, 231, 232
Estrophiles. *See* Estrogen, receptors
Estrous cycle, 225, 228, 233, 293
diestrus, 227, 318, 320
estrus, 227, 294, 318, 336, 337
serum prolactin during, 292, 293
Etiocholanolone, 158, 159

Factor
corticotrophin releasing (CRF), 327
epidermal growth, 6
follicle stimulating hormone releasing (FSHRF), 327
growth hormone releasing (GHRF), 327
luteinizing hormone releasing (LRF), 327
nutritional, 349, 350, 351
prolactin inhibitory (PIF), 327
serum, 115
Function, of binding protein, 101

Gene, 4
activation, 16, 97
derepression, 19
expression, 14, 69, 78, 101, 111, 112
repression, 69, 72, 97
structural, 18
transcription, 12, 14, 15, 79, 108
Genome, 19, 73, 97, 120
Gland
apocrine, 241
sebaceous, 241
mammary (*see* Breast)
Glucagon, 74, 76
and histone phosphorylation, 96
Glutamic acid, 210
Glycine, 210, 231
Growth
estrogen-induced, 12, 307
estrogen-mediated, 4, 5, 7, 12, 16, 18
target tissue, 5
Growth hormone, 6, 117, 260–62, 268, 269, 270, 276, 278–82, 288, 303, 328, 333

Hexestrol, 23
in breast cancer patients, 34
Histidine, 210
Histone, 69, 90, 96, 97
acetokinase, 91–95, 98
effect of aldosterone on, 93
effect of estradiol on, 86, 89
estrogen-mediated increase, 86
in mammary gland, 90
in rat uterus, 86
acetylation, 85–88, 94, 95, 121
amino acid sequence, 70, 71, 103
arginine-rich, 87–89
deacetylation, 87, 88
DNA binding, 73
DNA-histone F1, 72
F1, 71, 75
F2a1, 70
F2a2, 77
glycine-arginine-rich, 70, 71, 88, 96, 108
hormonal regulation of, 74
kinase, 71, 72, 74
lysine-rich, 70, 75, 87, 88, 89, 91
phosphatase, 73
phosphorylation of, 71–75, 78, 79, 81, 96, 121
repressor activity of, 72, 73
synthesis in mammary epithelial cells, 75
Hormone
conversion of steroid
by mammary cancer tissues, 237, 240
by skin, 238
-dependent
endothelial cells, 109
mammary epithelial cells, 79
mammary tumors, 31, 33, 60, 103, 110, 239, 257, 263, 276, 287, 334
tissues, 24, 30
follicular stimulating, 351
-independent
mammary tumors, 33, 102, 103, 238, 257
luteinizing, 351
neuro-, 327
ovarian, 243, 260
receptor complex (*see* Receptor protein)
responsive, 25, 287, 288, 326

Hormonal regulation
  of gene expression, 69, 78, 111
  of growth, 18
  of histone phosphorylation, 75, 76
  of histone synthesis, 75–76
  of RNA synthesis, 69
Hybridization, DNA-RNA, 16, 17, 79–81
Hydrocarbon, polycyclic aromatic, 263, 333, 334
  and serum prolactin, 347
Hydrocortisone. See Cortisol
6α-Hydroxyestradiol-17β-sulfate, 222
Hydroxylases, steroid, 127, 164, 173, 176, 178
16α-Hydroxylation, 127, 153
  in breast cancer, 252
p-Hydroxymercuribenzoate, 27, 103
Hyperplastic alveolar nodule, 258
  induction, 258, 262, 263, 268, 270
  maintenance, 260–62, 264, 266, 269, 270
  preneoplastic, 257, 259, 263, 265, 267, 270, 315, 356
  transplanted, 262
Hypophysectomy, 33, 34, 55, 117, 253, 261, 262
Hypothalamus, 317, 323, 326, 327, 345

Insulin, 114, 116
  phosphorylation of histone, 74–76
  stimulated mammary epithelial cells in vitro, 73
Isoleucine, 210
Isomerase, 127
Isozyme, 205, 207, 208, 211–13, 215, 216, 340

Lactation, 260, 285, 303, 339
Lamina propria, 109
Leucine, 210
Leukemia, 317
  carcinogen-induced, 333, 334, 338, 341
  spontaneous, 334
Lipase, 216
Lymphocytes, 85
  phytohemagglutinin-stimulated, 73, 74
Lysine, 210
Lysozyme synthesis, 4, 5

Macromolecule, 102, 307
  cytoplasmic intracellular, 4
  fraction, 103, 104
  receptor, 119
Mammary gland. See Breast
Mastectomy, 34, 52, 252
  radical, 140, 189, 191, 192, 198
  simple, 189, 191, 198
3-MC, 328
Median eminence, 276, 317–28
  lesion, 276, 278, 346, 348, 349, 351
    mammary tumor growth, 318, 319, 323, 324
    prolactin secretion, 319, 324, 325, 326
Metabolism, 125, 222, 228
  cholesterol, 169, 177
  DHEA, 127, 128, 130, 133, 168, 171, 177
  DHEA sulfate, 131, 168, 177
  estrogen, 221, 222, 229, 239, 244, 245
  estrone, 172, 177
  pregnenolone, 127, 128, 130
  testosterone, 128, 130, 165, 170, 177, 240
  testosterone sulfate, 167, 177
Methionine, 210
2-Methoxyestrogen, 222
3-Methylcholanthrene. See 3-MC
Mevalonate, 136
Mineralocorticoids, 86, 93–95
  and kidney acetokinase, 94, 95
  receptor, 307
Mucopolysaccharide, 197, 198, 245
  biosynthesis, 125
Myometrium, 109

Nodulogenesis. See Hyperplastic alveolar nodule
Novikoff hepatoma, 70
Nuclear-myofibrillar fraction, 27
Nuclear protein, 18, 69, 81
  phosphoprotein, 71
  phosphorylation of, 78, 79, 81
Nucleic acid, synthetic and natural, 13
Nucleotide sequence, DNA, 108

Oophorectomy, 52, 55, 139, 146, 169, 176, 178, 334
Organ culture, 114, 115
  effect of insulin in, 115
  of mammary gland, 75, 76

Index

Ornithine decarboxylase, 5, 6
    activity in prostate, 6
    cell growth, 5, 6
    effect of partial hepatectomy, 6
    oviductal, 5
Ovalbumin, 4, 5
Ovariectomy, 32, 53, 55, 103, 110, 111, 243, 261–68, 275, 278, 280–83, 346–49, 355
    and nodulogenesis, 263, 265, 267, 268
    and serum prolactin, 275, 293, 297, 300, 348
    and tumorigenesis, 262, 264
Ovary, 126, 262, 263, 268, 282, 287, 348
Oviduct, 3, 4, 16, 86
    avidin, 109
    content of ribosome, 7
    as model system, 3
    mRNA, 12, 17
    nuclear RNA, 13
    polyribosomes, 7
    RNA, 15
16-Oxoandrostenediol, 139, 140

Paraendocrine, 125, 145, 248, 249, 252
Perfusion, of breast cancer, 155
Permissive action of hormone, 102
Perphenazine, 297, 351
    effect on mammary tumor growth, 294, 295, 296, 297, 302
    effect on serum prolactin, 294, 296, 297, 302
Phenothiazine, 294, 352
Phenylalanine, 12, 210
Phosphatase, alkaline, 335, 336, 339, 340, 342
Phospholipids, 71
Phosphorylation of histone, 81
O-Phosphoserine, 71
Phosphotransacetylase, 93
Phytohemagglutinin, 85, 87
Phylogeny, 108
Pituitary, 59, 102, 287, 288, 298, 303, 308
    anterior, 260, 262, 275, 279, 280, 307, 314, 326, 327, 329, 345
        as target tissue, 23
        uptake of hormones in, 26
    transplants, 275, 276, 346, 352
    tumor, 275-79, 303, 328, 347, 349

Polyamines, 6, 122
Polynucleotide, 119
Polyphenylalanine, 12
Polyribosome
    isolation and characterization, 7, 9
    protein biosynthesis by, 10, 15
Polysome, 8, 9, 18, 113
    mRNA-directed synthesis, 17
    peptide synthesis by, 11, 14
Poly U, 12, 13
Postmenopausal women
    DHEA, 140, 142
    estriol, 136
    16-hydroxy DHEA, 140, 142
    16-oxoandrostenediol, 140, 142
Pregn-4-en-17α, 20α-diol-3-one, 135
Pregn-4-en-17α, 20β-diol-3-one, 135
Pregnenolone, 127, 128, 133, 182, 252
    metabolism in breast cancer, 127, 130
Premenopausal women
    DHEA metabolites in, 141
Progesterone, 17, 63–65, 127, 128, 234, 243, 268, 285
Prolactin
    endogenous, 282, 299
    exogenous, 269, 285, 289, 290, 298, 300
    and mammary growth, 113, 114
    pituitary, 76, 102, 117, 260–62, 268, 270, 271, 275, 276, 278–80, 284, 288, 289, 290, 307, 315, 317, 319, 327–29
    relation to estrogen, 282, 284, 301
    serum, 112, 251, 268, 274, 276, 282, 284, 288, 290–96, 301, 315, 320, 322, 324–26
Proline, 210
Prostatic tissue, 6, 122, 155, 156
Protein
    chromosomal, 72, 97
    estrogen-induced synthesis of, 8, 9, 85
    intracellular, 19
    kinase, 96
    ribosomal, 13, 129
    structural, 5, 20
    synthesis of, 7, 8, 10, 120, 231, 232, 351
    synthesis of in mammary gland, 93
Protein kinase
    cyclic AMP activated, 24

Protein phosphate phosphorylation, 216
Puromycin, 24
Putrescine, 6

Radioimmunoassay, 319
  prolactin, 288, 290
Receptor protein, 25, 28, 112, 120, 307.
  See also Estrogen, receptors
  competition for, 63, 65, 114, 243, 248
  cytoplasmic, 19, 26
  5α-dihydrotestosterone, 65, 157
  effect of ovariectomy on, 110
  mineralocorticoid, 93
  progesterone, 65, 107, 114
  two-step interaction, 27, 30, 101
5α-Reductase, 157
Ribosome, 7–10, 232
RNA, 3, 6, 12, 14–17, 232, 314, 315
  chromosomal, 97
  derepressor RNA, 20
  DNA-like sequence, 79
  messenger RNA, 12–15, 17, 18
  nuclear RNA, 12–14, 16, 17, 75, 79, 85, 96
  oviductal, 15
  periribosomal, 75
  ribosomal, 14, 18, 20, 75, 122
  synthesis of
    effect of prolactin on, 76
    estrogen-initiated, 85
    hormonal regulation, 69
    in lymphocytes, 74
  transfer RNA, 20
RNA polymerase, 12, 14, 15, 17, 76, 86, 108
  chromatin associated, 75
  DNA-dependent, 72
  effect of estrogen on, 15
  effect of histone on, 73
  nucleolar, 75
RNase, 103

Sebaceous gland, 241
  tumor, 334
Serine, 206, 210
Somatotrophin. See Growth hormone
Spermatogenesis, 74
Spermidine, 6
Steroid conjugation
  enzyme systems, 181, 186, 189
  in liver, 186
  in normal breast, 185
  in mammary cancer, 181, 186, 190
  in metastatic liver, 186, 187, 189
  and response to adrenalectomy, 189, 191
  sites, 181
  and sulfate metabolism, 195
Steroid conversion
  by bacteria, 238
  in liver, 145, 178, 240
  by skin, 145, 237, 238
  by uterus, 239, 240
Steroid glucuronide, 181, 243
  estradiol, 243
Steroid sulfate, 125, 181, 187, 190, 192, 193, 197, 198, 199, 201, 221
  in mammary cancer, 182, 183, 186, 190, 192–94
  in normal and metastatic liver, 187–89
  in primary and metastatic breast cancer, 194
  in primary breast cancer, and incidence of recurrence, 192
Steroid sulfotransferase, 126, 184, 191–96, 198, 201
  adrenal, 218
  DHEA, 126, 184
  estrogen, 184, 195, 201, 202, 210, 231, 234, 247
  3β-hydroxy, 195
  17β-hydroxy, 195
  21-hydroxy, 195
  microsomal, 232
Stromal, 109, 241, 356
Sulfatase, 129
Sulfate-activating enzymes, 195
  synergistic effect, 198
Sulfate adenylyl transferase, 195, 242
  and synthesis of steroid sulfate, 196, 197
Sulfurylation of
  deoxycorticosterone, 182, 183
  DHEA, 126, 182, 183, 190, 198
  estradiol, 182, 183, 190, 198, 243
  estriol, 182, 183
  estrone, 126, 182, 183, 243
  19-nortestosterone, 182
  pregnenolone, 182, 183
  testosterone, 182, 183

Index

Template activity, 85, 108
Testosterone, 6, 53, 63, 65, 113, 128, 132, 154, 155, 164, 167, 169, 170, 176, 178, 238, 248, 351
  conversion to estrogen, 163, 165
  16α-hydroxy, 132, 167, 168, 170, 171, 176, 177
  metabolism in breast cancer, 130, 153, 155–57, 177
  metabolism in liver tissue, 169
  metabolism in prostate, 156
  sulfate, 165, 178
    conversion of, 167, 177
Thermovac Autopulverizer, 107
Threonine, 206, 210
Thymidine, 114
Thyroidectomy, 350
Thyroxin, 350, 351
Tissue culture. *See* Organ culture
7,8,12-TMBA, 333–35, 337, 338, 341
7,8,12-Trimethylbenz(a)anthracene. *See* 7,8,12-TMBA
Tryosine, 210
  amino transferase, 109
Tumor extract, mammary, 184
Tumorigenesis, mammary
  DMBA-induced, 269, 280, 288, 291, 311, 318, 320, 328
  hormonal influence, 259, 262, 270, 280, 288, 289, 345
  inhibition by estrogen, 282, 284
  inhibition of, 351, 352

Urinary steroid
  effect of mastectomy on, 140, 143
  estriol, 136
  estrogens, 144
  3β-hydroxy-Δ^5 steroids in postmenopausal women, 140, 143
  in women with breast cancer, 248, 249
  in women with breast disease, 158, 159
Uterotrophic, 59, 145
Uterus, 44, 59, 86, 227, 230, 233, 234, 307, 312, 314
  embryogenesis of, 4
  estrogen-stimulated, 85
  fate of estrogen in, 223, 233
  as model system, 3
  oxidation of estradiol in, 228
  protein synthesis in, 231, 232
  as target tissue, 23
  uptake of hormone in, 26, 39, 109, 223–25

Vagina, 59, 307
  as target tissue, 23
  uptake of hormone in, 26
Valine, 210
Virus, 115, 116
  DNA-tumor, 116
  mammary tumor, 258, 261, 262
  Rous sarcoma, 333

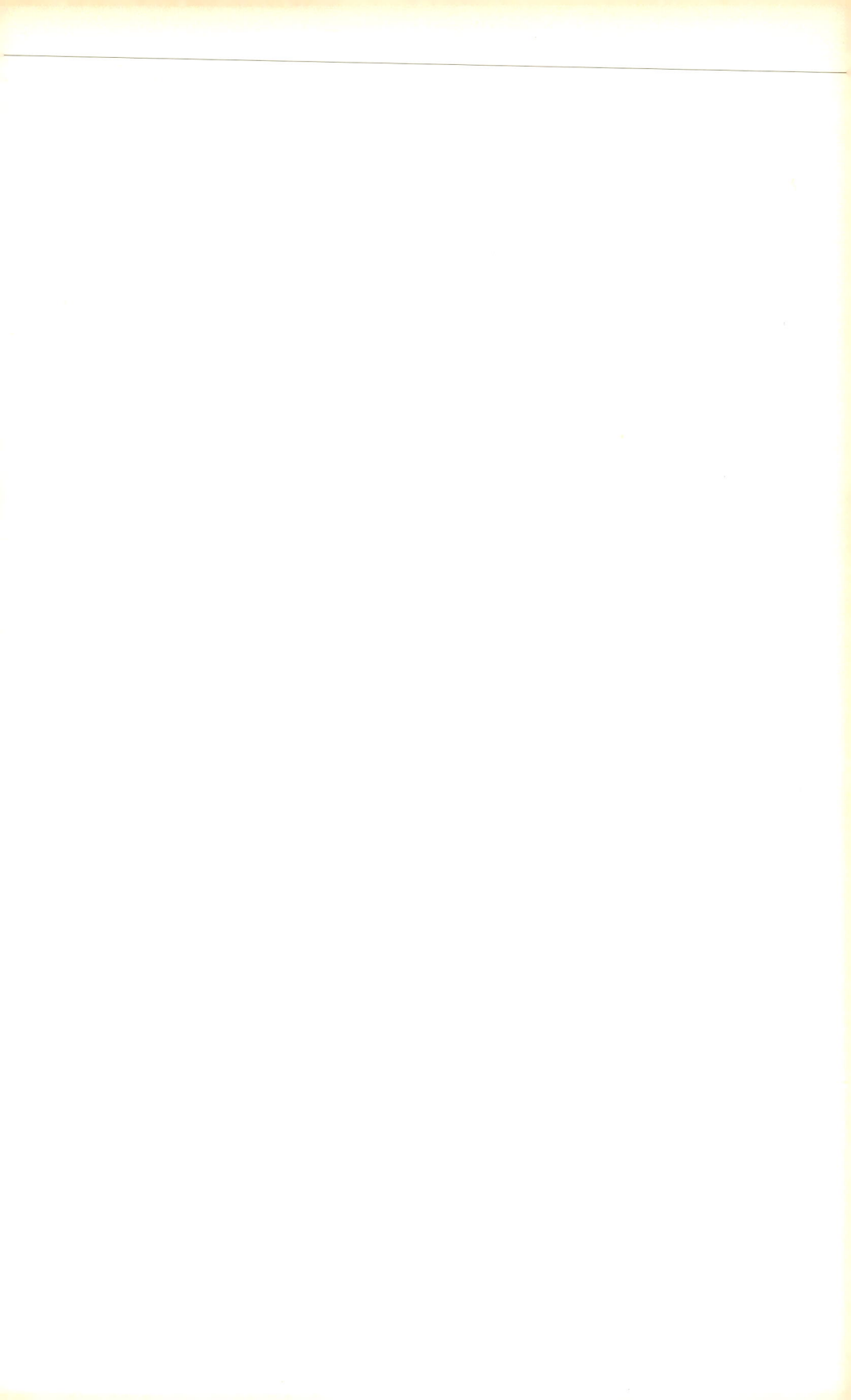